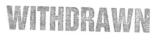

# Practical Audiology for Speech-Language Therapists

Janet Doyle PhD

with contributions from
John Bench, Nicola Daly and Christopher Lind

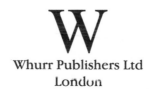

**W**

Whurr Publishers Ltd
London

© 1998 Whurr Publishers Ltd
First edition published 1998
by Whurr Publishers Limited
19b Compton Terrace, London N1 2UN, England

Reprinted 1999 and 2000

**British Library Cataloguing in Publication Data**
A catalogue record for this book is available from the
British Library.

ISBN 1 86156 059 1

Printed and bound in the UK by Athenaeum Press Ltd,
Gateshead, Tyne & Wear

For Jane, my sister

# Contents

# Contributors

**John Bench** is audiologist and psychologist in the School of Human Communication Sciences at La Trobe University, Victoria, Australia. He has a special interest in the study of communication processes in children. Parts of Chapter 9 were written when he was Honorary Research Fellow, Department of Phonetics and Linguistics, University College, London.

**Nicola Daly** is a sociolinguist and audiologist who has recently completed doctoral studies concerning gender differences in speech-reading at La Trobe University, Victoria, Australia.

**Janet Doyle** is Honorary Associate (Research) Associate at La Trobe University, Victoria, Australia. Until December 1996 she held the position of Associate Professor in the School of Human Communication Sciences, Faculty of Health Sciences, La Trobe University. She is also Principal of Janet Doyle & Associates, Research Consultants, Canterbury, Victoria, Australia.

**Christopher Lind** is lecturer in Audiology in the Department of Speech Pathology and Audiology at the University of Queensland, Australia. He has a particular interest in adult aural rehabilitation and communication therapy.

# Chapter 1
# Introduction

JANET DOYLE

The aim of this book is to assist in the provision of quality services to clients with communication disorders, by providing an accessible and very practically oriented description of aspects of audiology relevant to the clinical practice of speech-language therapy.

## Professional role and responsibilities

The scope of practice in the profession of speech and language therapy is increasing in a number of settings. Many speech-language therapists now have roles in health administration, multidisciplinary clinical teams, quality assurance, community education, public health planning, client advocacy and consultancies to health, education and business bodies. Increasingly these activities are seen as natural extensions of traditional clinical work with clients who have communication disorders. In addition, speech-language therapists have an emerging role in the enhancement of normal communication. Speech-language therapists may work with business to enhance staff communication performance (see, for example, Schwartz, 1997), with singers to maximise vocal performance and maintain voice health, and with teachers and other professional speakers to reduce voice stress. Some of these expanding roles demand a basic knowledge of room acoustics, signal-to-noise ratios, the masking effects of environmental noise, hearing conservation and other audiological concepts to a degree that was perhaps less necessary when the work role was confined to traditional speech therapy carried out in purpose-designed rooms. Further, speech-language therapists may be members of cochlear implant teams, a role that certainly requires a sound audiology base.

A discussion of professional boundaries in relation to the application of audiology knowledge is deliberately avoided in this book. Around the world there are many professional groups dealing with clients whose communication function may be impaired because of hearing problems. These professionals include audiologists, audiological physicians, audiological scientists, audiometrists, aural rehabilitationists, educators of the deaf, hearing therapists, otolaryngologists, paediatricians and speech-language pathologists/therapists. The ways these persons work together can vary to a great extent, as can the views of individuals and organisations as to the professional groups best-suited to perform various tasks. Having said that, the content of this book reflects this author's own appreciation of what the speech-language therapist in Australia can be expected to embrace as part of their professional knowledge, and what could be useful to speech-language therapists in other countries. It is acknowledged that some professional preparation programmes may expect more, or less, knowledge of audiological principles and practice among their speech-language therapy graduates than is provided in this book. Although some speech-language therapists may not consider some of the content to be relevant to their practice, at least some of the contents are relevant to all speech-language therapists.

Some professional organisations provide formal statements of the responsibilities and scope of practice of entry level speech-language therapists in relation to the hearing care of clients. For example, the American Speech-Language-Hearing Association (ASHA) has stated that screening of auditory function and appropriate referral is one of the roles of the speech-language therapist (ASHA, 1990a). The Speech Pathology Association of Australia (formerly the Australian Association of Speech and Hearing, AASH) has stated that the speech-language therapist must be able to integrate information such as audiological reports with the speech knowledge base to choose intervention strategies (AASH, 1994). Additionally, the role of the speech-language therapist in treating clients with hearing loss has been discussed in the literature (see, for example, Brackett, 1985; Garrard & Smith Clark, 1985).

These statements of professional responsibility underline what is, in reality, a pragmatic requirement of speech therapy practice. As speech, language, voice and cognition are all intimately related to hearing it is necessary for speech-language therapists to have a firm understanding of basic audiology theory, and to carry forward and augment that knowledge beyond the time of their graduation from university. Speech-language therapists need to be informed consumers of audiological data such as screening results, pure tone audiograms, middle ear function tests, speech perception tests and perhaps other more technical data relevant to their particular clinical situation. If one is attempting to assist the communication development of a child with congenital sensorineural hearing loss it is vital to be able to interpret aided audiograms so that appropriate therapy that neither pushes the child beyond their speech perception abilities nor underestimates their potential may be designed. If one is deciding whether or not a suspected hearing loss involves middle-ear pathology it is helpful to be able to read a tympanogram. The overall level of loss depicted in audiometric data will help determine appropriate room set-up so as to maximise communication and therefore the effectiveness of therapeutic intervention. In these and other ways a knowledge of basic audiology is needed for the practice of speech-language therapy.

## Teamwork in speech and hearing science

The client with hearing problems has four basic problems. The first is loss of hearing sensitivity and/or clarity to some degree. The second is the effect of that loss on the ability to communicate in a range of life situations. The third is the sometimes less than optimal ability and/or willingness of communication partners to assist in making communication more successful. The fourth, which applies largely to adult clients, is the fact that in general, society, and sometimes the client's own family, sees hearing loss as the responsibility of the person with the hearing loss. The latter two problems have been discussed by Erber (1988), among others.

Given these four major problems, the client is likely to need a range of services that may include:

- audiometric assessments;
- informational counselling about hearing loss;
- referral for medical services;
- rehabilitative technology (such as hearing aids, assistive listening devices, cochlear implants);
- advice on coping in various difficult communication situations (for example, rooms with poor lighting, noisy social occasions);
- assessment of perceptual and conversational abilities;
- advice to help communication partners become clearer and/or more responsible conversationalists;
- therapy to assist development and/or maintenance of speech, language and voice;
- advice on various educational, health, vocational and safety issues associated with having a hearing problem;
- advocacy in matters of access and decision-making.

Speech-language therapists are well placed to work closely with audiologists, physicians and others in a team effort to ensure that such services are available to clients. The potential to work effectively with audiologists in the communication assessment and treatment of clients with hearing impairment is especially great.

# Key skills and knowledge

In this author's view there are four audiology-based skills that are required by the speech-language therapist. These are:

- the ability to conduct screening tests of hearing and middle-ear function;
- the ability to interpret audiograms to support therapy and referral decisions;
- the subjective checking and troubleshooting of hearing aids;
- the ability to assist the client with information, referral and access to hearing-related services.

These skills are addressed in some detail in various chapters of this book. For the purposes of this introductory chapter the four key skills are now briefly described in turn.

## Skill 1: Ability to perform screening tests of hearing and middle-ear function

This skill is extensively discussed in Chapter 5. Many speech-language therapists practice in situations where audiology services have long waiting lists or are not available in the local geographical area. Given that knowledge of a client's hearing status is necessary in the early stages of diagnosis and treatment, it is important that speech-language therapists in such situations are able to determine whether their clients' hearing is within normal limits or not. If a hearing screening test indicates hearing loss the therapist has grounds for a priority audiology referral, and has some very basic information about auditory function to guide therapy in the meantime.

Additionally, it is useful for the speech-language therapist to be able to screen for middle-ear disorders, especially in children. If a child client has a long history of middle-ear problems and fluctuating hearing it is useful to the speech-language therapist, and to other professionals, to have a longitudinal profile of middle-ear function. This profile may be easily obtained by screening tests in speech therapy sessions if the tests cannot be readily conducted elsewhere.

## Skill 2: Reading of audiograms to inform therapy and referral

Chapter 6 is devoted to the description and interpretation of audiograms. The audiogram is the most commonly available diagnostic description of hearing sensitivity. Read correctly, the audiogram yields information about:

- the individual client's hearing sensitivity in relation to normal threshold sensitivity for sounds important to speech perception;

- the relative hearing sensitivity of the two ears;
- whether the hearing loss is conductive, sensorineural or mixed;
- the need for further investigation of communication function;
- the need for medical referral;
- the likely general level of difficulty the client will have in spoken communication;
- the likely general level of difficulty the client will have hearing in quiet and in noisy situations;
- the degree of need for special support in the development and/or maintenance of oral communication.

The audiogram is a valuable source of information for speech-language therapists treating clients whose communication is compromised by hearing loss, and hence skill in reading audiograms is essential.

### Skill 3: Troubleshooting of hearing aids and assistive listening devices

Speech-language therapists treating clients who use hearing-aid amplification need to feel confident that the hearing aids are operational during therapy. It is therefore important that the speech-language therapist be able to carry out simple functional checks (troubleshooting) of aided hearing, to deal with basic problems (such as a flat hearing-aid battery), and to arrange appropriate audiological and/or technical assistance as needed. Similarly, it is important to be able to determine if a client's binaural amplified listener or amplified telephone do in fact need repair or are not being used correctly. Additionally, a current knowledge of available assistive listening devices is very useful. These issues are discussed in Chapter 7.

### Skill 4: Ability to assist with information, referral and access to services

Many clients do not know how to access various services. Some clients need an advocate to help improve employer or family understanding of communication difficulties associated with hearing loss. Other clients may not know they are eligible for assistance with the cost of hearing aids and communication devices. Clients may need referral to an audiologist, a medical practitioner, a remedial teacher, social worker or other professional. It is a key skill of the speech-language therapist to assist with these situations. The speech-language therapist needs to develop and maintain a suitable network of other professionals, and to keep current information about service options. Issues around this fourth key skill are discussed throughout the book.

This book also attempts to provide three types of knowledge to support and augment the four key skills already described.

*Knowledge cluster 1: Sound, hearing and speech perception*

Chapter 2 offers a basic description of: the nature of sound and how it is produced and measured, the way sound is perceived by the human ear and the anatomy of the auditory pathway. This is the classic underlying information for an understanding of normal spoken communication. Additionally, a brief discussion of room acoustics illustrates how speech perception may be influenced by ambient noise. This information is augmented by a discussion of speech-reading in Chapter 8, including how the gender of the speaker and the context in which the message is placed may influence how well the message is speech-read. Other aspects of speech perception are addressed in Chapter 4, which deals, among other things, with speech audiometry and the assessment of hearing sensitivity for audio frequencies important to hearing speech signals. Chapter 9 deals with central auditory processing problems, which are, for some clients, the reason for difficulties perceiving speech.

*Knowledge cluster 2: Types, etiologies and assessments of hearing loss*

In Chapter 3 the major forms of hearing difficulty are described, along with the diseases, syndromes and environmental events that may cause those hearing losses. Management approaches to the major types of hearing loss are also discussed briefly. Chapter 4 deals with subjective and objective tests of hearing and describes how test results assist the differential diagnosis of various hearing disorders. Chapter 6 illustrates how the major types of hearing loss appear on audiograms. Examples of pure tone audiograms, and elements of pure tone audiograms, are also given in various other chapters. Chapter 7 contains examples of how various hearing losses may be assisted via hearing-aid amplification and/or other technical approaches. Chapter 9 describes in some detail how central auditory processing disorders may be diagnosed. Chapter 10 includes an example of the integration of information about hearing loss in case assessment and management.

*Knowledge cluster 3: Technology for diagnosis and rehabilitation*

Throughout the book, reference is made to various aspects of technology as applied to hearing and hearing disorders. Thus, in Chapter 2 the operation of a sound-level meter is described. Chapter 4 contains brief explanations of the equipment used in audiological testing and what clients undergoing such technically based assessments are likely to experience. In Chapter 5 detailed advice about equipment and techniques suitable for screening hearing and middle-ear function is given. In Chapter 6 there is a description of the reference levels for various audiograms, which relates to earlier comments about audiometer calibration given in Chapter 4. Chapter 7 contains an overview of the operation of hearing aids, assistive listening devices and cochlear implants.

# Philosophy of approach

## The principle of client-centred practice

One of the underpinnings of this book is the notion that clinical practice with individual clients is likely to be most effective when it is client-centred. Given the particular boundaries imposed by available resources, and the necessity to act in accordance with what professional knowledge indicates is in the client's best interests, the best plan for the client is one that addresses needs as agreed with the client. Clients are probably more likely to go through with therapy and follow various other recommendations if they see that they deal with what they consider to be the primary problem. The individual client will have a life setting that will interact with their hearing loss in particular ways. Therefore therapy that considers those interactions in a client-centred approach is likely to be particularly useful. A client-centred approach is also useful in evaluation of treatment and programme effectiveness (see Chapter 5). Outcome variables that include clients' perception of services and of the gains made in therapy can augment other data, such as efficiency indicators (see Chapter 7). Importantly, individual hearing losses as depicted on audiograms are only a one-dimensional representation of a complex experience (see Chapter 6). Hence throughout this book speech-language therapists are advised to exercise caution over the manner in which test results are interpreted in relation to the individual client's hearing difficulties and their potential for auditory-based communication (see Chapter 3 for example). In general this book takes the perspective of the speech-language therapist who has contact with individual clients rather than, for example, responsibilities in large-scale public health management.

## Clinical decision-making is a dynamic system

Elsewhere (Doyle & Thomas, 1988; Doyle, 1995) clinical practice has been described as a dynamic system involving the four main elements of client, clinician, task and environment. The way speech-language therapists and others assist clients with communication disorders is a function of how the elements of this clinical decision-making system interact. For example, the knowledge base of the clinician and the resources of the particular clinical environment will interact to determine, at least in part, what options are open to the client. Individual clients may receive differing treatments for very similar problems. Individual clinicians may select different approaches to the same problem (for example, how to screen for hearing loss). There may be equally sound rationale for these different approaches in relation to particular clinical settings. Thus, in Chapter 5, for example, a suggested protocol for screening is provided, but it is acknowledged that other protocols may be equally suitable given the clinical decision-making systems experienced by individual speech-language therapists.

### Guided enhancement of clinical skills sensitive to the local situation

This is not a 'how to do it' book. The intention has been to provide information that will assist the speech-language therapist to make decisions appropriate to their individual clinical situation. Most of the following chapters contain a section entitled 'Clinical decisions for the speech-language therapist', in which attention is drawn to some key issues needing consideration when deciding how best to assist the client. Some broad guidelines are provided, but the particular approach taken by the individual speech-language therapist will need to be sensitive to the local situation and to the particular nature of their practice.

## Organisation of this book

Each of the following chapters may be read as stand-alone treatments of the topics covered. However, multiple cross references between chapters are made, to provide opportunity for integration of knowledge as the reader progresses through the book. For example, the treatment of conductive versus sensorineural hearing loss in Chapter 3 (causes and effects on speech perception) is built on in Chapter 4 (how various tests are used to detect and help differentiate between these two types of loss and their subgroups), Chapter 5 (interpreting screening results) and Chapter 6 (interpreting threshold audiograms). In general, the practical application builds as the book progresses, finishing with the integrative examples in the final chapter.

Chapters 2 to 9 each begin with a set of principles relating to the broad topic under discussion. These principles are intended to draw attention to the core issues in applying knowledge of that topic to the clinical practice of speech-language therapy. Each chapter also lists some important clinical decisions related to the chapter topics.

Case studies and other clinical examples are presented in most chapters. These examples have been selected with reference to specific problems likely to be encountered by speech-language therapists. Thus the clinical examples include, for example, the acoustic reflex results of an adult with VIIth nerve palsy (Chapter 4) and the auditory processing test results for a child with a suspected learning disorder (Chapter 9). It is hoped these examples will underline the relevance of basic audiology knowledge for the speech-language therapist and assist therapists to become informed consumers of the information supplied by audiologists and others.

The style of exposition is verbal rather than mathematically oriented. Reference to formulae and symbols has been kept to a minimum. Some topics (e.g. screening) have been treated in much greater depth than other topics (e.g. acoustics), reflecting this author's appreciation of the information needs of speech-language therapists. Again, it is acknowledged that not all speech-language therapists will consider that they need all the information presented, and some may wish for more information than is provided on some topics.

Each chapter concludes with a summary of key points of information. These key points are written with a clinical rather than a theoretical orientation.

Many different systems exist for recording the results of audiometric threshold tests. In this book the ASHA, British Society of Audiology (BSA, 1989) and Audiological Society of Australia (ASA, 1997) symbol systems are explained, as it is likely that the majority of clinical audiologists use one of these systems. However, the ASHA system is used in the examples provided, except for some of the sound field audiograms. The reader is reminded that any audiogram, regardless of the symbol system used, may be read if, as is usual, the code key is supplied. Appendix B provides the BSA, ASHA and ASA symbol codes. Audiograms are fully explained in Chapter 6, but are introduced in earlier chapters in association with discussion of various hearing disorders and hearing assessment techniques.

As the emphasis of this book is on clinical application, some information, which is useful for reference but not vital for understanding audiologic principles, is supplied in appendices rather than in the main text. Appendix A, for example, lists a range of disorders associated with hearing loss. Only relatively common causes of loss and/or causes highly relevant to the speech-language therapist are discussed in the main text.

I wish the reader a happy journey.

## Further reading

American Speech-Language-Hearing Association (1990) Scope of practice: Speech-language pathology and audiology. Asha 32(Suppl. 2): 1–2. (A succinct page and a half of information that informs ASHA members of the activities appropriate to their area of clinical certification (audiology or speech pathology) and can be used to educate professionals, consumers and employers about the services provided by speech-language therapists. Readers are advised to monitor ASHA for any updates.)

American Speech-Language-Hearing Association (1991) Issues in ethics: clinical practice by certificate holders in the profession in which they are not certified. Asha 33: 51. (Deals with speech pathology and audiology responsibilities.)

American Speech-Language-Hearing Association (1993) Preferred practice patterns for the professions of speech-language pathology and audiology. Asha 35(Suppl. 11): 3–96. (Deals with speech pathology and audiology responsibilities.)

Australian Association of Speech and Hearing (1994) Competency based occupational standards for speech pathologists: Entry level. Melbourne: AASH. (A document that guides recognition of overseas trained speech-language therapists seeking membership of Speech Pathology Australia (formerly the Australian Association of Speech and Hearing), and details standards expected by persons entering the profession after graduation from an Australian university course. Readers are advised to contact Speech Pathology Australia, 11–19 Bank Place, Melbourne, Victoria for update information.)

# Chapter 2
# Sound and hearing

JANET DOYLE

In this chapter some fundamental knowledge related to sound and the perception of sound by humans is presented. The particular acoustic concepts and the anatomical and physiological details presented are discussed in a way that attempts to meet the needs of the speech-language clinician. The emphasis is on sound as it travels through air and the reception of that sound by the normal human ear. Additional reading is recommended for those who want more detail than is provided in this chapter.

## Principles

1. *The perception of speech sounds is essential to the development of spoken language*. The connection between hearing and speech functions is intimate. It is therefore important for the speech-language therapist to understand how produced speech is fed back to the speaker and reaches the consciousness of other listeners. In cases where hearing is not normal and/or the acoustic environment is inadequate, speech perception and production are compromised.

2. *A knowledge of acoustic concepts assists in the development of appropriate therapy for individuals with communication problems*. The complex acoustic signals that comprise speech can be described in terms of simple attributes that assist the speech-language therapist to understand how well individual clients will perceive spoken messages. The way sound travels within confined spaces can be influenced to improve listening environments and therefore the chances of successful communication. The selection of devices to aid hearing and speech needs an understanding of the way those devices can alter and deliver sound. In these ways basic acoustic concepts are important to the speech-language clinician.

3. *A knowledge of auditory anatomy and physiology is highly relevant to the speech-language therapist.* Some of the clients who consult speech-language therapists have anatomical abnormalities as a result of congenital conditions, have acquired damage to the auditory system or have a higher-than-average risk of experiencing ear disease. For example, children with Down's syndrome, cleft palate or cranio-facial disorders are at risk for middle-ear disorders. Persons with head injury may have sustained damage to the middle and/or inner ear. Many individuals with cerebral palsy have hearing loss. The speech-language therapist who treats such individuals needs to understand how auditory function may be compromised.

## The sound and hearing model

Speech-language therapists will be familiar with the classic 'speech chain' of communication described by Denes and Pinson (1973). The chain begins at the linguistic level as a speaker formulates thoughts. The second link in the chain is at the physiological level as the speaker produces a spoken message by the movements of the vocal organs. The third link, at the acoustic level, is provided by sound waves travelling in air from the speaker's mouth and across the space between speaker and listener. The fourth link, again at the physiological level, is the perception of sound by the listener's auditory system. The final link in the chain, if the speaker and listener share the same language, is the listener's linguistic recognition of the speaker's message. The speaker and listener need to have adequate language function, the speaker adequate articulation skills and the listener adequate hearing skills, and the background noise needs to be at an adequately low level, if the communication chain is to be effective. The chain begins and ends at the linguistic level, but could not occur without the acoustic transmission of sound waves, and without auditory anatomy and physiology, the subjects of this chapter.

Similarly, if one considers the 'speech circle' of Perkins and Kent (1986), communication begins with the neural impulses, associated with thought, which are transmitted to the speaker's respiratory system. The respiratory system provides air pressure, which is applied to the phonatory system and then to the articulators of the vocal tract. The speech sounds thus produced travel through air and are perceived by the auditory system, which, at its highest level, decodes the speech message so that it can be understood by the listener's brain. The listener's brain can then formulate thoughts in response to that message and so the circle continues. This speech circle could not occur without the acoustic waveforms of speech travelling from speaker to listener, and without auditory physiology. Thus sound and hearing are crucial to oral language communication.

# Sound waves

Sound waves are a travelling disturbance produced by a vibrating body, such as, for example, the vocal folds. Sound waves are variations in air pressure over a period of time. Table 2.1 explains some important terms, related to sound waves, which will be used in this chapter. Figure 2.1 illustrates waveforms of the most simple sound, a pure tone, which is used in audiometric hearing tests, and of a complex sound, which is the result of several pure tones occurring simultaneously. Both waveforms show variations in pressure (which is related to the strength or intensity of the sound and the amplitude of the sound wave) and variations in how often the pressure changes occur (which is related to the pitch or frequency of the sound). The complex sound of speech is made up of many different tones occurring simultaneously and interacting with the characteristics of the vocal tract in a way that produces the particular qualities recognisable as the speech of an individual.

**Table 2.1:** Some useful acoustic terms

| | |
|---|---|
| Attenuation | Reduction in the level of a sound. For example, ear protection used in a noisy workplace attenuates the noise before it reaches the worker's ear |
| Frequency | The frequency at which air particles vibrate. How rapidly the pressure changes in a sound occur. The number of cycles per second of a sound wave The unit of frequency is Hertz (Hz). One cycle is equal to 1 Hz. A property of sound that can be objectively measured |
| kiloHertz | A unit of frequency. One kiloHertz (kHz) is equal to 1000 Hz. Audiologists often use this term as an abbreviation when discussing hearing test results and hearing aids. 1 kHz = 1000 Hz, 2 kHz = 2000 Hz, 4 kHz = 4000 Hz, etc |
| Fundamental frequency | The lowest frequency component of a sound comprised of a number of frequencies |
| Pitch | The subjective correlate of frequency. High-frequency sounds are perceived as high pitched sounds |
| Intensity | Basically the strength or energy level of a sound. The human ear is sensitive to a very large range of intensity |
| Decibel | A useful way of expressing the intensity of a sound. Abbreviated to 'dB'. A logarithmic ratio scale that indicates the intensity of a sound in relation to some reference intensity |
| Loudness | The subjective correlate of intensity. More intense sounds are generally perceived as louder than sounds with low intensity |
| Sound pressure level | Abbreviated to 'SPL'. Can be measured by a sound-level meter. dB SPL indicates the intensity of a sound in reference to the minimum sound pressure required for a normally hearing adult to perceive that sound |

(contd)

**Table 2.1:** (contd)

| | |
|---|---|
| Pure tone | A sound comprised of a single frequency e.g. 2000 Hz. Also known as a sine wave. Most audiometric tests of hearing sensitivity use pure tones as stimuli |
| Minimal audible field | The average threshold of hearing for normal listeners in a sound 'field', such as a room, for a range of frequencies. Expressed in dB SPL. Used as a reference during hearing tests |
| Minimal audible pressure | The average threshold of hearing for normal listeners when the sound is presented directly to the listener's ear. Expressed in dB SPL. Used as a reference during hearing tests under headphones |
| Complex sounds | Sounds, such as speech, which contain more than one frequency. Complex sound waves can be broken down into their component frequencies by Fourier analysis |
| Signal-to-noise ratio | The relationship of a signal, such as speech, to the noise present at the same time. During audiological tests, particularly for central auditory processing disorder, speech materials may be presented at various signal-to-noise ratios |
| Reverberation | An effect of sound reflections in a room, in which sound can persist after the sound source has stopped producing the sound. A room with reflective surfaces is more reverberative than a room with absorptive surfaces, and will have a longer reverberation time. A reverberation time is the time taken for a sound to reduce by 60 dB after the sound source has stopped |

Some sounds are periodic; that is, the waveform repeats itself at regular and equal intervals. The simple pure tone shown in Figure 2.1 is a periodic sound. Complex sounds (e.g. a telephone ring) may also be periodic. Many sounds in the natural world, however, are aperiodic; that is, the waveform varies over time and does not repeat itself at regular and equal intervals. One aperiodic sound used in some audiometric procedures is white noise.

The frequency range detectable by the young, normal hearing listener is 20–20,000 Hz. The range of frequencies commonly tested in audiometric diagnosis (described in Chapters 4 and 6) is 250–8000 Hz, as this frequency range covers sounds involved in human speech. In screening tests of hearing (described in Chapter 5), the frequency range used is even less, commonly 1000–4000 Hz. The ear is most sensitive to sounds in the frequency range 500–4000 Hz, sounds within this range being detected at much lower intensities than sounds of lower or higher frequency.

The intensity range detectable by the young, normal human ear is very large, so large that it would be awkward to record in physical units such as pascals (Pa, the unit of sound pressure). It is much more convenient to indicate the strength of a sound by using decibels.

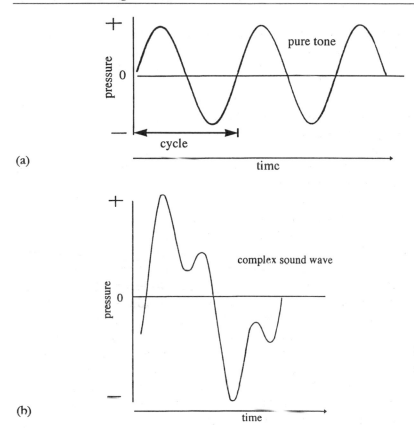

(a)

(b)

**Figure 2.1:** Waveforms of (a) pure tone and (b) a complex sound made up of several pure tones.

## Decibels

The decibel (dB) is a logarithmic ratio scale that indicates the intensity of a sound in relation to some reference intensity. It is important to understand that the decibel scale is not linear in the way that, for example, inches or kilograms are. Ten inches is a length ten times the length of 1 inch, 50 kg is twice the weight of 25 kg, but 30 dB is *not* three times the sound level of a 10 dB sound, or 30 times greater than 0 dB. Rather, because it is a logarithmic scale, 30 dB is 1000 times greater than 0 dB. This use of a logarithmic scale means that the difference between a just perceptible sound and the loudest sound we can tolerate can be dealt with by a range of about 140 dB.

The decibel is not a fixed unit. It is a means of expressing something (in this case the strength of a sound) with reference to another sound. The reference is usually the softest sound that can be detected by humans.

When listening with both ears to sounds travelling through the air (i.e. in an audible field), humans with normal hearing can, on average, detect sounds with a sound pressure of about 0.00002 Pa at frequencies around 2000–4000 Hz. This pressure is termed 0 dB SPL; 0 dB SPL therefore is not the absence of sound, but the presence of the smallest sound-pressure variation that is audible to normal listeners. At other frequencies, normal hearing is less sensitive. To perceive sound at those frequencies greater SPL levels are necessary. This is illustrated in Figure 2.2, which shows the minimum audible field curve (MAF). The monaural MAF values are slightly higher than the binaural values.

When testing hearing it is usually more convenient to present sounds via headphones, and to each ear separately, rather than in a sound field. The SPL necessary to detect sounds when listening through headphones and with one ear is greater than that required when listening in a sound field, but can still be expressed with reference to 0.00002 Pa. The differential hearing sensitivity curve in this condition is called the minimum audible pressure curve (MAP). This curve is also shown in Figure 2.2. Both MAF and MAP are expressed in dB SPL as a function of frequency.

If we wanted to compare the hearing sensitivity of an individual client to the average normal hearing sensitivity shown in Figure 2.2, we would have that individual listen to sounds through headphones and derive their hearing thresholds (those levels of sound, in dB SPL, which were just audible to the person for various frequencies). We could then compare the MAP value for each frequency (because those are normal values for listening through headphones) with the threshold obtained for the individual, the difference representing any deviation from normal hearing sensitivity. For example, the MAP value at 1000 Hz is 7 dB SPL for commonly used headphones. If the client's threshold for 1000 Hz was 23 dB SPL, then their hearing for that frequency would be 16 dB poorer than normal (23 – 7 dB), and they could be said to have a 16 dB hearing loss for 1000 Hz. They required the 1000 Hz tone to be 16 dB greater than the level normally required for perception by a listener with normal hearing.

Although it is clear that hearing loss is the difference between an

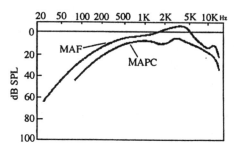

**Figure 2.2:** Minimum audible field (MAF) and minimum audible pressure (MAP) curves for average normal threshold hearing. The actual values that make up those curves depend on the measurement procedures used and the particular 'normal' subjects used to derive norms (see Durrant & Lovrinic, 1984, pp. 217–9, or Schubert, 1980, pp. 44–7 for readable discussions of this issue). The point here is to note the differential sensitivity of the ear and the greater sound levels required for detection of sounds delivered monoaurally via earphones (MAP) in comparison to sounds delivered binaurally via loudspeakers, and that both curves serve as references to which the hearing sensitivity of an individual listener may be compared.

individual's threshold response and the known average threshold SPL levels for persons with normal hearing, it is cumbersome to calculate hearing loss in dB SPL. It is much simpler to work in dB hearing threshold level (dB HTL), also known as dB hearing level (dB HL).

Decibels HTL is a concept relevant to audiometric testing of hearing and only applies to hearing procedures using calibrated audiometers to deliver test tones via headphones or insert earphones. Audiometers are calibrated so that 0 dB HTL equals the normal MAP value at each frequency. Thus if the audiometer dial is set at 0 dB HTL, the level of sound presented will be that amount of SPL necessary for a normal listener to perceive the tone. At 1000 Hz, 7 dB SPL will be produced when the audiometer dial is set at 0 dB HTL, as 7 dB SPL is the MAP value at that frequency. At 2000 Hz, 9 dB SPL will be produced when the audiometer dial is set at 0 dB HTL, and so on. Thus 0 dB HTL does not mean no sound, but that minimum level of sound audible to persons with normal hearing. It can be thought of as 'zero hearing loss', and is also known as audiometric zero. Figure 2.3 shows audiometric zero and indicates an individual's thresholds in dB HTL at three frequencies. Such a graph of thresholds expressed in dB HTL is called an audiogram, which is described more fully in Chapters 4 and 6.

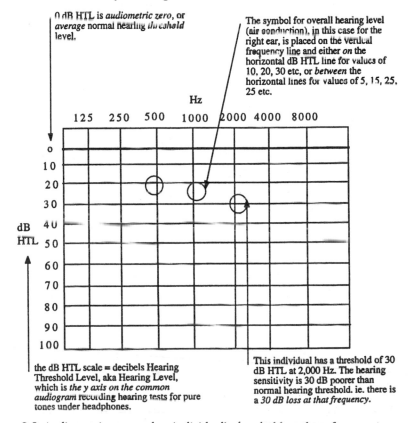

Figure 2.3: Audiometric zero and an individual's thresholds at three frequencies.

Sometimes it is useful to refer to sound as a level above an individual listener's threshold (rather than as a level above average normal hearing threshold as has just been discussed). The term 'sensation level' (SL) is used in these circumstances. Therefore dB SL refers to the number of decibels above an individual listener's threshold. If an individual had a threshold of 0 dB HTL at 1000 Hz for example (i.e. normal hearing sensitivity), and we presented a 1000 Hz tone to that person at 50 dB HTL, the tone would be 50 dB above their threshold and hence 50 dB HTL is equal to 50 dB SL for that individual. If another individual had a threshold of 40 dB HTL at 1000 Hz (i.e. hearing sensitivity 40 dB poorer than average normal for that frequency), and we presented the same 50 dB HTL 1000 Hz tone, that tone would be 10 dB greater than the individual's threshold and therefore would be a 10 dB SL tone. For the first individual 50 dB HTL = 50 dB SL, but for the second individual 50 dB HTL = 10 dB SL. The dB SL concept is useful in some audiometric procedures, such as speech audiometry (see Chapter 4), and is also sometimes used by audiologists when discussing, for example, aspects of hearing-aid rehabilitation.

Another reference for decibels relates to the measurement of environmental sounds via a sound level meter. dB A is a value in decibels of a sound, for example, industrial noise, measured by a sound-level meter with a special filter.

## Sound-level meters

Sound-level meters (SLMs) are instruments that provide readings of the level of a sound. Most commonly used SLMs have a system of weighting networks or filters. When set in linear mode, the SLM will measure the sound in dB SPL and is, for practicable purposes, almost equally sensitive to all frequencies up to about 10,000 Hz. When set to external octave band filter, the SLM will provide information on the dB SPL levels at each of several frequencies that make up the sound. When set to A network the meter measures dB SPL values and puts these values through the filter, which is designed to resemble the response of the human ear to low-level sounds. Thus dB A is a kind of adjusted dB SPL value. There are other similar filters, used to produce dB B or dB C when sounds are more intense, and dB D when sounds are extremely high level, such as jet noise, but these are less relevant to this discussion.

## Summary

In summary, decibels are useful for indicating the level of a sound, but it is crucial that a reference (SPL, HTL, SL, A) be specified, as a value in dB is not meaningful without that reference. It is particularly important to distinguish between dB SPL, dB HTL and dB SL, as these are all frequently used to describe the audiometric test responses of individual clients yet they mean quite different things. Table 2.2 summarises the meaning of the various dB references. We can refer to a change in decibel level (e.g. the sound reduced by 40 dB), or to a signal-to-noise ratio (e.g. the signal-to-noise ratio was 10 dB) without specifying a reference, but the information given by these statements is limited.

**Table 2.2:** Decibel references

| | |
|---|---|
| dB SPL | dB sound pressure level. A value in decibels with reference to 0.00002 Pa, the minimal sound pressure that is audible to persons with normal hearing. dB SPL values may be used in testing hearing in a sound field via loudspeakers, in some speech audiometry tests, to indicate the level of environmental sounds, and in measures associated with hearing aids. dB SPL can be used to refer to the level of a single frequency sound or to the level of a complex sound. dB SPL can be measured with a sound-level meter |
| dB HTL | dB hearing threshold level. A value in decibels with reference to average normal hearing. 0 dB HTL at any frequency represents normal hearing sensitivity. Used in audiometric tests under headphones to indicate hearing threshold for individual frequencies. The value in dB HTL is the amount by which the individual's hearing differs from normal and is therefore the degree of hearing loss. dB HTL may be used by some audiologists in speech audiometry to indicate the levels at which speech material was presented |
| dB SL | dB sensation level. A value in decibels with reference to an individual listener's threshold. A value in dB SL cannot be related to the actual level of sound without knowing which listener is involved. dB SL may be used by audiologists to indicate a level at which speech audiometry materials were presented, or in discussions about a client's dynamic range of hearing |
| dB A | dB A is a value in decibels of a sound, for example industrial noise, measured by a sound-level meter with a special filter. The meter measures dB SPL values and puts these values through the filter, which is designed to resemble the response of the human ear. dB A is a kind of adjusted dB SPL. dB A is used extensively in industrial settings |

# Sound in clinic rooms, classrooms, hospitals and workplaces

Communication is significantly affected by the overall level of background noise (called ambient noise) in the area in which people are conversing. Persons who have hearing loss, those who are easily distractable and those with voice or speech disorders may be particularly disadvantaged in a noisy situation. Many clinic rooms are designed to keep noise levels down, but classrooms can be a particular problem for the individual with communication problems. Background noise may come from activities within the classroom, from hallways and through windows, and from mechanical noises within the building. The American Speech-Language-Hearing Association (ASHA) recommends that the noise level in an unoccupied classroom not exceed 30 dB A, and that signal-to-noise ratios (see Table 2.1) at the listener's ear should be better than +15 dB (ASHA, 1995). Further ASHA recommends that the reverberation time (see Table 2.1) within classrooms be limited to less than 0.4 seconds. These are optimal goals and are difficult to achieve in practice. Where it is not practicable to reduce noise by locating the classroom away from noise sources, acoustically treating hard surfaces in the classroom or using landscaping to reduce external noises entering the room, it will be necessary to ensure that speaker–listener distance is reduced.

**Table 2.3:** Ways of dealing with noise in communication situations

- Relocate the communication situation (e.g. classroom) away from the noise source (e.g. large assembly hall)
- Plant trees, use earthworks and walls as a barrier between the communication situation (e.g. classroom) and the noise source (e.g. traffic noise from a main road)
- Apply sound reduction engineering (e.g. a muffler system) to particularly noisy equipment
- Decrease the sound reflection and generation in the room (e.g. hospital ward, meeting room) by use of absorptive materials such as curtains and carpets, and possibly acoustic tiles
- Reduce the distance between the speaker (e.g. teacher, therapist) and the listener (e.g. child with communication difficulty). This will provide a better signal-to-noise ratio
- Use technical aids such as FM communication systems (see Chapter 7) to provide excellent signal-to-noise ratio over considerable distance
- Use a binaural amplified listener (see Chapter 7) or similar device for the client (e.g. hospital inpatient) who needs to hear important information in a poor acoustic situation. This is especially useful for older clients who do not have personal hearing aids, and is inexpensive
- In therapy groups, use turn-taking protocols to reduce the number of persons speaking simultaneously and to increase alertness in listeners. Use small groups
- Carry out communication at a time when the noise level is known to be less (e.g. have a therapy session at lunch time or after 5 pm when certain noisy equipment is turned off)
- Increase the availability of visual cues by appropriate lighting and seating. For example, make sure the light from a window(s) provides adequate illumination of the speaker's face and is not shining in the eyes of the listener. Round tables are preferable to rectangular tables for meetings

Hospitals and nursing homes can be a real problem for effective communication because of a large number of hard surfaces and interconnecting spaces, the use of trolleys and public address systems, and the often high level of activity. In hospitals an ambient level of 34–47 dB

A is recommended by Lipscomb and Taylor (1978). Workplaces vary greatly in the level of noise. In some (e.g. some large building sites) effective communication is often simply not possible for much of the day. In others (e.g. open offices) an individual's existing communication problems may be exacerbated by a poor acoustic environment. In these cases it is important to assess the situation thoroughly. An audiologist or acoustic consultant may be able to assist with recommendations. Table 2.3 gives suggestions for dealing with the ambient noise within various communication situations.

## How the ear perceives sound

The next two sections present a basic overview of normal auditory anatomy and physiology. Table 2.4 lists and explains the anatomical and physiological terms related to the ear that are likely to be most relevant to speech-language therapists. Figure 2.4 is a schematic diagram of the ear structures.

The transmission of sound from the external ear through to the auditory cortex of the brain is a complex process involving several different kinds of energy. The external ear (Figure 2.4) accepts acoustic energy in the form of airborne sound waves. Sound reaching the auricle is funnelled into the external auditory meatus via the concha. The concha has resonant properties that amplify slightly sounds around 5000 Hz by about 10 dB. When the sound travels the length of the external auditory meatus those sounds in the frequency range 2500–4000 Hz (usually around 3500 Hz in particular) are slightly amplified, also by about 10 dB. The slightly altered acoustic signal then contacts the tympanic membrane (TM), which vibrates in response. The acoustic energy thus transformed into vibrations of the TM results in vibrations of the middle-ear ossicles (malleus, incus and stapes) to which the TM is articulated. The ossicles function to transmit the energy across the air cavity of the middle-ear space in a way that further amplifies the incoming signal, by about 25 dB, before it is transferred to the inner ear. This amplification in the middle ear occurs because the area of the TM is much larger than the area of the oval window (a membrane on the lateral wall of the inner ear), which is contacted by vibrations of the stapes, the most medial of the ossicles. The areal ratio of the TM to the oval window is about 17:1 if the whole area of the TM is considered and about 14:1 if the most efficient area of the TM is considered. The pressure at the oval window is therefore about 17 times greater than that at the TM, so the sound reaches the entrance to the inner ear with greater force. Additionally, it is thought that the ossicles have a lever action that adds yet more force and thus contributes to the amplification of sound as it travels across the middle-ear cavity. This amplification (or 'transformer action' of the middle ear) is necessary because the inner ear contains fluids. Sound travelling through air and contacting a fluid surface will mostly be reflected back into the air. Thus if the sound hitting the TM were to be directly transmitted to the perilymph (see Table 2.4) in the cochlea, almost none of the incoming acoustic signal would be perceived. The middle-ear transformer action largely overcomes this.

**Table 2.4:** Some useful terms related to auditory anatomy and physiology

| | |
|---|---|
| Auricle | Also known as the pinna. The visible part of the external ear. The auricle should be lifted up and back during auroscopic inspection of the ear |
| Concha | The depression in the centre of the auricle that leads to the opening of the ear canal. Persons who wear hearing aids need the aid or earmould to fit securely in the concha |
| External auditory meatus | Abbreviated to 'eam'. The channel that conducts sound from the auricle to the middle ear. About 25 mm long in adult ears. The lateral, cartilaginous portion contains glands that produce cerumen (ear wax) |
| Tympanic membrane | Abbreviated to 'TM'. The membrane at the end of the eam. Consists of three layers, the inner layer being continuous with the mucous lining of the middle-ear cavity |
| Cone of light | Also termed 'light reflex'. A reflection (not an anatomical feature) of the light shone on the tympanic membrane during auroscopic inspection. If the cone of light is visible you are looking at the tympanic membrane |
| Ossicles | The three bones that bridge the middle-ear cavity and conduct sound from the tympanic membrane to the inner ear. The most lateral, the malleus, is attached to the tympanic membrane. The incus connects the malleus to the most medial ossicle, the stapes, which sits at the entrance to the inner ear |
| Stapedial muscle | A muscle attached to the stapes, which contracts in response to loud sounds. Integral to the acoustic reflex, an important diagnostic phenomenon (see Chapter 4). The stapedial muscle is innervated by a branch of the VIIth cranial nerve |
| Eustachian tube | A tube that extends from the middle-ear cavity to the nasopharynx, angled downward in adults but flatter in children. Functions to drain the middle ear of excess fluid and to provide air to the middle-ear cavity. In adults the Eustachian tube is approximately 3.5 cm long. Commonly involved in hearing disorders in children |
| Temporal bone | That portion of the skull that houses the ear. Consists of squamous, mastoid, tympanic and petrous portions. Some hearing tests are carried out by placing a vibrator on the mastoid portion of the temporal bone. The cochlea is housed in the petrous portion of the temporal bone |

(contd)

**Table 2.4:** (contd)

| | |
|---|---|
| Cochlea | The portion of the inner ear that houses the sense receptors for sound. A spiral cavity within the petrous portion of the temporal bone |
| Basilar membrane | A membrane that extends the length of the cochlea, and varies in width and stiffness, being most narrow and stiff at the basal end of the cochlea adjacent to the middle-ear cavity |
| Organ of Corti | An arrangement of receptors and supporting structures that sits on the basilar membrane throughout its length |
| Hair cells | Important receptors contained within the Organ of Corti. Hair cell damage is frequently the cause of permanent hearing loss especially in adults |
| Perilymph | One of two fluids that are contained within the inner ear. The perilymph is found in the areas between the bone bordering the inner ear cavity and the membranes within that cavity which enclose the sense receptors for hearing and balance |
| Endolymph | The second of the two fluids contained within the inner ear. Endolymph is found in the membraneous portion of the inner ear. Disorders of endolymph and/or perilymph are involved in some diseases such as Ménière's disease |
| Semicircular canals | Three tunnels, each in a different plane, that contain some of the sense receptors for balance. Intimately connected with the cochlea, and containing perilymph and endolymph |
| VIIIth nerve | The bundle of cochlear and vestibular fibres that transmit impulses from the inner ear to the brain |
| Internal auditory meatus | A canal in the temporal bone through which passes the VIIIth nerve, the facial nerve, and the internal branch of the anterior inferior cerebellar artery. A narrow channel of communication between the inner ear and the brainstem |
| Superior olivary nucleus | An important neural terminus in the brainstem, where afferent impulses from left and right ears are compared. Involved in the acoustic reflex arc |
| Inferior colliculus | A neural terminus in the mid-brain, important in the processing of auditory cues in localisation |
| Anterior | Towards the front (e.g. towards the face) |
| Posterior | Towards the back (e.g. of the head) |
| Lateral | Towards the side (e.g. of the head) |
| Medial | Towards the middle (e.g. of the head) |
| Superior | Towards the upper surface (e.g. of the middle ear) |
| Inferior | Towards the lower surface (e.g. of the middle ear) |

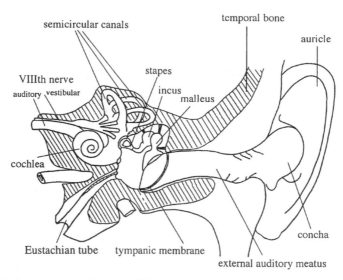

**Figure 2.4:** Schematic diagram of the ear.

The mechanical vibrations of the stapes in the oval window mark the transmission of sound from the middle ear to the inner ear. At this point the energy is transformed into hydraulic energy. The movements of the stapes in and out at the oval window set up hydraulic waves in the perilymph. The stapes is able to exert movements against the perilymph because the round window (a membrane in the lower portion of the lateral wall of the inner ear) moves in and out correspondingly and so relieves the pressure exerted by the stapes. These structures are described more fully in the next section. The point here is that pressure waves are set up in the cochlear fluids. These hydraulic waves carry forward the frequency and intensity characteristics of the incoming sound energy (e.g. high frequency sounds will be associated with hydraulic waves that have a high number of compressions per second; low frequency sounds will cause hydraulic waves with fewer compressions per second). The wave motion set up in the perilymph of the cochlea (the portion of the inner ear associated with hearing) causes excitation of the sense receptors of hearing housed inside a closed system of membranes, (membranous labyrinth), which is surrounded by the perilymph. The sense receptors inside the cochlear portion of this membranous labyrinth are bathed in a fluid called endolymph (which closely resembles cerebrospinal fluid).

The stimulation of the sense receptors of the cochlea mean that the hydraulic energy associated with sound is converted into a set of neural impulses. These are conducted, via the auditory portion of the VIIIth cranial nerve, from the inner ear to the brainstem. A system of neural pathways (the afferent auditory pathway) transmits the signals from the brainstem through several important stages to the auditory cortex, where the impulses are further organised and interpreted as meaningful sounds.

This complex process of hearing normally occurs as a result of airborne (i.e. air-conducted) sound. The common clinical test of hearing through headphones is called air conduction audiometry. However, there are occasions when the cochlear sense receptors are stimulated by vibration of the bones of the skull rather than by sound that has travelled through the middle ear to reach the cochlea. Hearing can therefore also occur by bone conduction. Hearing by bone conduction is not very useful in real life, and does not work very effectively. Clinically, however, it is a useful process to exploit. There is a clinical test of hearing that employs a vibrator placed on the mastoid process of the temporal bone. This is called bone conduction audiometry (see Chapter 4).

There are two situations in which hearing by bone conduction can occur. First, if sound is sufficiently intense it will vibrate the skull. Second, if a vibrating body (e.g. a tuning fork) is placed against the skull, hearing by bone conduction can result. The difference between hearing by air conduction and by bone conduction is that the external- and middle-ear systems are effectively bypassed in bone conduction, the cochlea being directly stimulated via vibrations set up in the skull. Skull vibrations cause hearing principally in two ways. Compressional bone conduction occurs mainly for high-frequency sounds, and involves alternate compressions and expansions of the skull bones. The cochlea is subject to these compressions and expansions, which in turn cause the cochlear fluids to be displaced and the cochlear sense receptors for hearing to be stimulated. Inertial bone conduction occurs mainly for low frequencies, and results from the relative inertia of the ossicular chain and the cochlear fluids in comparison to the skull. As movements of the ossicles and cochlear fluids lag behind movements of the skull, the effect is the same as if the ossicular chain was vibrating in response to an air-conducted sound, i.e. the stapes is displaced inwards in the oval window and the round window is displaced outwards and so on. It is important to note that whether hearing occurs by air conduction (as it normally does) or by bone conduction, the sense receptors in the cochlea of the inner ear are stimulated in the same way, i.e. by movements of the cochlear fluids and associated movements of the membranous system that houses the sense receptors.

## Important structures involved in hearing

Some of the structures indicated in Figure 2.4 deserve a relatively detailed discussion. This section will describe more fully parts of the middle ear and inner ear, and will note some features of the ascending auditory pathway.

## Middle ear

Figure 2.5 is a schematic diagram of the TM. Several features are worth noting. First, the cone of light that is seen when a light is shone on the membrane angles down from the umbo in an anterior–inferior direction. Therefore if looking at a right ear drum, the cone of light will normally angle down to the right (roughly at 5 o'clock) and in a left ear it will normally angle down to the left (roughly at 7 o'clock). Second, the handle of the malleus, which is integrated with the middle fibrous layer of the TM, angles in an anterior–superior direction (roughly 1 o'clock in a right ear and 11 o'clock in a left ear). If the TM is retracted, as can occur with middle-ear disorders, the handle of the malleus may appear very prominent because the TM is pulled medially over it. Third, the TM in a healthy ear appears a pearly grey colour. If the middle ear is infected, the TM can appear pink or red and distended. In severe cases it may be difficult to discern landmarks such as the handle of the malleus. If there is a collection of largely sterile fluid in the middle-ear cavity a fluid line and/or the presence of air bubbles in the fluid may be seen through the TM, or the TM can appear darker than normal.

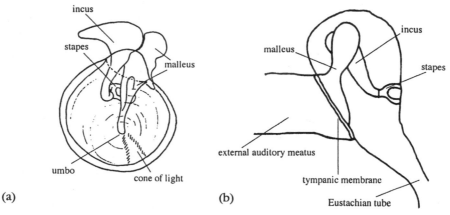

(a)                                        (b)

**Figure 2.5:** Schematic diagram of the tympanic membrane and middle ear: (a) lateral view; (b) coronal view.

The middle-ear cavity normally contains air and is kept aerated by the Eustachian tube, which connects the anterior wall of the middle-ear cavity to the nasopharynx. The Eustachian tube is lined with mucous membrane continuous with the lining of the middle ear. The diameter of the Eustachian tube is variable, being greatest at the pharyngeal end, where it is connected to the levator veli palatini and tensor veli palatini muscles. The Eustachian tube is normally closed at the pharyngeal end but opens on swallowing and yawning, and in this way keeps the middle ear aerated. In adults the Eustachian tube is about 3.5 cm long, but it is only half this length in children. It is also more horizontal in children.

The stapes, the most medial link in the ossicular chain, and the attached stapedial muscle, shown in Figure 2.6, are particularly interesting for two reasons. First, the stapes is a crucial point of transfer of sound energy from the middle to the inner ear. It is driven by the vibrations of the more lateral incus and correspondingly moves in the oval window to which it is attached by a ligament. Some adults can develop otosclerosis (see Chapter 3), a condition in which the footplate of the stapes and/or the annular ligament becomes ossified, reducing the ability of the stapes to move and hence causing a hearing loss. The stapedial muscle is very important in a phenomenon called the acoustic reflex (see Chapter 4). The acoustic reflex involves a contraction of the stapedius in response to very intense sounds (another muscle, the tensor tympani, which is attached to the malleus, is also involved). This contraction reduces the ability of the stapes to vibrate effectively in the oval window, and hence momentarily reduces the level of sound reaching the cochlea. This reflex is thought to have a protective effect and helps to reduce transmission of low-frequency sounds associated with breathing and speech. The acoustic reflex is often absent in facial palsy, because the stapedius is innervated by a branch of the facial nerve.

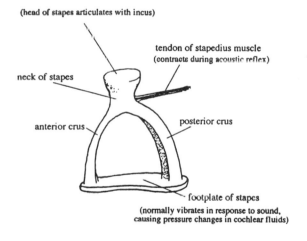

Figure 2.6: Schematic diagram of the stapes.

### Inner ear

Several features of the cochlea, the portion of the inner ear concerned with hearing, are now described. The cochlea is formed as a hollow space within the petrous portion of the temporal bone. Within this hollow space is contained a system of membranes (the membranous labyrinth), which does not quite fill the cochlear space. Within the membranous labyrinth is the collection of sensory cells called the Organ of Corti, which are bathed in endolymph, a fluid high in potassium and low in sodium. That part of cochlear space between the temporal bone and the membranous labyrinth contains the fluid perilymph, which is high in sodium and low in potassium.

Figure 2.7 shows a schematic view of the Organ of Corti in cross section. The hair cells, which are frequently discussed in cases of inner-ear hearing loss (e.g. hearing loss caused by excessive noise), are a key feature of the Organ of Corti. The steriocilia, or hair-like projections, emerging from the tops of the outer hair cells contact the overlying tectorial membrane. The base of the Organ of Corti is formed by the basilar membrane. The hydraulic waves set up in the perilymph as a result of the movement of the stapes in the oval window cause the basilar membrane to move in a wave-like response. The mechanical travelling wave in the basilar membrane transmits the sound energy in a way that preserves the frequency and intensity features of the sound received. High-frequency sounds will cause a wave that peaks near the basal end of the basilar membrane and low-frequency sounds will cause a wave-like motion that peaks closer to the apical end of the basilar membrane. This is important to note because the basilar membrane, which extends the length of the cochlea, varies in width and stiffness along its length in a way that means it is 'tuned' to receive sounds of particular frequency at various places (a feature called tonotopic organisation). The peak of the incoming travelling wave occurs at the place most sensitive to sounds of that frequency. The basilar membrane movement will then cause movement of the tectorial membrane and this in turn causes a bending of the steriocilia of the hair cells. In this way the hair cells are stimulated to produce a neural impulse that is then carried by nerve fibres to form the auditory nerve. There are approximately 30,000 nerve fibres in each ear.

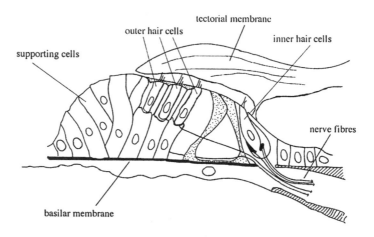

**Figure 2.7:** Schematic diagram of the Organ of Corti.

## Neural afferent pathways

Once neural impulses from the cochlea reach the auditory nerve, they are transmitted to the cochlear nucleus (see Figure 2.8), where most of the nerve fibres cross to the other side of the brain. One of the features of the ascending auditory pathway is that most of the information from one ear is transmitted to the contralateral side. Another feature of the ascending auditory pathway is that there is direct communication between the left and right sides of the brain in three places. Aside from the cochlear nucleus, there is communication from the contralateral ear at the superior olivary nucleus, also at brainstem level. The superior olivary nucleus has an important role in the acoustic reflex mentioned earlier (see Chapter 4). The third point of direct communication is at the inferior colliculus, in the mid-brain. Thus information from both ears reaches the cortex on both sides of the brain, and the information is directly shared at a number of levels.

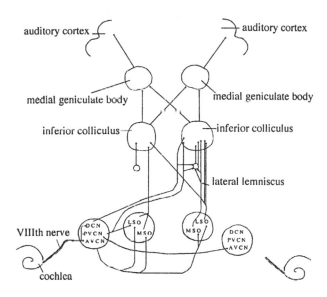

**Figure 2.8:** Schematic diagram of the afferent auditory pathways. DCN = dorsal cochlear nucleus; PVCN = posterior ventral cochlear nucleus; AVCN = anterior ventral cochlear nucleus; LSO = lateral superior olive; MSO = medial superior olive.

# Hearing with two ears

Having two ears is useful for a number of reasons, but it can cause diagnostic difficulties during hearing assessments. Binaural hearing allows comparison of the information arriving at one ear with the signals arriving at the other ear. This helps us to determine the direction from which a sound is coming, and thus is critical to localisation. Hearing with two ears is also slightly more sensitive than hearing with one ear (see the discussion on MAF versus MAP on p. 16). Binaural hearing helps when listening to important signals like speech in noisy situations. Many audiologists encourage persons with bilateral loss to wear a hearing aid in each ear, for these reasons.

However, during hearing assessments it is often necessary to prevent the sounds presented to one ear from being perceived by the other. Diagnostic hearing assessments (see Chapter 4) rely on being able to describe accurately the separate performance of the left ear and the right ear. During air-conduction hearing tests when sounds are presented to separate headphones it is often easy to distinguish the response of the left and right ear. If, however, one ear is very much less sensitive than the other a situation called cross-hearing can occur. This is discussed in Chapter 4, but essentially it means that loud sounds presented to an ear with very poor hearing are perceived by the opposite ear, which has much better hearing. The test sound, presented to one ear, has crossed the skull to stimulate the other ear. The sound will have reduced or attenuated somewhat in crossing the head (the amount by which the sound is reduced is called interaural attenuation), but it is still sufficiently loud to be perceived by the non-test ear. Cross-hearing is more often a problem during bone-conduction hearing tests than with air-conduction tests. If cross-hearing is suspected, a process called masking is used, in which a sound is produced into the non-test ear to occupy it and prevent it perceiving the tones presented to the poorer ear. Masking is described in Chapter 4.

## Some observations for speech-language therapists

Some features of the anatomy and physiology of hearing have particular clinical relevance for speech-language pathologists, and these are discussed briefly below.

The external ear can indicate the presence of congenital abnormalities associated with hearing loss (see Chapter 3), and so a quick visual inspection of the auricle is useful. The external auditory canal can become occluded with cerumen, which can adversely affect the use of hearing aids and other assistive listening devices (see Chapter 7). Additionally, an occluded external auditory canal can preclude screening tests of middle-ear function (see Chapter 5). An auroscopic inspection of the external auditory canal and the tympanic membrane is therefore a useful part of a first assessment for every client.

The middle ear is particularly prone to disorders in young children because of the incompletely developed Eustachian tube. These problems can occur even in the absence of obvious symptoms such as pain. Monitoring of middle-ear function (see Chapter 5) is useful especially for children. Clients with Down's syndrome are prone to problems involving middle-ear aeration and drainage.

Abnormalities of facial nerve function can be in part tested and monitored by acoustic stimulation sufficient to cause contraction of the stapedial muscle in the middle ear. Such stimulation involves the acoustic reflex (see Chapter 4), which can give very useful diagnostic results.

The inner-ear structures are sometimes compromised in congenital hearing loss of sufficient degree to cause difficulties acquiring oral language. Head trauma and vascular disorders can also cause cochlear hearing loss.

Because the highest neural centres for hearing lie in the temporal lobe, head trauma can be associated with auditory processing problems (see Chapters 4 and 9). Tests of the neural activity of the ascending auditory pathway may also be able to inform on auditory processing abilities in children with learning disorders (see Chapter 9).

## Summary of key points

The perception of speech sounds is essential to the normal development of spoken language. The normal human ear can detect sounds in the frequency range 20–20,000 Hz and is sensitive to a large range of intensity or sound pressure levels (SPL). The ear is differentially sensitive, being much more sensitive to sounds in the range 2000–4000 Hz than to sounds of higher or lower audio frequencies.

The decibel (dB), a logarithmic ratio scale, is used as a convenient way of indicating the strength or intensity of a sound. There are various references used with the decibel scale, two of the most important being 0.00002 Pa (dB SPL) and average normal hearing threshold values (dB HTL). Communication and hearing testing are both adversely affected by high levels of background noise.

The normal ear perceives sounds via a complex system of energy transfer involving the effective funnelling of sound by the external auditory meatus, the transformer action of the middle ear, the stimulation of the Organ of Corti in the membranous labyrinth of the cochlea and the transmission of neural impulses to the temporal lobe via the ascending auditory pathways.

## Further reading

Perkins WH, Kent RD (1986) Textbook of functional anatomy of speech, language and hearing. London: Taylor & Francis. (An extremely clear description of concepts relevant to the clinician. Includes helpful schematic diagrams, glossaries and self-assessment questions.)

# Chapter 3
# Forms of hearing difficulty

JANET DOYLE

This chapter describes the major forms of hearing loss, and gives examples that are of particular relevance to the speech-language therapist. The discussion is focused on the effects of various hearing losses on spoken communication, and on the clinical decisions facing the speech-language therapist who encounters clients with these forms of hearing difficulty.

## Principles

1. *Any hearing loss can be described in terms of (a) anatomy and physiology, (b) audiometric test results and (c) client symptoms.* That is hearing loss is associated with (a) some changes to the physical functioning of the auditory system, (b) the client's ability to process sound in comparison to known norms, and (c) the physical and/or communication difficulties noted by the client or other persons with whom they interact. Client symptoms are usually the first set of data available. While symptoms alone can give the speech-language therapist valuable information to support communication therapy, they also indicate the need for physical and audiometric examinations.

2. *Hearing loss should be considered in terms of both client communication and client health.* The client with hearing difficulty has, by definition, got a communication problem that the speech-language therapist will need to consider. However, the speech-language therapist also has a responsibility to arrange audiological and/or medical evaluation so that the health issue may be addressed. Likewise, clients who consult medical practitioners about hearing health ought to be questioned about the possible effects of the aural problem on communication, and referral made if necessary.

3. *Hearing loss can have significant effects on other individual characteristics.* Hearing loss can adversely effect psychological wellbeing, social functioning, and communication behaviour (Thomas & Herbst,

1980; Meadow-Orlans, 1985; Nowell, 1985; Wall, 1995). For example, it is possible that a child who presents with severe behaviour problems and poorly developed language skills may have a level of functioning that fluctuates with episodes of middle-ear disease, or even more unfortunately, may display these symptoms entirely because of undiagnosed hearing loss. Because of these possibilities the speech-language therapist needs some knowledge of hearing status in every client they treat. Where a loss is known to be present the speech-language therapist will benefit from an understanding of the nature of that loss so that therapy can be appropriately tailored to the client's needs.

4. *It is possible for an individual to have more than one type of hearing problem.* A client who has inner-ear hearing loss is not immune from developing middle-ear problems and vice versa. A person with a long-standing diagnosis of one type of hearing loss may, over time, develop additional and different problems. Hence knowledge of current hearing status is important. This is particularly important in the case of children with congenital hearing impairment, because their hearing function may, on occasions, be further impaired by transient middle-ear disorders.

# Disruptions to normal hearing

Chapter 2 explains how the sensation of hearing normally involves receiving airborne (air-conducted) sound waves, which are then transmitted, via the middle ear and the inner ear, to the ascending auditory pathways where the signals from the two ears are integrated and then ultimately received at the auditory cortex. A disruption to this normal reception of airborne sounds will result in a loss of normal hearing function. That is, a disruption to the normal workings of the external ear, the middle ear, the inner ear or the auditory nerve (VIIIth cranial nerve) will result in a loss of hearing by air conduction. The magnitude of hearing loss is determined by comparing an individual's threshold sensitivity to the threshold sensitivity known to exist in persons with normal hearing. The difference is expressed in decibels. For example, an individual with an average 40 dB HTL hearing loss can detect sound only when it is 40 dB greater than that required for detection by persons with normal hearing. Sounds of less intensity will not be perceived. A discussion of reference norms for various audiograms is given in Chapter 4.

Chapter 2 also notes that sound can be transmitted to the inner ear by vibrations of the skull bones. In this instance the external and middle ear are bypassed, the sound being directly received by the inner ear and subsequently ascending the afferent auditory pathways. Such bone-conduction vibrations do not normally play a significant role in natural hearing. They are, however, very useful in helping to determine the type of hearing loss.

Where there is a loss of hearing for air-conducted sounds and yet bone-conducted sounds are perceived at normal levels, then the hearing loss must be the result of an external- and/or middle-ear disorder, because normal bone conduction indicates normal hearing in the inner ear. That is, when the conductive mechanisms of the external and/or middle ear are impaired, there is a conductive hearing loss. When neither air- or bone-conducted sounds are heard normally, inner-ear dysfunction must be at least partially responsible for the hearing loss. If there is an equal degree of hearing loss for air- and bone-conducted sounds then the conductive mechanisms of the external and middle ear cannot be responsible for the loss. The loss must be caused by problems in the inner ear (which contains sensory receptors and transmits sounds to the neural pathways). In this case there is a sensorineural hearing loss. If there is a loss for both air- and bone-conducted sounds and yet bone-conducted sounds are heard more easily than air-conducted sounds, then there must be problems in both the external- and/or middle-ear conductive mechanism and in the sensorineural function of the inner ear. In this case there is a mixed hearing loss.

Regardless of the type of hearing loss, hearing by air conduction describes the overall degree of hearing loss and reflects the hearing function experienced in real life.

## Conductive hearing loss

A conductive hearing loss occurs when the cause of the loss lies in the external or middle ear. In purely conductive loss, the inner ear is always normal. The common feature of all conductive losses is a change to the normal mechanics of the external and/or middle ear. Medical treatment of conductive loss is in many, but not all, cases effective, and can often restore hearing to normal or near normal levels.

These mechanical changes can result from, for example:

- congenital deformities of the auricle, external auditory meatus and/or middle ear;
- wax (cerumen) blockages in the external auditory meatus;
- infections of the external and/or middle ear;
- trauma to the tympanic membrane and/or the ossicular chain;
- calcification of the ossicles.

Congenital deformities of the auricle and the external auditory meatus mean that the normal funnelling effect of the external ear is absent. Clients who have craniofacial defects can in some cases also have atresia (an absent or partially formed external auditory meatus) or microtia (very small and malformed auricles). Persons with atresia and/or microtia may also have deformities of the middle ear. In severe cases the middle ear can be absent. Many clients with Down's syndrome have narrow external auditory canals. Some genetic syndromes (e.g. Alport syndrome and Treacher Collins syndrome) involve fixated or incompletely developed middle-ear structures and hence conductive hearing loss (Fritsch & Sommer, 1991).

Wax blocking the external auditory meatus can result in conductive hearing loss. The resulting hearing loss is usually slight, although if the individual already has hearing loss due to other causes, the additional slight reduction in perceived volume associated with wax occlusion can cause significant listening problems. Use of cotton buds for cleaning the ear should be discouraged as this stimulates the cerumen glands and can in fact increase wax production. Further, there is the danger of causing trauma to the skin of the external auditory meatus, of pushing the wax down into the osseous portion of the external auditory meatus and even of perforating the tympanic membrane. Foreign objects inserted into the external auditory meatus can lodge there and cause subsequent conductive loss.

Infection of the external auditory meatus is termed otitis externa. This can be extremely painful and because of the associated swelling of the skin lining the external auditory meatus, can result in a stenosis (narrowing) of the canal and subsequent conductive hearing loss. This is a particular problem if the client regularly uses hearing aids, insert earphones, stethoscopes or similar devices. Such clients may have their occupation, recreation and communication disadvantaged by the inability to use any such devices while the infection is present. Otitis externa can be caused by local trauma to the skin of the external auditory meatus, by bacterial, fungal or viral infections, or by eczema and dermatitis (Hammond, 1987).

Conductive loss as a result of trauma to the tympanic membrane and middle-ear structures can occur with head injury involving longitudinal fractures. For example, the ossicular chain may be disrupted. The loss is usually unilateral, and for this and other reasons may not be evident immediately post trauma. The facial nerve may also be affected in some cases. The speech-language therapist who is treating a head-injured client is wise to check that hearing has been assessed.

Two further causes of mechanical change to the conductive system of the ear will now be described in more detail. These causes are otitis media, which is very common in children, and otosclerosis, which usually occurs in adults. Otitis media and otosclerosis both affect the middle ear and can result in similar levels of conductive hearing loss. However, they involve very different etiology and management.

## Otitis media

Otitis media is inflammation of the middle-ear cavity (Bess & Humes, 1990), commonly involving the presence of fluid in the middle ear. Although otitis media does occur in adults, it is much more common in children (Haggard & Hughes, 1991). At least 70 per cent of all children are likely to have experienced otitis media at least once before the age of 6 years, with 6–18 months of age being a time of peak incidence (Teele, Klein & Rosner, 1989; Haggard & Hughes, 1991; Northern & Downs, 1991). Otitis media appears to be more common in male than female children. Some populations, such as Australian Aboriginal and Native American children, in comparison to non-Aboriginal children, have a higher risk of developing otitis media (Nelson & Berry, 1984; McPherson, 1990; McPherson & Knox, 1992). Children with Down's syndrome and children with cleft palate also have an increased risk of otitis media (Bluestone et al., 1972; Davies & Penniceard, 1980; Wilson, Folosom & Widen, 1983; Young, 1985; Kemker & Zarajczyk, 1989). In some senses it is probably 'normal' to have otitis media in early childhood. Nevertheless, the presence of otitis media in child clients who consult speech language therapists is very important to understand and manage, as it has the potential to seriously exacerbate communication difficulty and compromise therapy.

Otitis media can have dramatic symptoms, but equally can be a relatively covert condition. This is because the disease varies in terms of the degree of bacterial infection, amount and type of fluid present in the middle-ear cavity, onset time and duration. The principal means of distinguishing between the different expressions of otitis media is to consider the type of fluid present and the duration of the disease. Table 3.1 records one system of understanding the common terms for various types of otitis media in relation to these two factors. There are, however, many classification systems, a situation that needs resolution. Indeed any classification is difficult to apply to otitis media because otitis media can be viewed as a complex continuum (Payne & Paparella, 1976).

The condition known as *acute otitis media* is frequently responsible for ear pain of fairly sudden onset. The mucous membrane of the middle-ear cavity is inflamed and usually contains a purulent fluid with a high bacteria content. The tympanic membrane may be distended and will appear red and bulging on auroscopic inspection. Acute otitis media is usually obvious because of rapid onset (often following an upper respiratory tract infection) and associated pain, which is the most common symptom. In some cases the tympanic membrane may rupture. This is because the mucosa of the Eustachian tube has become swollen, preventing drainage and causing the purulent fluid trapped in the middle-ear cavity to exert pressure on the tympanic membrane. If the tympanic membrane is perforated in this way pain is usually relieved because the fluid can be discharged from the ear. Most tympanic membrane perforations resulting from acute otitis media heal spontaneously (Shah, 1981). With repeated perforations that have healed, white plaques may form in the tympanic membrane, a condition known as tympanosclerosis.

If untreated, possible complications of acute otitis media include chronic otitis media, cholesteatoma (a growth of squamous epithelium into the middle ear, usually as a result of a retraction pocket in a flaccid tympanic membrane), facial paralysis, adhesions of the middle-ear cavity, meningitis, mastoiditis and infection of the inner ear. Dalebout (1995a) provides good brief descriptions of each of these complications.

The hearing loss associated with otitis media is caused by the increased mass of fluid in the middle-ear cavity. If infection is unilateral, hearing loss may not be reported as a symptom. Hearing loss is difficult to measure in acute otitis media because the condition makes the ear(s) painful. Audiometric headphones may not be tolerated by the client and client concentration for the listening task may be affected.

Acute otitis media generally resolves within 3–6 weeks (Bess & Humes, 1990; Bluestone & Klein, 1990), but much more rapidly if effective antibiotic treatment is applied (Pender, 1992). Treatment of acute otitis media is more controversial if many episodes are involved (Bridges-Webb, 1993), because options include antibiotic prophylaxis, that is, the use of antibiotics in anticipation of infection. Antibiotic prophylaxis has potential side effects, such as diarrhoea. There are also concerns that the routine use of certain medications (e.g. ampicillin) to treat otitis media may lead to resistance problems (see, for example, Qvarnberg & Valtonen, 1995).

**Table 3.1:** Classification of otitis media

| | Fluid | |
|---|---|---|
| | Purulent | Non-purulent |
| Acute | Acute otitis media (AOM). Also known as: <br>• acute suppurative otitis media<br>• acute bacterial otitis media<br>• acute purulent otitis media | Acute non-suppurative otitis media (ANSOM). Also known as:<br>• acute non-bacterial otitis media<br>• acute non-purulent otitis media |
| Chronic | Chronic otitis media (COM). Also known as:<br>• chronic suppurative otitis media<br>• chronic bacterial otitis media<br>• chronic purulent otitis media | Chronic non-suppurative otitis media (CNSOM). Also known as:<br>• chronic non-bacterial otitis media<br>• chronic non-purulent otitis media<br>• chronic serous otitis media |

If the infection persists for several months, then it is termed *chronic otitis media* (Table 3.1). Chronic otitis media is frequently associated with large central perforations of the tympanic membrane and, in some cases, damage to the middle-ear structures. If the infection in chronic otitis media is active, there is a purulent discharge from the middle ear. If the infection is not active, discharge is much less likely (Paparella, Adams & Levine, 1989).

In non-suppurative or *serous otitis media* the fluid in the middle ear contains little or no bacteria, and the client will report little or no pain. The problem can last months or, in some cases, years (Sade, 1979). The tympanic membrane looks dull on auroscopic inspection, and can appear a bluish colour if the fluid in the ear is very thick. Bubbles can sometimes be seen; these are little pockets of residual air in the middle-ear cavity. Serous otitis media usually develops because of poor middle ear ventilation, which in turn results from Eustachian tube dysfunction. This latter may be associated with enlarged adenoidal tissue and/or tonsil enlargement. The air in the middle-ear cavity is gradually absorbed and, following this, the middle-ear mucosa begins to secrete fluid by a process of transudation (Cohen, 1981). The fluid is very like blood serum. If the fluid becomes very thick and glue-like, the condition is known as 'glue ear'. Serous otitis media may also develop as a result of acute bacterial otitis media that has been successfully treated with medication. The infection is controlled, but the fluid, sterilised by the application of antibiotics, may remain (Teele, Klein & Rosner, 1980).

Measurement of hearing loss in serous otitis media is not hampered by pain, but fluctuations of hearing sensitivity can occur. These fluctuations can make accurate threshold assessment difficult (Walker & Lamb, 1989).

In general, treatment for otitis media basically involves a choice between no action, medication and surgery (NSW Health Department, 1993). Each of these options has advantages and disadvantages (Vorrath, 1993). Selection of treatment will usually be based on consideration of the details of the individual case, including degree of hearing loss, persistence of the disease and whether or not infection is present. In addition to medication with antibiotics, surgery is carried out in many cases, especially if there is persistent bilateral otitis media with significant associated hearing loss. Surgery commonly involves myringotomy, in which the tympanic membrane is incised. This permits drainage of middle-ear fluid. A hollow ventilation tube (also known as a tympanostomy tube, pressure-equalisation tube or grommet) may be inserted in the tympanic membrane. This tube performs the ventilation and drainage functions normally provided by the Eustachian tube. In children with cleft palate, ventilation tubes may be inserted at the time of palate repair (Morris, 1993). Ventilation tubes commonly remain in the tympanic membrane for up to 12 months before they are extruded. Surgery may also include adenoidectomy and/or tonsillectomy, although the benefit of the latter procedure is questionable. As with all surgery, there are some risks, and the client is advised to discuss these fully with the surgeon before a decision about treatment is reached.

### Otosclerosis

Otosclerosis is a progressive conductive hearing loss, which in some cases can develop into a mixed hearing loss because of otosclerotic-like

processes in the cochlea. Unlike otitis media it never resolves spontaneously and if untreated it progresses to cause significant hearing loss
over time. The defining feature of typical otosclerosis is fixation of the
footplate of the stapes by the development of unorganised bone, which
is thicker and more highly vascularised than normal bone (Schukneckt,
1974; Booth, 1981). Because of stapes fixation, the compliance of the
middle-ear system is reduced, its transformer function is compromised
and sound waves arriving at the tympanic membrane are no longer
conducted as effectively across the middle ear to the cochlea.

The majority of clients who develop otosclerosis have bilateral
involvement. Females with otosclerosis often experience a marked
decline in hearing during and/or soon after pregnancy (Beales, 1987).
Otosclerosis is more common in females than males (Ginsberg et al.,
1979 Derlacki, 1984). The disease tends to run in families; many clients
with otosclerosis will have a parent, aunt, uncle or sibling with the
disease.

In otosclerosis the initial phase of the disease involves a slight hearing
loss and the advanced stage is associated with hearing loss sufficient to
make conversation very difficult without the assistance of hearing aids
and/or other amplification devices.

Treatment options for otosclerosis are surgery and/or the use of
amplification. Surgery involves stapedectomy, in which all or part of the
fixated stapes is removed and replaced by a prothesis. Useable hearing is
restored in 80–95 per cent of cases (Caltlin, 1981). There are surgical
risks, and these include facial palsy, severe or total hearing loss and
perilymphatic leaks. Otosclerosis can reoccur, and the prothesis may
become dislodged. If the ear with otosclerosis is the client's only hearing
ear then surgery is contraindicated. Where otosclerosis is bilateral,
surgery is performed first on one ear, and the situation monitored for at
least one year before an operation on the second ear is considered.
Hearing-aid amplification and assistive listening devices are an option
for persons who do not wish to undergo surgery and for those cases in
which surgery is contraindicated for other reasons.

### Effects of conductive loss on speech perception and language development

The principal effect of conductive hearing loss is a reduction in the
perceived volume of sound. If a particular signal (e.g. recorded music)
is made loud enough, then the signal is usually perceived quite clearly,
because the inner ear, which is responsible for interpretation of
signals, is normal. Purely conductive hearing loss does not exceed
60–70 dB HTL, because when sound reaches this level it is sufficient to
vibrate the skull, allowing sound to be perceived by bone conduction
(see Chapter 2).

Conductive hearing losses typically vary from an average of 20–30 dB HTL in otitis media to greater levels in advanced otosclerosis, severe glue ear and trauma to, or erosion of, the middle-ear structures. If the loss is bilateral and greater than 25 dB HTL, there will be at least some degree of difficulty hearing conversation in some situations, especially in distinguishing low intensity phonemes such as /ʃ /, /s/, /p/ and /t/. (There is some evidence that speakers of tonal languages such as Cantonese may be able to tolerate this level of loss without communication problems; Doyle & Wong, 1996.) If the conductive loss exceeds 45 dB HTL there will usually be difficulty understanding speech at normal levels in most situations, although understanding may be assisted to some extent by visual information if the speaker and listener are in face-to-face communication. If the conductive loss is unilateral, the individual will experience difficulties localising sound and is likely to have inconsistent hearing ability in conversational situations, depending on the position of conversational partners.

There is considerable discussion about the possible effects of conductive loss on the development of language and speech and on childrens' educational progress (Haggard & Hughes, 1991; Bench, 1993). It is probably fair to say that recurrent otitis media, for example, associated with inconsistent auditory input, can have sequelae for language development and educational progress, but that the size of the effect may be overestimated because of the difficulty of designing studies that address issues of internal and external validity (Ventry & Schiavetti, 1986; Menyuk, 1992; Bench, 1993). Additionally, many children who are identified as having learning problems may not have had hearing assessments (Dwyer, 1993) and hence the data that could link episodes of conductive loss with developmental problems are simply not available in some cases. This may in part be due to parents and teachers not suspecting hearing loss and/or middle-ear dysfunction when it is present (Haggard & Hughes, 1991; Pollard & Tan, 1993). What is clear is that children attending for speech therapy may be more likely than other children to have a history of recurrent middle-ear problems (Pollard & Tan, 1993), and that some children who have had otitis media have shown difficulty with particular aspects of auditory perception, such as understanding speech in noise (see, for example, Schilder et al., 1994). Additionally, very mild hearing losses (≤ 25 dB) caused by conductive problems may be associated with delays in language, especially vocabulary development (see later section on unilateral, chronically fluctuating and mild hearing losses). The possible connections between conductive hearing loss due to otitis media and central auditory processing problems are discussed in Chapter 9.

## Clinical decisions for the speech-language therapist

The three main decisions facing the speech-language therapist whose client has suspected conductive hearing loss are likely to be:

1. How should I refer the client for medical and for audiological opinions?
2. How will I monitor and/or follow up the client's progress after referral?
3. How does this client's hearing problem inform my assessment and therapy?

These decisions are now briefly discussed in turn.

Referral for medical opinion and treatment of conductive losses should always be made, and in the case of suspected acute otitis media referral should be immediate. The speech-language therapist should help the client to get the earliest possible appointment. Referral for audiological assessment is a secondary concern in acute otitis media. It is generally sufficient to refer for audiological opinion after medical treatment has resolved the infection. However, it is necessary to establish the client's hearing status after the episode is over, because it cannot be assumed that hearing has returned to pre-infection levels. In cases where the client is suspected of serous otitis media, and where there is no pain, medical referral may seem a less urgent matter but must be followed through, particularly where client history and/or hearing tests indicate a long-standing problem. Audiological referral may be made at the same time, and ideally should take place before medical examination, as audiometric information will be of value to the practitioner making the medical examination. In this author's experience a workable formula is this: for suspected acute otitis media refer for medical assessment first and audiology later; for suspected serous otitis media refer for audiological assessment first and medical second, but in the same close time frame. An overriding rule is this: if there is pain, discharge, vertigo or other serious symptoms always refer urgently for medical opinion.

There is usually less time pressure in referral of clients with other suspected causes of conductive hearing loss (for example otosclerosis), especially where clients are adults. The speech-language therapist may take the lead in arranging appointments, or may advise the client to arrange these personally, as seems appropriate. In the latter case the speech-language therapist is wise to provide the client with a written referral.

It is not always easy to follow up what happens to the client after referral. However, it is important that the speech-language therapist establishes if the client was examined as recommended and records the result of those examinations.

Deciding what to do with the information received about the client's conductive hearing loss will generally revolve around ensuring that the client receives reasonable and consistent sound input for important signals. If the audiological evaluation shows hearing loss in excess of 25 dB, then it is important to reduce distance between therapist and client in therapy sessions and to advise other relevant persons, such as parents and teachers, to do the same. As the principal problem in conductive losses is loss of volume, this simple tactic can often make a significant difference to the quality of communication and the effectiveness of therapy. Seating positions of conversational participants are important if the loss is unilateral, or if the average hearing level in the two ears differs by more than 20 dB. It may be necessary to use slightly louder speech in some cases (for example, where a child has a 40 dB bilateral loss and is awaiting surgery for long-standing glue ear). It is also important to give the client opportunities to use visual information during spoken communication, and to get their attention before speaking, especially in the case of children. Therefore seating positions and room lighting need consideration (for more detail, see Chapter 7). These tactics are absolutely vital if the client is a child with congenital hearing loss who has subsequently developed otitis media, particularly if the otitis media is persistent. The child in this situation is experiencing highly unreliable auditory input, and the effectiveness of previously prescribed hearing aids may be reduced significantly.

It may be necessary to provide the client with informational counselling about the technical and other options available (see Chapter 7) and to encourage the client to discuss these with their audiologist and/or otologist, especially if the client is weighing up surgical and non-surgical ways of resolving the hearing problem, or if medical or surgical treatment is not possible.

## Sensorineural hearing loss

A sensorineural hearing loss occurs when the cause of the loss lies in the cochlea and/or auditory nerve. In purely sensorineural hearing loss the external- and middle-ear function is normal. The common feature of all sensorineural hearing loss is disruption to the highly complex process of coding the frequency and intensity of incoming signals, of converting those signals to neural impulses and of transmitting those signals to the higher auditory pathways. The particular effect of problems in the inner ear/auditory nerve varies very greatly. Persons with sensorineural hearing loss may have unilateral or bilateral loss, the degree of loss may be very slight or total and the effect on speech perception may be mild or highly disruptive. In general, medical or surgical treatment of sensorineural hearing loss is not effective in restoring hearing.

Causes of sensorineural loss include:

- genetic transmission;
- neonatal disease;
- maternal rubella;
- Rhesus incompatibility;
- noise exposure;
- ageing of the cochlea structures;

- head injury;
- Ménière's disease;
- neurological disorders such as multiple sclerosis, motor neurone disease or tumours of the auditory nerve.

A fuller listing of disorders that are associated with sensorineural loss is given in Appendix A.

### Sensorineural loss present at or around birth

Genetic transmission of hearing loss is possibly responsible for half of the cases of sensorineural hearing loss present at or shortly after birth (Bess & Humes, 1990; Wall, 1995). Many of these cases of genetic hearing loss are due to autosomal recessive inheritance (Northern & Downs, 1991), in which both parents have a single recessive gene on one of the 22 pairs of autosomes (non-sex chromosomes), the other gene of the pair being normal. Because the abnormal gene is recessive (i.e. weaker than the normal half of the gene pair), the parent will be normal, yet carry the potential to transmit the abnormal gene. Children of such parents have a 25 per cent chance of being born with a gene pair made up of two abnormal genes, in which case they will exhibit the genetic hearing loss.

A much smaller percentage of genetically inherited sensorineural hearing loss is caused by autosomal dominant inheritance, in which there is a 50 per cent chance of the abnormal gene occurring in the child of a parent with that gene. Because the gene is dominant (i.e. stronger than the normal half of the gene pair) the parent with that gene will always exhibit the hearing loss.

Genetically determined sensorineural hearing loss is sometimes associated with other anomalies in a recognisable syndrome. Examples of such syndromes are:

- Pendred syndrome, in which sensorineural hearing loss, goitre and some vestibular anomalies occur;
- Turner syndrome, in which sensorineural hearing loss is associated with truncal obesity and abnormalities of the fingers and toes;
- Waardenburg syndrome, which includes heterochromia of the eyes and a white forelock in addition to sensorineural hearing loss;
- Usher syndrome, in which sensorineural hearing loss is progressive, and visual problems due to retinitis pigmentosa develop during childhood or early adulthood (Fritsch & Sommer, 1991; Silman & Silverman, 1991).

Some 10 per cent of children with Down's syndrome may have congenital sensorineural hearing loss.

A child may experience sensorineural hearing loss because of prenatal diseases in the mother, the best known of these being maternal rubella, in which the fetus is infected with the virus via the placenta. The chances of this occurring are greatest in the first trimester. The child may then be born with considerable bilateral sensorineural hearing loss as well as other problems, including visual and heart defects (Northern & Downs, 1991). Figure 3.1 shows the hearing loss of a child whose mother had rubella in the first month of pregnancy.

Rhesus incompatibility can result in cerebral palsy with sensorineural hearing loss. High frequency sensorineural hearing loss may occur with athetotic cerebral palsy, for example.

Postnatal diseases such as measles and bacterial meningitis can also cause bilateral sensorineural hearing loss. Mumps is the cause of many unilateral sensorineural hearing losses, which may not be obvious in early life because of normal hearing in the unaffected ear.

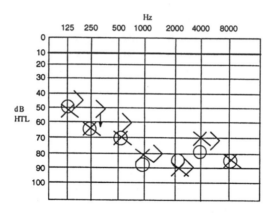

**Figure 3.1:** Audiogram from a child with sensorineural hearing loss caused by maternal rubella. The air conduction sensitivity of the right ear (shown by circles) is very similar to that of the left ear (shown by crosses). The loss is sensorineural because the bone-conduction thresholds (shown by arrowheads) are no better than the air-conduction thresholds.

## Noise-induced hearing loss

Hearing loss due to noise can occur as a result of short-term exposure to intense noise, such as an explosion. This situation is termed acoustic trauma. The loss is immediately obvious, and probably occurs because the physiological limits of the ear have been exceeded. The tympanic membrane and ossicular chain may be damaged, and the structures of the Organ of Corti disrupted (Pender, 1992). Acoustic trauma can occur at any age and may be unilateral or bilateral.

In contrast to acoustic trauma, noise-induced hearing loss (NIHL) occurs as a result of long-term exposure to noise, and is usually gradual in onset. The mechanisms involved in the development of noise-induced hearing loss probably include: changes to the cochlear blood supply, repeated microtrauma to the Organ of Corti and metabolic changes in the stria vascularis (Wenthold et al., 1992). Noise-induced hearing loss is one of the most common causes of hearing loss in adults (Gilad & Glorig, 1979), and it occurs primarily because of noise in the workplace and noise associated with certain recreational activities. However, children are not immune to noise-induced hearing loss. Indeed, some children may be at risk due to noisy toys (Hellstrom, Dengerink & Axelsson, 1992), and students in technical schools may be exposed to hazardous noise levels (Allonen-Allie & Florentine, 1990). Recreational noise such as music can also be a problem. For example, persons who use personal cassette players at high volume for more than 7 hours each week and/or attend more than two rock concerts each month may be more likely to suffer noise-induced hearing loss than persons without those recreational habits (Meyer-Bish, 1996). Some individuals may be more susceptible than others to noise-induced hearing loss (see, for example, Chung et al., 1982; Barrenas & Lindgren, 1991).

The greatest impairment in noise-induced loss almost always occurs at 4000 Hz or at the adjacent frequencies of 3000 Hz or 6000 Hz. There is usually recovery at 8000 Hz. The loss is initially limited to the 3000–6000 frequency band, but with repeated exposure this 'noise notch' will deepen and widen to involve other frequencies. After very long-term exposure it may not be easy to distinguish noise-induced hearing loss from loss associated with ageing, especially in females (Rosenhall, Pedersen & Svanborg, 1990), although there are mathematical methods proposed for dealing with this problem (see, for example, Dobie, 1992; Macrae, 1992). Figure 3.2 shows audiograms typical of the development of noise-induced hearing loss. Noise-induced loss is commonly bilaterally symmetrical. Exceptions are truck drivers, in whom the loss tends to be greater in the ear exposed to traffic noise via the driver's side window (Dufresne, Alleyne & Reesal, 1988), and rifle shooters, in whom the loss may be greater in the ear opposite handedness.

The client with noise-induced loss may report that speech doesn't sound very clear and/or that they have difficulty hearing speech in background noise. Tinnitus, or ringing in the ears (covered later in this chapter) may be the initial, or even the only, symptom of noise-induced hearing loss. Again, this is usually bilateral (Patuzzi, 1992). In the early stages of noise-induced loss, and in some cases of acoustic trauma, at least part of the loss may be temporary (temporary threshold shift or TTS), with the hearing recovering after several hours. With repeated exposures the loss becomes permanent (permanent threshold shift) and slowly progressive.

Treatment for noise-induced hearing loss involves conserving remaining hearing and enhancing communication where necessary. Ear protection, informational counselling, monitoring of hearing levels, and

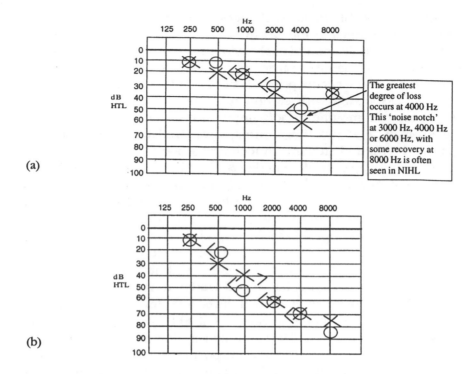

(a)

(b)

**Figure 3.2:** Audiograms in two cases of noise-induced hearing loss. (a) Audiogram from an adult with sensorineural hearing loss caused by long-term industrial noise exposure. The air conduction sensitivity of the right ear (shown by circles) is very similar to that of the left ear (shown by crosses). The loss is sensorineural because the bone-conduction thresholds (shown by arrowheads) are no better than the air-conduction thresholds. (b) Audiogram from an adult with sensorineural hearing loss caused by noise exposure over 30 years. No ear protection was worn until the last few years. The thresholds now have a sloping configuration which is similar to that seen in sensorineural loss due to presbycusis, for example. In the earlier stages of the hearing loss recovery at 8000 Hz was evident, as in (a).

assessment of needs for amplification and/or communication therapy are important. If the loss is related to noise exposure at work, ear protection and monitoring of hearing levels may be best provided at the workplace. Communication therapy can be effectively provided by the speech-language therapist. Erber (1988) provides an excellent, practically oriented discussion of therapy appropriate for persons with noise-induced hearing loss, and indeed many other forms of acquired sensorineural loss in adults.

## Presbycusis: sensorineural loss associated with ageing

Many persons develop sensorineural hearing loss as they grow older, with possibly up to 40 per cent of Western populations over 75 years of age having presbycusis (Bess, Lichtenstein & Logan, 1991).

Although some of the presbycusic changes to the cochlea may be similar to those seen in noise-induced hearing loss, presbycusis is also seen in persons who have had no significant exposure to noise. Presbycusis is possibly best considered a term to describe hearing loss in older adults that cannot be explained by other than what are assumed to be slowly degenerative changes in the afferent auditory pathways, especially in the cochlea. The hearing loss is usually very slow in onset, tends to be at least roughly symmetrical and more severe in the higher frequencies. Tinnitus is present in many cases. As many older people also develop visual problems, such as cataracts or macular degeneration (reducing the ability to compensate for hearing loss by the use of visual information), the impact of presbycusis on communication can be considerable.

## Head injury

Sensorineural hearing loss can result from transverse fractures of the temporal bone, but may also occur without any apparent skull fractures. Severe or total hearing loss may result if the fracture runs through the cochlea. The facial nerve may be affected in many cases of transverse fracture involving hearing loss. The relative contribution of cochlea hearing loss and central auditory problems in sensorineural loss following head injury can be difficult to discern (Sakai & Mateer, 1984; Lukas & Genchur-Lukas, 1985; Mueller, 1985; Musiek, 1985). Because the client may also have sustained conductive hearing loss as a result of the head injury, the symptoms and the level of loss may be unstable for the first month or more after injury. If the client reports otalgia, discharge, dizziness or changes in hearing, they should be referred for audiological and medical opinion, even if hearing was reportedly checked earlier.

## Ménière's disease

Ménière's disease is usually an unfortunate combination of sensorineural hearing loss, tinnitus and rotational vertigo, although not all three symptoms need be present. The symptoms occur in episodic attacks during which vertigo and nausea are often the most obvious and distressing symptoms. Because the disease is thought to be associated with problems in the regulation of endolymph it is also termed endolymphatic hydrops. The hearing loss tends to fluctuate, being worse around the time of an attack, and the audiogram will often show a sensorineural loss that is either fairly flat or with greater impairment in the low frequencies. The loss is more often unilateral than bilateral (Barber, 1983). Over time, with increased number of episodes, the loss is slowly progressive. The hearing loss in Ménière's disease often involves the lower frequencies first, giving a rising configuration to the audiogram (see for example, Paparella, MacDermott & de Sousa, 1982). As the disease progresses the audiometric configuration tends to flatten.

Treatment for Ménière's disease usually involves medication to control the vertigo, and changes to the diet, especially reduction of salt and fluid intake. In severe cases surgery to introduce an endolymphatic shunt may be performed. In cases where the hearing loss is very profound, and the symptoms are sufficiently distressing, labyrinthectomy (in which the inner ear is destroyed) or vestibular nerve section may be appropriate. Hearing-aid amplification and other aural rehabilitation may be necessary.

## Neurological disorders

Sensorineural hearing loss can occur with multiple sclerosis, although there are no reliable figures on the incidence of sensorineural hearing loss specifically caused by the disease (Hall, 1992). Sensorineural hearing loss is also seen in many, but not all, tumours of the auditory nerve. The most common of these tumours is the Schwannoma (also referred to as acoustic neuroma, acoustic neurinoma or acoustic Schwannoma), a growth of the Schwann cells, usually arising on the vestibular portion of the nerve. These progressive, benign tumours can invade the cerebellar pontine angle and develop to compress other cranial nerves and the cerebellum. The hearing loss is unilateral, progressive and of variable configuration, although higher frequencies are often the first to be involved. Symptoms may be unilateral tinnitus, hearing loss and/or vertigo, a triad of symptoms very similar to those of Ménière's disease. Any client with unilateral sensorineural loss, even in the absence of other symptoms, should be referred for investigation to exclude Schwannoma. Radiographic techniques such as computerised axial tomography (CAT) scans, magnetic resonance imaging (MRI), and electrophysiological tests of the auditory brainstem response (see Chapter 4) are most useful in diagnosing Schwannoma (Turner, Shepard & Frazer, 1984).

Treatment usually involves surgery to remove the Schwannoma, although in some cases, due to the slow growth of the tumour, the decision may be to monitor the condition. If surgery is carried out, hearing may or may not be preserved, depending largely on the size of the tumour at diagnosis. The facial (VIIth cranial) nerve may or may not be affected. There are support associations available to assist people who have had Schwannoma.

## Effects of sensorineural loss on speech perception and language development

The influence of sensorineural hearing loss on the development and maintenance of oral communication varies greatly among individuals, depending on the degree and configuration of the hearing loss, age at onset of the hearing loss, age at diagnosis, the life experiences and communication needs of the affected individual, their other attributes and the support they receive. However, in general, sensorineural loss means both a reduction in volume of sound perceived and the presence, to some extent, of distortion in what sounds may be heard. This latter problem is the case even when hearing-aid amplification is worn, although technical advances mean that it is now possible to provide much clearer aided sound than was previously possible.

Most children with congenital or pre-lingually acquired sensorineural loss have some measurable hearing, and hence potential to perceive at least some aspects of the auditory signals of speech. As with conductive hearing problems, an average hearing loss in excess of 45 dB HTL will cause obvious difficulties in hearing speech in most situations, and even minimal losses may be associated with speech and language delay in some individuals (see section on unilateral, chronically fluctuating and mild hearing losses). However, there is also the problem of the inability to hear one's own speech clearly, because of impaired hearing by both air conduction and bone conduction. Unless aided, and supported as necessary with speech therapy and lots of auditory input, the child's own speech will reflect very closely what he or she hears, that is, a distorted version of normal speech (Hudgins & Numbers, 1942; Smith, 1975; John et al., 1976; Gold, 1980). Where the hearing loss is very great, there may be additional problems with speech production, including movement of the articulators and respiration during speech (McGarr & Harris, 1983; Whitehead, 1983; Tye-Murray, 1991), despite hearing-aid amplification. The speech problems will usually include both suprasegmental (prosody and intonation) errors (see, for example, McGarr & Osberger, 1978) and segmental (phonemic) errors (see, for example, Monsen, 1978). Further, impaired speech perception contributes to problems in the development of cognitive skills and language abilities. Markides (1983), for example, suggested that intelligible speech may enhance the linguistic development of the child with hearing impairment because of the greater ease of communication it allows. Conversely, opportunities for communication may be reduced by poorly intelligible speech. The impact of this general situation has been comprehensively discussed by Bench (1992a).

It is clear that most children with sensorineural hearing loss require assistance with speech and language development, and plenty of auditory language input if they are to maximise their potential for oral–aural communication. Where the hearing loss is profound (> 90 dB), children may use residual aided hearing to assist lipreading, although some individuals with this level of loss can communicate primarily through audition. Early diagnosis has the advantage of providing the child with better audition via hearing aids and hence better input for language and speech development (see reviews by

Bader, 1992a,b; Ling, 1992), although in some, hopefully few, cases it may have the disadvantage of causing parents and others to reduce the auditory language input they offer the child, precisely because of the knowledge that their child is 'deaf' (Williams, 1970). There is recent evidence that for some hearing-impaired children provision of hearing-aid amplification before 6 months of age allows development of vocal and linguistic skills at an age comparable to normally hearing children (Robinshaw, 1995).

Most adults with sensorineural loss have developed their hearing loss in adulthood, and many such persons have hearing loss limited to high frequencies. With normal or near-normal low-frequency hearing the primary effect of such a loss is to make difficult the perception of low-intensity, high-frequency speech sounds, which are largely voiceless consonants such as /s/ and /t/ in English. This often leads to the mishearing of words (for example, 'shed' may be heard as 'head', or 'heel' as 'feel') and the typical complaint 'I can hear but people don't seem to speak clearly anymore'. This is particularly a problem in noisy situations, because the background noise masks low-intensity, high-frequency speech sounds and reduces the ability of the listener with the hearing loss to use their residual hearing. Erber (1988) provides examples of typical instances of mishearing associated with such a situation. As mentioned previously, speakers of tonal languages may be less affected by high frequency loss than speakers of languages such as English (Doyle & Wong, 1996). Adults who have acquired very profound or total hearing loss may develop articulation errors, such as fricative and affricate distortions and deletion of final consonants, and may suffer difficulties in maintaining normal voice (see, for example, Leder & Spitzer, 1990). Persons who have suddenly acquired profound or total hearing loss, as for example via a head injury, may speak with a very loud voice in an attempt to hear their own voice via bone conduction, and because they have not yet learned other ways of monitoring voice level.

In sensorineural hearing loss the loss may involve all audiometric frequencies fairly equally, but more commonly the loss is greater at higher frequencies. This is the case for both congenital and acquired hearing losses. In Chapter 6 some practical guidelines are given for interpreting audiograms of persons with sensorineural hearing loss. At this point it is sufficient to note that if an individual has some measurable aided or unaided hearing at frequencies up to and including 1000 Hz, they can usually perceive at least the suprasegmental aspects of speech. The first formant of all vowels should be perceived. If there is useful hearing for frequencies up to and including 2000 Hz then first and second formants of most vowels are probably discernible, as are many of the voiced consonants. The place of articulation of consonants should be perceived. If there is useful hearing up to and including 4000 Hz, then voiceless consonants may be perceived to some extent. Of course, if the hearing loss is very severe then there may be great difficulty using audition because of high levels of distortion and because very little of the signal may be perceived. If the loss is acquired after the development of speech and language, the individual has the benefit of previous experience of what he or she is now attempting to hear.

In addition to problems around speech perception and production, the adult with acquired sensorineural hearing loss may experience depression, frustration and a sense of loss associated with greatly reduced ability to communicate via previously habitual means (such as conversation from other room or over the telephone) and loss of the previous ability to enjoy the experience of music, theatre or television (see Kaplan, 1992).

Because sensorineural hearing loss can reflect changes in the auditory nerve and central auditory pathways in addition to cochlea damage, persons with similar audiograms can experience very different levels of communication difficulty. Some persons with sensorineural loss may have difficulty processing or even recognising speech if part of their loss is due to damage in the central auditory pathways. This is discussed in Chapter 9.

A problem experienced by many children and adults with sensorineural hearing loss is intolerance to suprathreshold sounds that would be comfortably loud to persons with normal hearing. This problem is due to an abnormal growth of loudness and is termed recruitment (Fowler, 1936). This can be problematic for the fitting of hearing aids (see Chapter 7). Another difficulty associated with sensorineural hearing loss is monitoring speech level. If the client is unaided, the presence of a significant sensorineural hearing loss may cause them to speak with a louder than normal voice, because they do not have the benefit of normal bone-conduction hearing by which they can monitor the level of their own speech.

## Clinical decisions for the speech-language therapist

The variation in problems and symptoms associated with sensorineural hearing loss is great. However, the basic cluster of issues for children with sensorineural hearing loss is often different from those for adults with sensorineural loss.

The principal decisions to be made by the speech-language therapist whose client is a child with sensorineural loss are probably:

1. How does my role fit into the programme of support to be given to this child?
2. How do the particular features of this child's hearing problem inform my assessment and therapy?
3. When do I need to refer for medical and/or audiological review?

These decisions are now discussed in turn.

It is important that the hearing-impaired child is supported by effective and efficient services, and that the roles of all the various persons involved are clearly understood and agreed. This may be difficult to achieve if different funding agencies are involved, if there is not an agreed person with responsibility for overall coordination and/or if there are differences in opinion about the child's potential or the methods best applied to the development of that potential. Nevertheless, every effort should be made to achieve a well coordinated system of support for the child. In this author's opinion parents are the most appropriate persons to coordinate support for their child, but they will often appreciate the backup of a clinician who can assist them with information, provide advocacy in negotiating bureaucracies and be available for telephone support. The speech-language therapist may be the person who is asked to provide such backup.

To act most effectively as part of the team, it is essential to have regular communication with the child's teacher, otologist, audiologist and other professionals. The particular form and frequency of that communication will need to be decided after consideration of the nature of the information to be shared, parental consent and available resources.

Among other data, the features of the child's hearing loss can inform therapy and help set treatment goals. Where the speech-language therapist has been consulted about a child with sensorineural loss, it is highly likely that the parents wish the child to develop functional oral communication, and particularly to develop speech that is sufficiently intelligible to allow effective interaction with normal hearers. In order to develop a plan aimed at achieving these goals, a basic knowledge of audiograms, hearing aids and assistive listening devices is essential. These are discussed in Chapters 6 and 7. However, two basic considerations are:

1. Always have access to the child's aided, as well as unaided, audiograms. If therapy goals are set according to unaided audiograms potential may be underestimated.
2. Use the audiogram from a developmental communication perspective, that is, assess and plan for the development of voice, prosody and turn-taking skills before working on articulation (see Clezy, 1984).

In a good professional team, routine reviews by audiologists and otologists are likely. However, there are occasions when the speech-language therapist may need to arrange additional consultations. These are:

- if the child's behaviour or hearing abilities have appeared to deteriorate;

- if there is suspicion of middle-ear disease;
- if the rate of progress in therapy appears to be less than would be expected given the clinical data available.

Adults with sensorineural loss may consult the speech-language therapist directly, seeking aural rehabilitation therapy, but often the client with the hearing loss may be referred for other reasons, such as communication problems following head injury or stroke. The hearing loss may only become evident on closer examination.

If the adult client has been referred for apparent receptive language problems, it is essential to know hearing status. Because damage to auditory structures and processes can occur with head injury (Shulman, 1979) and vascular accidents (Goodhill & Harris, 1979), and because many persons experiencing stroke are likely to be older adults and thus in turn likely to have some degree of hearing loss associated with ageing (Willot, 1991), it is possible that peripheral hearing problems could be misinterpreted as part of a higher order language dysfunction. For example, phonological confusions on the Psycholinguistic Assessments of Language Processing in Aphasia test (Coltheart & Lesser, 1991) may be interpreted as breakdown of receptive language at the phonological level, when in fact the confusions are due to peripheral hearing loss. Additionally, hearing loss can affect test performance due to misheard instructions. It is vital that no long-term plans are made without management of the hearing loss.

The two main dilemmas faced by the speech-language therapist whose client is an adult with sensorineural loss are likely to be: How do the features of this client's hearing loss inform my assessment and treatment? and What action, if any, do I need to take with regard to the hearing loss?

If the hearing loss is on average greater than 40 dB HTL, therapy is very likely to be compromised unless particular attention is paid to providing eye contact, appropriate seating and multiple opportunities for clarification. Interpretation of particular audiometric patterns is discussed in Chapters 6 and 10. The reader is referred to Chapter 7 for advice on clinic room arrangements suitable for adults with sensorineural hearing loss.

The principal action required when it is discovered that an adult client has sensorineural hearing loss is to ensure that medical and audiological assessment is provided. Referral is especially important in cases with unilateral sensorineural hearing loss, vertigo and/or severe tinnitus, because these conditions can be associated with retrocochlear disorders.

## Mixed loss

Where both conductive and sensorineural components are present, the individual has a mixed hearing loss. This can occur as a result of, for example: various traumas that damage both the middle and inner ear, middle-ear infections that have progressed to involve the inner ear, otosclerotic processes in both the middle ear and cochlea structures, and where a pre-existing sensorineural loss is overlaid by a conductive problem or vice versa. The principal clinical decision to be made in cases of suspected mixed hearing loss is how to ensure that the client's hearing loss is managed appropriately. In this author's experience the best course of action is to help the client to gain access to a good audiologist–otologist team who can work closely with the client and keep the speech-language therapist informed.

## Unilateral, chronically fluctuating and mild hearing losses

Persons who have unilateral hearing loss will experience problems with sound localisation and other communication problems in a range of social situations, because of the lack of binaural hearing. Children with unilateral loss, whether conductive or sensorineural, may experience difficulty in the classroom and delay in educational progress (Bess & Tharpe, 1984, 1986; Bess, 1985; Klee & Davis-Dansky, 1986). Children with fluctuating otitis media, unilateral sensorineural loss or bilateral sensorineural loss less than 30 dB have been termed 'minimally hearing-impaired' by Bess (1985), who suggested that the problems of these children had been greatly underestimated, particularly with regard to speech perception. Therefore, the client with one normally hearing ear, or with minimal levels of hearing loss, cannot be assumed to be free of communication difficulties although they may well be.

## Central auditory processing problems

Some persons may have a normal ability to detect the presence of sound (i.e. normal thresholds for pure tones) yet have difficulties using auditory information because of central auditory problems. Such persons may pass a screening test and have a normal audiogram, because these tests assess peripheral auditory function. An individual with central auditory problems may, for example, be able to hear perfectly well in quiet situations, but become effectively hearing-impaired when conversing in background noise. Central auditory processing disorder is characterised by difficulties manipulating and using sound at the level of the central nervous system (Lasky & Katz, 1983), and involve aspects of both perception and cognition. In Chapter 9 the assessment of these central auditory processing problems is reviewed in some detail. The cause of such problems is not clear in many cases, but central auditory processing problems can occur in conjunction with learning disorders, traumatic brain injury, cerebral vascular accidents, multiple sclerosis and delay in maturation of the higher auditory pathways (Baren & Musiek, 1995). This last problem may possibly be related in some cases to chronic otitis media, additionally, HIV/AIDS has been associated with central auditory disorders in a number of case reports (see for example, Hart et al., 1989).

## Tinnitus

Tinnitus is the term for noises in the ears and/or head. Tinnitus can occur in persons with conductive hearing loss, with sensorineural hearing loss and even with normal hearing. It may be constant or intermittent, involve one or both ears and can vary greatly in the type of sound perceived (Slater & Terry, 1987). Tinnitus is almost always subjective, i.e. evident only to the person experiencing the tinnitus. In a very few cases the tinnitus is objective and may be heard by other persons.

Tinnitus can be associated with potentially serious problems, such as tumours of the auditory nerve (Ginsberg & White, 1985) and lesions of the central auditory system (Musiek, 1985), but most often it is not. It can be considered an indication that the auditory system is somehow irritated or overloaded. Thus, tinnitus is common after noise exposure (Axelsson & Barrenas, 1992; Melnik, 1995), in persons who are on certain medications (Lassman & Aldridge, 1985) and in persons with vascular disorders (Ginsberg & White, 1985). Tinnitus may also occur in a range of systemic disorders, such as multiple sclerosis, diabetes and autoimmune diseases (Slater & Terry, 1987). Persistent tinnitus should always be investigated, particularly if it is unilateral, to exclude problems such as Schwannoma or Ménière's disease, which require medical treatment. Additionally, audiological evaluation and informational counselling can help the client to understand the problem and develop ways of coping with it (Hallam, 1989). If the client also has a hearing loss, the use of a hearing aid may help, as this allows the individual to focus on external sound rather than the noises in their own head. Tinnitus masking or desensitisation devices may also be used (see Chapter 7).

The level of distress experienced by persons with tinnitus can vary from none at all to severe stress and thoughts of suicide. Medical treatment of tinnitus is generally not effective, hence treatment is often aimed at understanding and controlling the individual's reaction to, and perception of, the tinnitus (Erlandsson et al., 1991; Jastreboff & Hazell, 1993; Vesterager, 1994; Dineen, Doyle & Bench, 1997b) by means of relaxation, counselling, coping therapy and/or tinnitus maskers. There are support associations for people with tinnitus (e.g. the Australian Tinnitus Association), and some audiologists and otologists specialise in assisting clients with tinnitus.

# Non-organic hearing loss

Non-organic hearing loss (NOHL) is this author's preferred term for hearing loss that cannot be attributed to physiological causes. Other commonly used terms are pseudohypacousis and functional hearing loss. The terms psychogenic deafness and malingering are also sometimes used, although they are not encouraged as they imply an unconscious or conscious motivation (see Martin, 1985, for a discussion of terminology and the causes of NOHL). Occasionally, a client presents with apparent hearing difficulties yet there is no discernible problem in the afferent auditory pathway. This may be a conscious attempt to gain, by a feigned hearing loss, a situation reflecting an unconscious need for attention or other reward, or theoretically at least, a real problem that is simply not detectable by currently available techniques. NOHL may, in some cases, indicate underlying psychological and other problems (Brooks & Geoghgan, 1992). Tests to check for NOHL are described briefly in Chapter 4.

# Summary of key points

Hearing difficulty is an individual experience. The difficulty may be associated with changes to any portion of the afferent auditory pathway, but most commonly with dysfunction of the middle ear (resulting in a conductive hearing loss) or the inner ear (resulting in a sensorineural hearing loss). The principal hearing problem experienced in conductive loss is reduced volume of sound. This problem is also experienced in sensorineural hearing loss, but in sensorineural loss there is the added difficulty of distortion in the signal received. Difficulties developing and/or maintaining speech, language, voice and educational progress are commonly experienced when sensorineural hearing loss is severe or profound. Psychological and social difficulties may be experienced, especially by adults who have acquired significant levels of hearing loss. Otitis media (causing conductive loss) is very common in children, especially children with Down's syndrome or cleft palate. Presbycusis and noise-induced hearing loss (causing sensorineural hearing loss) are common in adults. Clients with head injury, a history of vascular accidents or neurological disorders may have sensorineural hearing loss and/or central auditory processing problems, which are important to detect if communication therapy is to be effective. The clinical decisions facing the speech-language therapist whose client has a hearing loss concern referral, monitoring of hearing status, team functioning and the interpretation of audiograms to inform therapy.

# Further reading

Bench RJ (1992) Communication skills in hearing impaired children. London: Whurr Publishers. (A comprehensive review of early assessment and intervention procedures, of speech reception, speech production and literacy in children with pre-lingual hearing loss. The first chapter provides an excellent overview of processes in human communication.)

Dalebout S (1995) Disorders of hearing in children. In Wall LG (Ed.), Hearing for the speech-language pathologist and health care professional. Boston: Butterworth-Heinemann, pp. 39–70. (Provides additional detail about a range of disorders and syndromes, including various complications of otitis media.)

Pender DJ (1992) Practical otology. Philadelphia: JB Lippincott Co. (A readable coverage of clinical tests used by physicians and an excellent basic coverage of ear disorders. There are a large number of helpful drawings to aid understanding.)

# Chapter 4
# Forms of hearing assessment

JANET DOYLE

This chapter presents an overview of the audiological techniques most commonly used to assess hearing. The test procedures described are diagnostic, i.e. they provide information that (a) confirms and quantifies hearing loss, (b) differentiates between conductive, sensorineural and mixed losses, (c) assists in the search for the cause of the hearing loss, and (d) documents aspects of hearing function. Other test procedures, aimed at the more fundamental task of screening for hearing loss (i.e. identifying persons who may have a hearing loss) are discussed in Chapter 5.

## Principles

1. *Audiological hearing assessments can be described in terms of (a) the aim of the test, (b) the level of client cooperation required, (c) the equipment and training needed and (d) the information yield.* Although there are several tests that are very routinely used, the particular assessment procedures applied in a given case will be selected with reference to these factors.
2. *Individual tests have a particular, and sometimes variable, level of accuracy.* Any diagnostic test has a certain 'power' or chance of giving valid information, for example, of correctly diagnosing a Schwannoma. Readers interested in the power of individual diagnostic tests are referred to Hyde, Davidson and Alberti (1991) and to the work of Turner and colleagues (Turner & Neilson, 1984; Turner, Frazer & Shepard, 1984; Turner, Shepard & Frazer, 1984; Turner, 1988). The accuracy of a test is also dependent on correct calibration of equipment, the expertise of the tester and the level of subjectivity involved in the client's responses and the tester's interpretation of the results. Therefore, although it is not commonly a

problem, it is possible for various audiological tests to give apparently conflicting results.

3. *The results of individual audiological tests describe auditory functioning relative to a standard set of results that represent 'normality'. They do not necessarily describe very well the degree to which a particular individual is handicapped by his or her hearing problem.* Hence while test results may be usefully applied in differential diagnosis and in technical decisions associated with hearing-aid amplification, they are somewhat less useful in arriving at detailed estimates of an individual client's ultimate communication potential, particularly when the hearing loss is prelingual. This is because other factors (e.g. family support) and characteristics (e.g. intelligence) interact with the hearing loss to influence communication ability.

4. *The speech-language therapist has a responsibility to understand information yielded by the common hearing tests for purposes of planning speech and language therapy, counselling and referral.* In particular, unaided and aided pure tone audiograms and tympanograms are useful to the speech-language therapist, as they provide practical information useful for planning both individual treatment sessions and longer-term goals.

5. *Normal hearing must be proven, not assumed.* It is important to exclude hearing loss as a contributing cause of communication problems in clients consulting speech-language therapists. It is wise to ensure hearing has been checked, even when there is no complaint of hearing difficulties and even when another cause is overtly linked to the presenting problems. The proof of normal hearing sensitivity is a normal audiogram and not the absence of the complaints about hearing.

## Overview of tests

Any audiological test is either subjective or objective. Subjective tests (such as the very common unaided pure tone audiometry with headphones) require the client's active cooperation, and the resulting data are based on clients' judgements of various stimuli presented. Objective tests (such as tympanometry or acoustic reflex testing) require only passive cooperation from the client, and the resulting data are based on various electrophysiological responses. (Objective tests, however, can involve a degree of subjectivity in interpretation). Table 4.1 lists a range of audiological tests, showing for each whether they are subjective or objective procedures, the approximate time involved in the procedure, the equipment used, the nature of the information yielded and what the client is likely to experience. The most commonly used of these tests are now described.

**Table 4.1:** Range of audiological tests

| Test | Usual application | Subjective or objective | Information yield | Client experience |
|---|---|---|---|---|
| Pure tone audiometry under headphones | Adults and children of 3 years or more, who can give an unambiguous signal such as hand-raising | Subjective | Unaided air-conduction thresholds in dB HTL for 250–8000 Hz, and bone-conduction thresholds for 250–4000 Hz, for each ear. Fewer frequencies may be tested in the case of some children. Results are plotted on an audiogram with 0 dB HTL reference norm | Client is seated in a sound-treated room or booth with headphones over both ears, or insert earphones placed in ear canals, and asked to indicate each time a tone is heard. Some uncertainty in judgements is common. Adults may or may not be alone during the test. Children are usually asked to give a play response. If masking is used, the client will be asked to ignore any broad-band noises presented and to respond only to pure tones |
| Sound field audiometry | Adults and children wearing hearing aids. Infants and other clients who cannot cooperate with headphone audiometry | Subjective | Unaided binaural air-conduction thresholds, or aided binaural or monaural thresholds, in dB SPL for 250–8000 Hz. When testing unaided binaural hearing, results generally do not exclude | Adults and children being tested for aided hearing levels are seated at a calibrated distance from a loudspeaker in a sound-treated room, wearing their hearing aid(s). Adults and older children are |

| | | | Procedure | Results |
|---|---|---|---|---|
| | | | asked to indicate each time they hear a warble tone. Infants and young children being tested for aided or unaided hearing are conditioned to respond (usually with a head turn) to warble tones. This is achieved by initially pairing the tones with a pleasant visual stimulus (such as a puppet in a lighted window or above the speaker) and later presenting the visual stimulus as a reward for head turns in response to the warble tones | the possibility of a unilateral loss. Fewer frequencies may be tested in the case of some children. Results are plotted on an audiogram with dB SPL reference norm or in tabular form |
| Speech audiometry under headphones | Adults and older children | Subjective | Clients seated in a sound-treated room, asked to listen to recorded syllables, words or sentences and indicate their understanding by repeating what they heard or pointing to a picture. Sometimes live voice rather than recorded materials are used | Percentage correct scores, which indicate level of ability to perceive speech signals at various intensities. Speech-reception thresholds are recorded in dB HTL. Speech-discrimination scores are recorded as % correct at various dB HTL levels. Some audiologists record speech audiometry with other references |

(contd)

**Table 4.1:** (contd)

| Test | Usual application | Subjective or objective | Information yield | Client experience |
|------|-------------------|-------------------------|-------------------|-------------------|
| Tympanometry | Adults and children. Some difficulty with infants and young children due to requirement to remain reasonably still | Objective | Tympanic membrane compliance at various air pressures introduced into the ear canal. Separate data are obtained on each ear. Can detect abnormal middle-ear function | Client is asked to sit still. After auroscopic inspection a rubber plug and probe assembly is introduced into the ear canal. A low-pitched sound (probe tone) is usually heard and may change in loudness as pressure changes during the test |
| Acoustic reflex test | Adults and children | Objective | Acoustic reflex thresholds for each ear at frequencies 500, 1000, 2000 and 4000 Hz, with either contralateral or ipsilateral stimulation | This test is usually done after tympanometry. The client may hear brief loud pure tones either in the ear with the tympanometry probe in place, or via a headphone placed on the other ear |
| Real ear (insertion) gain measurements | Adults and children who are being fitted with hearing aids | Objective | The effective gain and frequency response of a particular hearing aid in an individual's ear | A small probe microphone is inserted into the ear canal and measurements taken in the open ear and also while wearing a hearing aid |

| | | | | |
|---|---|---|---|---|
| Auditory brainstem response (ABR) audiometry | Adults and children. Assists in detection of retrocochlear disorders, and in assessment of hearing in infants suspected of significant hearing loss | Objective | Traces that indicate the responsiveness of the auditory nerve and the brainstem. It is not frequency-specific below 1000 Hz | Surface electrodes are attached to the client's skull. A series of clicks or tone bursts are presented via headphones. Children and infants may need sedation or anaesthesia because of the need to remain still. The test is painless |
| Cortical evoked response audiometry (CERA) | Adults and children | Objective/subjective. Easily influenced by the client's state of alertness | Traces that indicate the responsiveness of the auditory pathways above the brainstem. It can give frequency specific information | As for ABR, but there are some differences in the nature of the sounds presented |
| Electrocochleography | Adults and children | Objective | Traces that record the potentials from within the cochlear and auditory nerve in response to sound. It is useful for differentiating between sensory and neural cochlea pathology. Gives limited information for frequencies below 1000 Hz | Surface electrodes are placed on the head and a needle electrode is placed either in the ear canal or (transtympanic) on the promontory in the middle ear. A series of clicks or tone bursts are presented via headphones. Anaesthesia is necessary |

(contd)

**Table 4.1:** (contd)

| Test | Usual application | Subjective or objective | Information yield | Client experience |
|------|-------------------|-------------------------|-------------------|-------------------|
| Electronystagmography | Usually adults | Objective/subjective. Easily influenced by the client's state of alertness, by various medications and alcohol | Traces that record spontaneous and evoked eye movements (nystagmus) and thus inform on the state of the vestibular system. Does not give information about hearing. Is useful in differential diagnosis of cochlear and retro-cochlear pathology | Surface electrodes are placed on the skin around the eyes. The ears are separately stimulated with warm and cold air or water. The client may also be given various visual and movement stimuli. Some dizziness is often experienced at times during the test |
| Otoacoustic emissions | Adults and children | Objective. The test is influenced by the presence of middle-ear fluid, limiting its application in children | A spectral display which reflects outer hair cell function of the cochlea, and hence a measure of the 'strength' of the cochlear emission | A probe apparatus is held in the client's ear canal. A series of clicks and or tones are presented |

# Tympanometry

Tympanometry is one of three principal subtests of immittance audiometry. Immittance audiometry is an objective procedure that assesses, in an individual ear, the relative impedance (resistance offered to the flow of energy in acoustic signals) and admittance or compliance (the reciprocal of impedance, and the ease with which the ear accepts the flow of energy in an acoustic signal). The other two subtests of immittance audiometry are static admittance/compliance (not discussed here) and the acoustic reflex test. The general term 'immittance' is used to indicate the principle of evaluating energy flow. Particular test equipment may measure either impedance or admittance.

Tympanometry assesses the ability of the tympanic membrane to accept sound, and is therefore a test of the conductive mechanism of the ear. It is a dynamic measure, meaning that the tympanic membrane is in motion during the test. The basic approach in tympanometry is to introduce a pure tone (usually 220 Hz or 660 Hz) into the external auditory meatus and to measure how much of that sound wave is accepted (admitted) or rejected (impeded) by the tympanic membrane. In a normal ear the tympanic membrane will accept most of the sound and will do this when the air in the external auditory meatus is at or very close to normal atmospheric pressure.

During tympanometry, air pressure, expressed in decapascals (daPa) or millimetres of water (mm $H_2O$), is varied continuously in the external auditory meatus from values greater than normal atmospheric pressure (usually +200 daPa/mm $H_2O$), through normal atmospheric pressure (0 daPa/mm $H_2O$), to values less than atmospheric pressure (usually –200 daPa/mm $H_2O$). This causes the tympanic membrane to move in response to the positive and negative pressures applied to it. As discussed in Chapter 2, in a normal ear the middle-ear cavity contains air, and that air is at or very close to atmospheric pressure. Thus, in a normal ear, pressure introduced into the external auditory meatus at values greater than normal atmospheric pressure will cause the tympanic membrane to be displaced medially, making it more reflective than accepting of sound presented to the ear. When pressure is introduced into the external auditory meatus at values less than normal atmospheric pressure the tympanic membrane is displaced laterally, thus again reducing the ability of the tympanic membrane to accept sound. In both cases, the impedance of the tympanic membrane has been increased and the admittance decreased by the artificial manipulation of air pressure in the external auditory meatus. Only when the pressure introduced into the external auditory meatus of a normal ear is at or very near normal atmospheric pressure will the impedance be relatively low and admittance relatively high, as in this situation the tympanic membrane is able to move freely in response to incoming sound, because the air pressure in the external auditory meatus is equal to the air pressure in the middle-ear cavity.

The tympanic membrane in an individual ear will always have optimum movement (greatest admittance/compliance and least impedance) when the air pressure is equal on both sides of the tympanic membrane, i.e. when the air pressure in the external auditory meatus equals the air pressure in the middle-ear cavity. Thus, if tympanometry shows that the tympanic membrane can accept most of the incoming sound, and does this when the pressure in the external auditory meatus is at or very close to normal atmospheric pressure, we can infer that the air in the middle-ear cavity is also at normal atmospheric pressure, and hence that the middle-ear system is normal. If tympanometry shows the ear to accept most of the sound when the air in the external auditory meatus is less than normal atmospheric pressure (i.e. at negative pressure), then this infers negative air pressure in the middle ear, as the pressure in the external auditory meatus has had to be reduced before peak mobility of the tympanic membrane is achieved (i.e. before the pressure in the external auditory meatus equals that in the middle-ear cavity). In some ears with significant middle-ear dysfunction, such as can occur with otitis media, tympanic membrane movement may be very restricted. In these cases the impedance of the middle-ear system is high, and pressure changes in the external auditory meatus during tympanometry will have little or no measurable effect on impedance or admittance.

Figure 4.1 provides a schematic illustration of the equipment used in tympanometry. An essential feature is that a rubber probe tip is introduced into the external auditory meatus, through which the stimulus probe tone is delivered, the atmospheric pressure changes are made and the measurement of sound reflected back from the tympanic membrane can occur. This probe tip must form an airtight seal in the canal before the test can proceed. For routine tympanometry an intact tympanic membrane is required.

Tympanometry results are plotted, either automatically or manually, on a tympanogram, a graph of impedance/admittance values against air pressure values. Figure 4.2 shows schematic tympanograms consistent with various middle-ear conditions. The diagnostic interpretation of tympanograms can not only distinguish normal from non-normal middle-ear systems, but can assist in the differentiation of various conductive disorders, such as Eustachian tube dysfunction, otitis media, ossicular discontinuity and otosclerosis. The indicators used are the actual admittance/compliance value at peak tympanic membrane mobility (the high point of the tympanogram), the width of the tympanogram and the air pressure at which the peak or peaks, if any, occur. Eustachian tube function may also be assessed in an ear with tympanic membrane perforation or pressure-ventilation tubes, by introducing negative pressure and asking the client to swallow. If the Eustachian tube is functioning normally swallowing will restore normal atmospheric pressure to the middle ear.

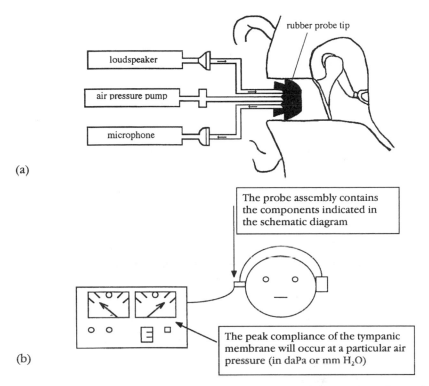

**Figure 4.1:** Schematic illustration of tympanometry equipment. (a) Shows detail of the probe that is inserted into the external auditory meatus. (b) Illustrates general set up. (In part, reproduced with permission from: Balthazor RJ and Cevette MJ (1978)).

Tympanometry is a sensitive procedure with the potential to detect middle-ear disorders before patient symptoms are obvious. For this reason there may sometimes be apparent inconsistency between the results of tympanometry and of visual inspection of the tympanic membrane (Haggard & Hughes, 1991).

Tympanometry may also be used as a screening procedure. Detailed guidelines for screening middle-ear function with tympanometry are given in Chapter 5.

## Acoustic reflex test

The acoustic reflex test is an objective test and the second principal subtest of immittance audiometry. It is carried out using the same equipment as used in tympanometry, in conjunction with a pure tone generator, which is normally integrated in the diagnostic immittance equipment. The test involves presenting brief (1–2 s) high-intensity tones at various frequencies (usually 500 Hz, 1000 Hz, 2000 Hz and 4000 Hz) and observing whether there is a corresponding decrease in admittance/compliance (i.e. an increase in impedance) for the duration

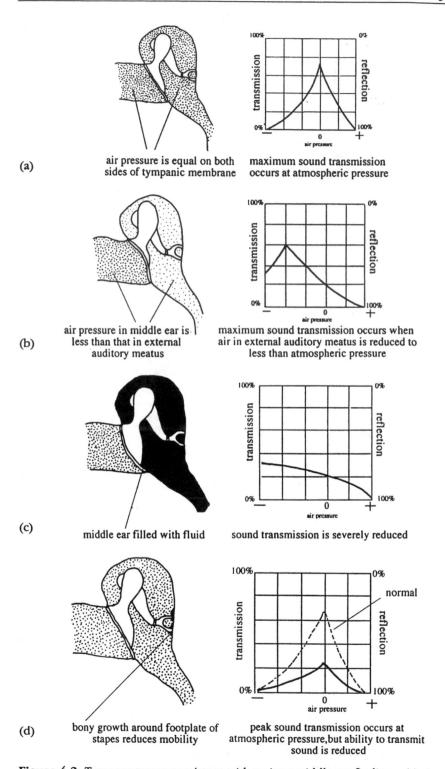

**Figure 4.2**: Tympanograms consistent with various middle-ear findings: (a) normal; (b) Eustachian tube dysfunction; (c) fluid in the middle-ear cavity; (d) otosclerosis. (Reproduced with permission from Cevette MJ, Balthazor RJ (1977)).

of the tone. Such a change in admittance in response to the pure tone stimulus indicates that the acoustic reflex arc is intact (see Figure 4.3).

The acoustic reflex arc shown in Figure 4.3 illustrates the arc for the stapedial muscle. (The tensor tympani is also involved, but to a much lesser degree. The tensor tympani muscle is supplied by the mandibular branch of the Vth (trigeminal) nerve.) The afferent pathway involves transmission of impulses from the cochlea via the VIIIth nerve to the dorsal and ventral cochlear nuclei. From there, impulses travel both ipsilaterally and contralaterally, via the medial superior olivary complex (the reflex centre) and the motor nucleus of the VIIth (facial) nerve, to stimulate a branch of the VIIth nerve, which in turn causes reflexive contraction of the stapedial muscle in both ears.

The normal acoustic reflex causes the stapedial muscle in the middle ear to contract, hence momentarily pulling the tympanic membrane medially and reducing the admittance of the middle-ear system. The acoustic reflex is bilateral. Normally, the reflex contraction of the middle-

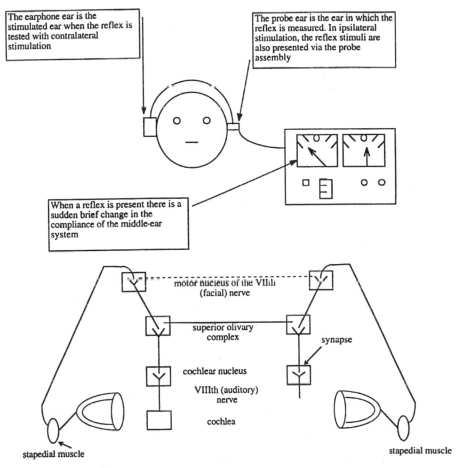

**Figure 4.3:** Schematic diagram of the equipment set-up for testing acoustic reflex and the reflex arc.

ear muscles occurs in both ears, regardless of which ear is stimulated. In diagnosis of a range of disorders, the amplitude, latency and rise/fall time of the reflex are examined.

The stimulus tones are delivered either via the probe tip used in tympanometry (ipsilateral stimulation) or via a headphone on the opposite ear (contralateral stimulation). The response is measured from the probe ear. Because in contralateral stimulation elements of the bilateral auditory system are assessed, it can be confusing to refer to either the probe ear or the stimulated ear as the 'test ear'. It has become more common practice to refer to an acoustic reflex result as having been obtained 'with probe left (or right) and stimulus right (or left)', although many audiologists still refer to the stimulated ear as the test ear.

Acoustic reflex results are commonly expressed as the minimum dB HTL of stimulus required to elicit the momentary decrease in admittance (although some equipment is calibrated in dB SPL). With a normal acoustic reflex arc, reflexes are usually seen when the stimulus is in the range 70–100 dB HTL (i.e. 70–100 dB SL for normal listeners).

Abnormal acoustic reflex results may comprise absence of reflexes, reflexes present at elevated levels of stimulation, reflexes present at lower than normal levels of stimulation and/or reflexes that display delay in onset, early decay or unusual changes to admittance. With contralateral stimulation, an absence of reflex can indicate any of the following:

- Hearing loss in the stimulated ear. In this case the loss reduces the sensation level of the stimulus to below that necessary to activate the reflex.
- Pathology of the VIIIth nerve in the stimulated ear. Damage to the auditory nerve fibres may mean that additional intensity of stimulation is required, or that the nerve is not capable of sustaining suprathreshold stimulation.
- Problems with the central portion of the acoustic reflex arc. Certain brainstem abnormalities may compromise the reflex.
- Problems with the VIIth nerve on the measured (probe) ear. An intact facial nerve is necessary to innervate the stapedius muscle.
- Problems in the middle-ear cavity in the probe ear. Conditions such as ossicular chain fixation or severe otitis media, for example, may prevent the tympanic membrane from moving reflexively.

The decision as to which of these situations pertains is made with reference to other information, such as ipsilateral reflex results and pure tone audiometry. Examples of acoustic reflex results in various pathologies are shown in Figure 4.4. The way in which such results are interpreted in conjunction with other tests is discussed in Chapter 10.

# Pure tone audiometry

Pure tone audiometry is a subjective test in which the client's ability to detect pure tones of various frequencies relevant to speech perception is assessed. The test indicates the sensitivity of the client's hearing. Certain inferences may be made about the effects of reduced sensitivity (such as which listening situations will be most difficult for the client), but pure tone audiometry does not directly measure the ease with which the individual processes sound.

The principle of diagnostic pure tone audiometry is to present pure tones at individual frequencies and ask the client to indicate when they hear the tone. The minimum level at which the client can reliably hear a given tone is considered to be their threshold or hearing level for that frequency. Thresholds for octave frequencies from 250 Hz to 8000 Hz inclusive are usually sought for each ear. Thresholds are recorded in dB HTL, i.e. the number of decibels above the level required by listeners with normal hearing to detect that tone. Chapter 2 explains the differential sensitivity of the normal ear and gives minimal audible pressure (MAP) values. Those MAP values (in dB SPL) constitute 0 dB HTL for all frequencies in pure tone audiometry, and clinical audiometers are calibrated accordingly. Thus, 7 dB SPL (the MAP value for average normal listeners at 1000 Hz) is the intensity that is produced at the headphone of an audiometer when the dials are set to 1000 Hz and 0 dB HTL. When the frequency of presentation is 2000 Hz, 9 dB SPL is produced at the headphone when the presentation level is 0 dB HTL. At 20 dB HTL, 29 dB SPL is presented, at 30 dB HTL, 39 dB SPL, and so on as long as the frequency remains 2000 Hz.

Therefore any reliable response at 0 dB HTL at any frequency will indicate the ability to detect the test tone at average normal sensitivity levels. In reality some individuals have hearing sensitivity slightly better than the average normal level (e.g. –5 dB HTL) or slightly poorer (e.g. +10 dB HTL). A level of 20 dB HTL is generally considered the poorer end of functionally normal hearing sensitivity, and the level beyond which hearing difficulties become obvious. If the test tone must be increased to say 30 dB HTL before the client gives a reliable response, then the client's hearing sensitivity for that frequency is 30 dB poorer than average normal threshold.

In pure tone audiometry the clinician varies the intensity of presentation in steps no smaller than 5 dB. If a client does not respond at 10 dB HTL, for example, the stimulus is increased to 15 dB HTL. For practical purposes there is no gain in working with smaller increments. Thus the recorded threshold will always be a multiple of either 10 (e.g. 10 dB HTL, 20 dB HTL, 30 dB HTL) or of 5 (e.g. 15 dB HTL, 25 dB HTL, 35 dB HTL).

The most common approach in seeking thresholds is to begin testing at 1000 Hz, as this frequency seems easiest for most clients to hear. If an

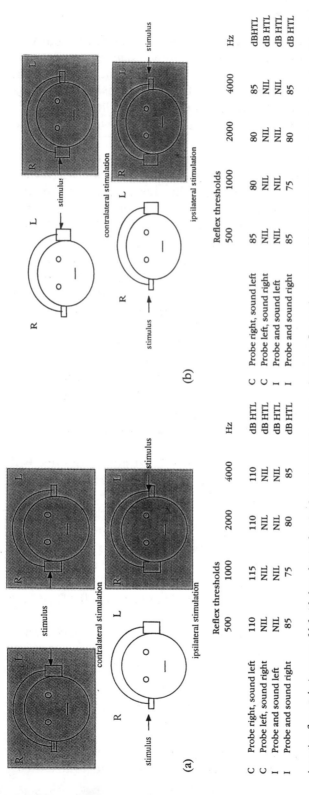

(a)

**Reflex thresholds**

| | 500 | 1000 | 2000 | 4000 | Hz |
|---|---|---|---|---|---|
| C   Probe right, sound left | 110 | 115 | 110 | 110 | dB HTL |
| C   Probe left, sound right | NIL | NIL | NIL | NIL | dB HTL |
| I   Probe and sound left | NIL | NIL | NIL | NIL | dB HTL |
| I   Probe and sound right | 85 | 75 | 80 | 85 | dB HTL |

Acoustic reflex results in a case of *left-sided conductive hearing loss*. Whenever the probe assembly is in the left ear (i.e. when the left middle-ear response is measured) there is no acoustic reflex seen because the abnormal middle-ear system has prevented the reflex. When the probe is in the right ear (i.e. when the right middle-ear response is measured) there are reflexes at normal levels in the ipsilateral condition, and reflexes present at elevated levels in the contralateral condition (i.e. sound in the left ear). The elevated reflexes are due to the elevated hearing levels in the left ear. Hence the right ear has hearing sufficient to produce a reflex at normal levels and a middle-ear system capable of responding. The left ear, however, has both a middle-ear problem and a hearing loss.

(b)

**Reflex thresholds**

| | 500 | 1000 | 2000 | 4000 | Hz |
|---|---|---|---|---|---|
| C   Probe right, sound left | 85 | 80 | 80 | 85 | dBHTL |
| C   Probe left, sound right | NIL | NIL | NIL | NIL | dB HTL |
| I   Probe and sound left | NIL | NIL | NIL | NIL | dB HTL |
| I   Probe and sound right | 85 | 75 | 80 | 85 | dB HTL |

Acoustic reflex results in a case of *left-sided facial palsy* where the lesion is medial to the stapedial branch of VIIth nerve. Whenever the probe is in the left ear (i.e. the response of the left middle-ear system is measured) there is no reflex. However, a significant hearing loss in the left ear is unlikely, as with sound left and probe right reflexes are present at normal levels. Results for the right ear are normal in both contralateral and ipsilateral conditions.

continued

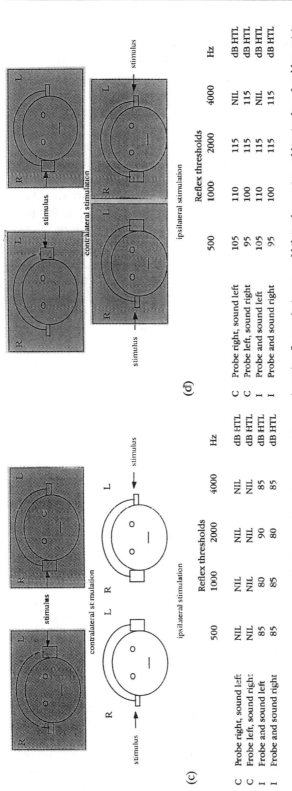

(c)

| | Reflex thresholds | | | | |
|---|---|---|---|---|---|
| | 500 | 1000 | 2000 | 4000 | Hz |
| C Probe right, sound left | NIL | NIL | NIL | NIL | dB HTL |
| C Probe left, sound right | NIL | NIL | NIL | NIL | dB HTL |
| I Probe and sound left | 85 | 80 | 90 | 85 | dB HTL |
| I Probe and sound right | 85 | 85 | 80 | 85 | dB HTL |

Acoustic reflex results in a case of *brainstem pathology involving the superior olivary complex*. Whenever the test is performed with contralateral stimulation, the reflex is absent. Yet the ipsilateral results are normal. As the middle-ear system in each ear is responsive and at normal levels, the lesion must involve the central portion of the reflex arc.

(d)

| | Reflex thresholds | | | | |
|---|---|---|---|---|---|
| | 500 | 1000 | 2000 | 4000 | Hz |
| C Probe right, sound left | 105 | 110 | 115 | NIL | dB HTL |
| C Probe left, sound right | 95 | 100 | 115 | 115 | dB HTL |
| I Probe and sound left | 105 | 110 | 115 | NIL | dB HTL |
| I Probe and sound right | 95 | 100 | 115 | 115 | dB HTL |

Acoustic reflex results in a case of *bilateral sensorineural bearing loss of cochlear origin*, with recruitment. Reflexes are present in both contralateral and ipsilateral conditions, but only at elevated levels. The presence of reflexes indicates a responsive middle-ear system in each ear. The elevated levels indicate the presence of hearing loss. As the middle-ear system is functional, the loss must be sensorineural. A sensorineural loss with recruitment will often be associated with reflexes at lower than normal sensation levels. For example, in this case the hearing threshold (known from pure tone audiometry) was 60 dB HTL at 1000 Hz in the right ear. As with sound in the right ear at 1000 Hz a reflex was seen at 100 dB HTL, the sensation level of the reflex stimulus was only 40 dB (100 dB - 60 dB = 40 dB SL). The 40 cB SL tone was perceived to be sufficiently intense to produce a reflex. As sensation levels of 70–100 dB are usually required, this individual must have recruitment (see Chapter 3).

**Figure 4.4:** Acoustic reflex results in various disorders: (a) left-sided conductive loss; (b) left-sided facial palsy; (c) brainstem pathology; (d) bilateral sensorineural loss. These results would normally be considered in conjunction with the results of tympanometry and pure tone audiometry (see Chapter 10). Shading indicates absent or elevated reflexes.

interaural difference is suspected, the better ear is tested first. The initial presentation is at a level presumed to be comfortably loud for the client (e.g. 30 dB HTL in the case of a client not suspected of having a significant hearing loss). If the client responds the tone is decreased by 10 dB. If the client does not respond the tone is increased by 5 dB. This '10 dB down, 5 dB up' technique is maintained until the minimum level of sound to which the client has responded two out of three, or three out of five times, is identified. This level is recorded as threshold. Thresholds are then sought for remaining frequencies, generally in the order of 2000 Hz, 4000 Hz, 8000 Hz, 500 Hz and 250 Hz. If the client has suspected noise-induced hearing loss, and/or where thresholds at adjacent octave frequencies differ greatly, intermediate frequencies (e.g. 3000 Hz or 6000 Hz) are also tested. Testing is usually completed for all frequencies of interest in one ear at a time. Tones are presented firstly by air conduction and then, if necessary, by bone conduction.

The air-conduction tones in pure tone audiometry are presented via headphones or insert earphones. Insert earphones are used by many audiologists because of their advantages in terms of noise reduction and client comfort, and because they reduce the need for masking (discussed later in this chapter).

When air-conduction tones are presented to the external auditory meatus they travel the normal air-conduction route of tympanic membrane, middle ear, VIIIth nerve and higher ascending pathways to be perceived, if hearing permits, in the auditory cortex. If a client responds to air-conduction tones at normal levels, then this entire pathway is essentially intact with regard to sound detection. If the level of the stimulus must be increased beyond normal levels before threshold is obtained, then some impediment to sound transmission exists somewhere along the pathway. In this case it is necessary to also test hearing by bone conduction.

The bone-conducted tones in pure tone audiometry are presented via a vibrator placed on the mastoid bone of the ear under test, or on the forehead. The sounds presented via the vibrator directly stimulate the skull, sending the signal to the cochlea. Once the cochlea receptors are stimulated the incoming signal is transmitted to the VIIIth nerve, higher auditory pathways and auditory cortex, as for air-conduction sounds. Because bone-conduction testing bypasses the middle ear, the comparison of air-conduction and bone-conduction responses allows the distinction between conductive and sensorineural losses. When air-conduction responses are poorer than normal levels and bone-conduction responses remain normal, then a conductive loss is indicated. When air-conduction responses and bone-conduction responses are both poorer than normal levels and essentially equal, a sensorineural loss is indicated. When both air-conduction responses and bone-conduction responses are poorer than normal, but bone-conduction responses remain to some extent better than air conduction responses, a mixed loss (partly conductive and partly sensorineural) is indicated.

Bone-conduction responses cannot be poorer than air-conduction responses because bone-conduction testing examines part of the system examined by air-conduction testing.

The thresholds for an individual client are plotted on an audiogram. Figure 4.5 displays sample audiograms for (a) normal hearing, (b) a unilateral conductive hearing loss and (c) a bilateral sensorineural hearing loss. The audiograms here and elsewhere in this book are charted with the symbols recommended by the American Speech-Language-Hearing Association (ASHA). Some clinics prefer to chart audiograms for left and right ears on separate audiograms, but this author is convinced that interpretation is facilitated by having the responses of both ears recorded on a single audiogram, as shown here. A further convention in many clinics is to record the threshold information for the right ear in red and that for the left ear in blue. This reflects the identifying colours of the right and left headphones or insert phones commonly used. A more detailed discussion of audiograms is given in Chapter 6.

Pure tone audiometry may be used for most adults and children over the age of 3 years. With children the clinician usually uses a form of play audiometry, in which the child is asked to place a ball on a stick, put a peg in a peg board or perform some other similar task, each time they hear a tone. The child is rewarded by praise for appropriate responses, which must be unambiguous and closely follow the presentation of the stimulus. Most children happily engage in the task. A skilled clinician can obtain valid audiograms from children as young as 2 years.

For some clients pure tone audiometry is carried out using operant conditioning techniques. One test technique that uses operant conditioning is tangible reinforcement conditioning audiometry or TROCA (Lloyd, Spradlin & Reid, 1968), in which the client receives a tangible reward (usually food) for appropriate behavioural responses. Such operant techniques may also be applied in sound field audiometry (see later section of this chapter).

## Masking

During pure tone audiometry it is possible for test tones presented to one ear to be perceived by the opposite ear, meaning that a client's response to such tones does not reflect the hearing of the ear under test. This can occur during both air-conduction and bone-conduction testing. This problem occurs when hearing in one ear is significantly better than in the other. The test tones presented to the poorer ear may be sufficiently intense to cause skull vibration, which then stimulates the better ear, causing the client to respond. This situation is termed 'cross-

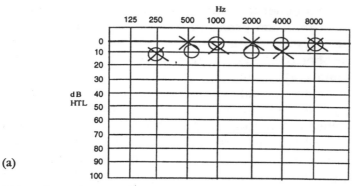

(a)

All air-conduction thresholds are at or better than 10 dB HTL. The three frequency (500 Hz, 1000 Hz, 2000 Hz) pure tone average is 6.7 dB HTL in the right ear (10 + 0 + 10 = 20/3 = 6.66) and 1.7 dB HTL in the left ear (0+ 5 + 0 = 5/3 = 1.66). As the air-conduction thresholds are normal and the bone conduction cannot be poorer than air conduction, bone conduction has not been performed in this case.

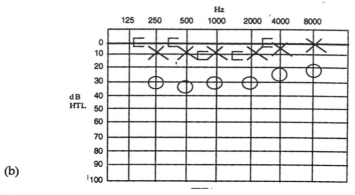

(b)

The air-conduction thresholds in the right ear (circles) are poorer than normal, showing an average hearing loss of approximately 30 dB. The bone-conduction thresholds of the right ear (bracket) obtained with masking in the better left ear, remain in the normal range. When bone-conduction thresholds are normal in an ear with hearing loss the loss is conductive.

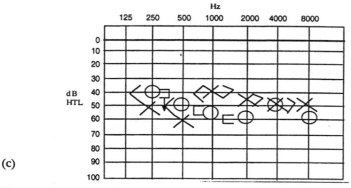

(c)

The air-conduction thresholds in both the right ear (circles) and the left ear (crosses) are poorer than normal. The bone-conduction thresholds (shown by the various arrowhead and brackets shapes) are at essentially the same level as the air-conduction thresholds. When air- and bone-conduction thresholds show similar levels of sensitivity loss, the hearing loss is sensorineural.

**Figure 4.5:** Audiograms charted with ASHA symbols, illustrating: (a) normal hearing sensitivity; (b) unilateral conductive hearing loss; (c) bilateral sensorineural loss.

hearing', and in such cases it is necessary to prevent the non-test ear from participation in the test. This is achieved by masking the non-test ear. Masking means presenting a masking noise (usually a narrow band of noise centred on the particular test frequency at issue) to the non-test ear while at the same time presenting the usual pure tones to the test ear.

Only certain sounds are likely to cause cross-hearing. This is because the intensity of an air-conducted sound presented through headphones to one ear will decrease (attenuate) by at least 40 dB before the signal reaches the other cochlea. Thus the interaural attenuation for air-conducted sounds is 40 dB. Interaural attenuation may be greater than 40 dB in certain individuals and for certain test frequencies, but the minimum value of 40 dB is assumed for clinical purposes. An air-conducted tone presented to one ear at 80 dB HTL will attenuate to at least 40 dB HTL before it reaches the other ear. If cross-hearing does occur, it is because the cochlea on the non-test side has sufficient sensitivity to detect the attenuated tone. When hearing is being tested by bone conduction, the signals are delivered via a vibrator placed directly on the skull, usually the mastoid process of the ear under test. This direct vibration of the skull means that the signal can easily reach both cochlea. Hence the interaural attenuation for bone-conducted sounds is assumed to be 0 dB. It may be greater in some individuals and at some frequencies, but it is safest to assume that a bone-conducted test tone of, say, 25 dB HTL, which is presented to the mastoid of one ear, will not attenuate at all before it reaches the other ear. Again, cross-hearing can occur if the non-test cochlea has sufficient sensitivity to perceive that tone.

The need for masking in any particular case depends on the inter-relationship between three factors. These are:

1. the bone conduction threshold of the non test ear;
2. the intensity of the test tone being delivered to the test ear;
3. the interaural attenuation.

Figure 4.6 illustrates the need for masking in pure tone audiometry for one frequency when the air-conduction hearing of the right ear is under test and Figure 4.7 illustrates the need for masking in pure tone audiometry for one frequency when the bone-conduction hearing of the right ear is under test. If cross-hearing has occurred, the introduction of masking noise into the non-test ear (the left ear in Figures 4.6 and 4.7) will result in an elevation of response to tones presented to the test ear. The level of the masking noise is chosen and manipulated in such a way as to allow the clinician to be sure when responses can be attributed to the test ear. Masking noise is presented by air conduction (via a headphone or an insert earphone) regardless of whether the test ear is being assessed for air-conduction hearing or bone-conduction hearing. The clinician who applies masking seeks a plateau of responses from the test ear. This plateau represents the true threshold of the test ear, as changes to the amount of masking presented to the non-test ear do not change the level at which tones presented to the test ear are perceived. In Chapter 6 examples are given of audiograms obtained with masking.

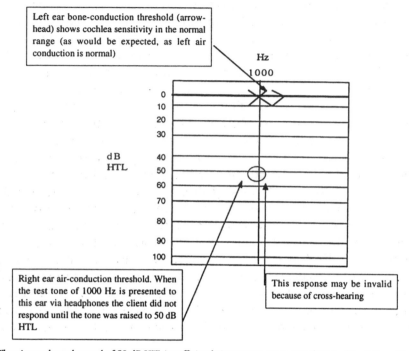

Left ear bone-conduction threshold (arrow-head) shows cochlea sensitivity in the normal range (as would be expected, as left air conduction is normal)

Right ear air-conduction threshold. When the test tone of 1000 Hz is presented to this ear via headphones the client did not respond until the tone was raised to 50 dB HTL

This response may be invalid because of cross-hearing

The air-conducted sound of 50 dB HTL is sufficiently intense to cause stimulation of the left cochlea. As air-conducted sounds attenuate 40 dB before stimulating the opposite ear, 10 dB HTL of the test tone presented to the right ear may reach the left cochlea. The left bone-conduction threshold of 0 dB HTL shows that the left cochlea is capable of perceiving such a tone. In this case then, the unmasked air-conduction threshold of 50 dB HTL for the right ear may simply be a reflection of cochlea sensitivity on the left. Therefore it is necessary to mask (occupy) the left ear, and re-present the test tone to the right ear

**Figure 4.6:** Partial audiogram showing the need for masking when the air conduction of the right ear is being assessed.

## Pure tone average

The results of pure tone audiometry can be summarised numerically by computing a pure tone average (PTA) for each ear. This indicator of the overall magnitude of the hearing loss is obtained by averaging pure tone air-conduction thresholds for 500 Hz, 1000 Hz and 2000 Hz (3-frequency PTA) or 500 Hz, 1000 Hz, 2000 Hz and 4000 Hz (4-frequency PTA). The PTA for the right ear in the normal audiogram shown in Figure 4.5 for example would be 6.7 dB HTL.

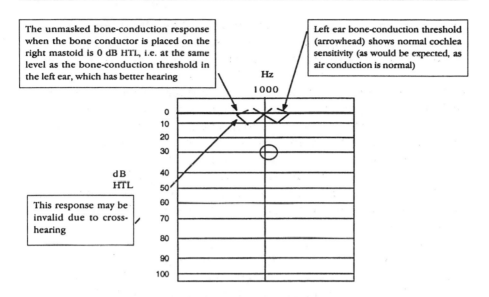

The unmasked bone-conduction response when the bone conductor is placed on the right mastoid is 0 dB HTL, i.e. at the same level as the bone-conduction threshold in the left ear, which has better hearing

Left ear bone-conduction threshold (arrowhead) shows normal cochlea sensitivity (as would be expected, as air conduction is normal)

This response may be invalid due to cross-hearing

The responses of the right ear indicate a possible conductive hearing loss at this test frequency because the bone-conduction response is normal while the air-conduction response is not. However, as the interaural attenuation for bone-conducted tones is 0 dB, the 0 dB HTL tone presented to the right mastoid can reach both cochleas. As the left cochlea at this frequency can perceive such a 0 dB HTL tone, it is possible that the apparent bone-conduction response from the right mastoid is a reflection of the hearing sensitivity in the left ear and not the right. Therefore it is necessary to mask (occupy) the left ear and re-present the bone-conducted sound to the right ear

**Figure 4.7:** Partial audiogram showing the need for masking when the bone conduction of the right ear is being assessed.

### Automatic pure tone audiometry

Pure tone audiometry may be performed by having the clients' responses to tones in effect control the presentation levels, via an automatic audiometer. This process yields various traces, which can be read to estimate threshold. An extension of this approach, called Bekesy audiometry (Jerger, 1960) can yield additional data helpful in the differentiation of cochlear and retrocochlear lesions. Automatic audiometry can also be applied in hearing screening. However, automatic audiometry is rarely used for routine diagnostic threshold audiometry because of various practical difficulties, such as problems in applying masking, a procedure frequently necessary when one ear has hearing significantly better than the other.

## Sound field audiometry

Sound field audiometry basically has two applications: (1) to assess hearing sensitivity in persons who are unable to cooperate with standard pure tone audiometry because of, for example, inability to give a voluntary response or reluctance to accept headphones; and (2) to assess hearing when the client is using hearing-aid amplification (additional techniques for hearing-aid assessment are discussed in Chapter 7).

In general the desire is to gain as close an approximation to an audiogram as possible (i.e. to obtain client responses to tonal stimulation centred on the same frequencies used in audiometry with headphones), or if that is not possible, to obtain responses to at least some sounds relevant to speech perception. In sound field audiometry pure tones are not used, because this would cause standing waves in the test room. Instead, warble tones are usually employed. These are tones in which the frequency varies slightly around the frequency of a pure tone. For example, a warble tone centred on 1000 Hz could vary from 950 Hz to 1050 Hz. Warble tones also sound more 'interesting' than pure tones to many people.

Tones (or other stimuli) are presented via one or more loudspeakers and the client is seated if possible in a calibrated position at which the sound levels relative to the audiometer dial are known. As the stimuli are presented in a sound field, and not through headphones calibrated with regard to normal sensitivity, the responses are recorded in dB SPL. The client's voluntary, involuntary or conditioned responses are noted.

Voluntary responses may include pressing a response button (e.g. in the case of an adult or an older child having their aided hearing assessed) or a play response similar to that used in standard pure tone audiometry (e.g. in the case of a younger child having an aided assessment). In the case of aided assessments, sound field audiometry may be conducted with, and without, the hearing aid(s), the difference in responses forming one functional measure of hearing-aid benefit.

Involuntary responses, such as turning the head or eyes towards the sound source, crawling towards the speaker, cessation of activity or vocalisation, may be the basis of the test in cases where the client is an infant or a multiply handicapped individual. In these cases stimuli other than warble tones may be used. These include tape-recorded everyday sounds (e.g. dog barking, baby crying, footsteps), live voice or noise makers. This form of sound field audiometry is usually termed behavioural observation audiometry (BOA). There are a number of BOA test protocols available that use portable tone generators, calibrated noise making toys and/or live voice. Great skill is required to judge involuntary responses in BOA, and it can be difficult to obtain repeatable responses (Primus, 1991). However, BOA can contribute significantly to test protocols for very profoundly handicapped individuals (Gans & Gans, 1993).

A third form of responses in sound field audiometry are conditioned responses. A commonly used technique is conditioned orientation response audiometry (CORA) also termed visual reinforcement audiometry (VRA), which is based on the conditioned orientation reflex (Suzuki & Ogiba, 1961). In CORA, visual reinforcement is given for a behavioural response to auditory stimuli. Typically, the technique is used for infants and young children who have developed a reliable and easily observed head turn. At the start of a CORA test, auditory signals (e.g. warble tones) are presented simultaneously with an interesting visual display (e.g. an illuminated puppet or toy in a window or on top of the speaker box), and the child's attention is drawn to the visual display. After several such paired presentations the auditory signal alone is presented. If the child has learnt (i.e. been conditioned) to associate the sound with the visual display, he or she will look for the visual display. This looking behaviour is the response to auditory stimulation, which is then, and on subsequent occasions when the child responds appropriately, rewarded with the presentation of the visual display.

Regardless of the general techniques employed and the type of responses assessed, when sound field audiometry is aimed at documenting unaided hearing sensitivity the resulting data are subject to several important limitations. First, the responses are assumed to reflect the hearing sensitivity of the better ear. Because the stimulus is presented into the sound field, rather than via individual headphones, the ears are not tested separately. Hence if normal responses are obtained the clinician generally concludes that there is 'normal sensitivity in at least one ear'.

Second, sound field audiometry indicates hearing levels by air conduction. This is useful because air-conduction testing reflects overall hearing sensitivity, but the lack of bone-conduction information reduces the ability to differentiate between conductive and sensorineural hearing losses.

Third, the lowest level (in dB SPL) of stimulus to which the client reliably responds is most appropriately considered a 'best level of response', rather than a threshold. This is because (a) young children may respond at suprathreshold levels; ( b) with infants less than 6 months of age and with developmentally delayed individuals it is often necessary to use stimuli considerably above threshold to elicit responses. An example is the intense tones needed to cause an auropalpebral or 'eyeblink' reflex (APR); and (c) there are many factors acting in the sound field situation (such as the client's degree of interest in visual reinforcement, the clinician's skill during presentation of noise-maker stimuli and the presence of recruitment in sensorineural hearing losses) that can influence the results obtained.

Finally, sound field audiometry results are not recorded on an HTL audiogram as for pure tone audiometry through headphones, even when frequency specific warble tones are used. This is because (a) in sound field audiometry the stimulus levels (and hence the responses) are expressed in dB SPL (or sometimes dB A), which has a different reference point to dB HTL; (b) in sound field audiometry it is not usually possible to be sure if the responses reflect the hearing of both ears or one ear. Therefore the standard audiometric symbols for headphone testing are inappropriate; and (c) the best levels obtained may be suprathreshold responses. For these reasons sound field audiometry responses are either noted in tabular form, or plotted on a sound field audiogram (explained in Chapter 6). Sound field audiograms may be usefully compared with HTL audiograms to assess, for example, the benefit of hearing aids. This is also discussed in Chapter 6.

# Speech audiometry

Speech audiometry is a general term for hearing assessment in which the stimulus material is speech. The material may be phonemes, words, sentences or connected speech. The task required of the client may be detection, recognition or demonstrated understanding. The particular combination of stimulus and response task will depend on the purpose of the test. The speech material may be presented via headphones or via loudspeakers in a sound field. Live voice presentation via the audiometer microphone is sometimes used, but recorded materials are much more common as they allow better control of calibration.

The two most common uses for speech audiometry are to establish the hearing threshold for speech (expressed in dB HTL or dB SPL) and to estimate the client's ability to understand, or discriminate, speech at suprathreshold levels (generally expressed as the percentage correct response at each of several dB presentation levels). This second application allows useful, if general, assessments of the effect of hearing loss on speech perception, assists in decision-making regarding hearing-aid amplification, helps in the differential diagnosis of hearing loss and can be useful in determining candidacy for surgery. Additional applications of speech audiometry are in the detection of non-organic hearing loss (discussed later in this chapter) and in the assessment of central auditory disorders (discussed in detail in Chapter 9).

### Decibel notation used in speech audiometry

Speech audiometry is usually carried out under headphones with the signals routed via a diagnostic audiometer. The audiometer is usually calibrated with reference to a 1000 Hz calibration tone on recorded speech materials, so that the level (in dB SPL) at which persons with normal hearing can detect correctly 50 per cent of the speech material equals 0 dB on the audiometer dial (i.e. 0 dB HTL). For spondaic words or 'spondees' (two syllable words with equal stress on each syllable) this equates to about 20 dB SPL. This level (20 dB SPL ± 2 dB) has become accepted as the reference equivalent threshold calibration level for speech audiometry by most audiologists. Therefore a speech signal delivered at, for example, 40 dB HTL would be a 60 dB SPL signal at the headphone (see Olsen & Matkin, 1979, pp. 150–152; Martin, 1987, pp. 291–292).

Some audiologists record speech audiometry results obtained via headphones in dB HTL, which has the advantage of being on the same decibel scale as that used in pure tone headphone audiometry. This is very useful in diagnostic hearing assessments. Other audiologists prefer to record speech audiometry results in dB SPL. This is particularly useful when speech audiometry is applied to hearing-aid fitting, as dB SPL is used in many hearing-aid related measurements. Speech audiometry presented via loudspeakers into a sound field is recorded in dB SPL. As a general and approximate rule, speech audiometry results may be converted from SPL to HTL by subtracting 20 dB, and from HTL to SPL by adding 20 dB.

As the actual intensity (in dB SPL) of speech material varies with the speaker, and to some extent the recording, some audiologists prefer to record speech audiometry presentation levels in dB speech reference Level (dB SRL). This is the SPL at which 50 per cent of the particular speech material used in that test can be detected without necessarily being understood (British Society of Audiology, 1981). However, the trend is increasingly to use dB SPL notation. Indeed many clinicians who work largely in hearing-aid rehabilitation consider that pure tone headphone audiometry results would also be usefully recorded in dB SPL. This is now possible with some new clinical audiometers.

## Speech threshold tests

It is often useful to establish the hearing threshold for speech material, as opposed to pure tones. This information provides a validity check on the pure tone audiogram and gives an indication of the lowest level at which speech may be perceived and/or partially understood.

The most common threshold for speech is the level, in dB (HTL or SPL), at which 50 per cent of the speech material (usually spondaic words, although other material may be used) is correctly identified. ASHA terms this level 'speech recognition threshold' (SRT). The term used by the British Society of Audiology for this threshold is the 'hearing level for speech' (HLS).

As with pure tone threshold testing the level of presentation in speech threshold testing is usually raised and lowered in 5 dB steps. Therefore an SRT (HLS) result will be, as for pure tone thresholds, either a multiple of 10 (e.g. 10 dB HTL, 20 dB HTL) or of 5 (e.g. 5 dB HTL, 15 dB HTL).

SRT testing usually follows pure tone audiometry. The client is usually familiarised with a list of test words and then asked to repeat each word subsequently presented through the headphones. The first test word is presented at an easily audible level (e.g. 30 dB SL, or 30 dB above the PTA for that ear). Following a correct response the level is lowered and the second test word is presented. The level of presentation is lowered after each correct response until the client begins to make errors. Several words are then presented at each subsequent level of presentation (which is varied in a 10 dB down, 5 dB up manner) until a level is established at which the client correctly perceives say, three of six words presented. This level is the SRT for that ear. The interested reader is referred to Silman and Silverman (1991) for more information about SRT techniques and test development.

The SRT obtained with spondee words will usually closely approximate the PTA in the same ear. An exception is the case of a steeply sloping pure tone loss, in which the SRT may be better than the PTA. Otherwise, when SRT and PTA results differ by more than 10 dB, the validity of each test must be questioned (Olsen & Matkin, 1979).

Another, perhaps less clinically relevant, speech threshold is the speech detection threshold (SDT), also called the speech awareness threshold (SAT), which is the level (in dB HTL or dB SPL) at which the client can detect the speech signal about 50 per cent of the time, without necessarily understanding it.

Not all clinics test for SRT or other speech thresholds, especially if there is no reason to query the validity of the pure tone audiogram. For example, SRT, SDT and SAT are less frequently used in Australia than in the USA. In Australia and the UK, some speech threshold information is often obtained during the process of speech discrimination testing, which is described in the next section. In the UK, for example, the half peak level (HPL), which is the intensity at which the individual scores 50 per cent of their maximum score (which may be less than 100 per cent), is often noted during speech discrimination testing.

## Speech discrimination tests

Speech discrimination tests are those aimed at estimating the client's ability to understand conversational speech, or aspects of it, correctly. These tests may be conducted in quiet, or in the presence of calibrated competing noises, the latter test situation giving some information about the ability to understand speech in difficult listening situations.

In speech discrimination tests the speech material is delivered, through headphones or loudspeakers, at various suprathreshold levels depending on the particular test protocol, but one of the presentation levels is likely to be the most comfortable listening level (MCL), which is generally about 30 dB above the average three frequency (500 Hz, 1000 Hz and 2000 Hz) pure tone average. The client is asked to repeat or to point to pictures of the test words, phrases or sentences, and a percentage correct score is calculated on the basis of the client's responses. In cases where the hearing in one ear is significantly poorer than the other, masking may be applied, as the potential exists for cross-hearing, as with pure tone audiometry.

Speech discrimination tests usually yield a performance-intensity function (PIF) or speech audiogram (previously called an articulation curve, to indicate the articulation or link between the speaker and the listener's ability to understand that speaker (Martin, 1975)). The PIF is a graph of percentage correct scores by presentation levels, as shown in Figure 4.8. The maximum score achieved by the client over this range of presentation levels is called the maximum discrimination score or MDS (British Society of Audiology, 1981), but it may be named to reflect the speech material used, as for example, PB max, the maximum discrimination score obtained when the material is phonetically balanced (PB) monosyllables (Eldert & Davis, 1951).

Because some speech materials (e.g. sentences) are easier to correctly identify at low intensities than others (e.g. nonsense syllables) due to phonemic, syntactic and/or semantic redundancy, the shape of the PIF will vary somewhat depending on the speech material used.

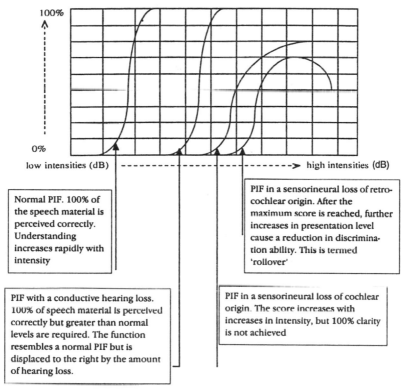

PIF in a sensorineural loss of retro-cochlear origin. After the maximum score is reached, further increases in presentation level cause a reduction in discrimination ability. This is termed 'rollover'

Normal PIF. 100% of the speech material is perceived correctly. Understanding increases rapidly with intensity

PIF with a conductive hearing loss. 100% of speech material is perceived correctly but greater than normal levels are required. The function resembles a normal PIF but is displaced to the right by the amount of hearing loss.

PIF in a sensorineural loss of cochlear origin. The score increases with increases in intensity, but 100% clarity is not achieved

Performance intensity functions for speech audiometry by general type of hearing loss. The actual slope of the functions will differ according to the materials used (e.g. words versus sentences) and the test conditions (e.g. quiet versus in competition with background noise) as well as the pathology and individual abilities

**Figure 4.8:** Schematic diagram of a performance intensity function (PIF) in speech audiometry.

Regardless of the material used, the clinician is primarily interested in the client's PIF in relation to the PIF for persons with normal hearing, for diagnostic purposes. Figure 4.8 shows a series of hypothetical PIFs for (a) normal hearing, (b) a conductive hearing loss, (c) a sensorineural hearing loss of cochlear origin, and (d) a sensorineural loss of retro-cochlear origin. PIF information is also useful in indicating, in a very general way, the possible benefit or otherwise of increased volume (amplification) to the client's speech understanding.

Materials used for speech discrimination tests include, for example:

- AB word lists (Boothroyd, 1968);
- the CID W-22 word lists (Hirsch et al., 1952);
- the California Consonant (CCT) test (Owens & Schubert, 1977);
- the Bench–Kowal–Bamford (BKB) sentences (Bench & Bamford, 1979);
- the BKB/A sentences (Bench, Doyle & Greenwood, 1987);
- the Manchester Junior (MJ) word lists (Ewing, 1957);
- the Synthetic Sentence Identification (SSI) test (Kalikow, Stevens & Elliot, 1977);
- the Speech Perception in Noise (SPIN) test (Bilgeret al., 1984);
- the Phonetically Balanced Kindergarten (PBK-50) test (Haskins, 1964);
- the Word Intelligibility by Picture Identification (WIPI) test (Ross & Lerman, 1970);
- the Common Objects Token (COT) test (Plant & Moore, 1992).

Each of these tests was developed with a particular population or clinical need in mind, but they may all be presented via an audiometer in the assessment of speech understanding. The percentage correct scores of individual tests may be based on scoring individual phonemes, whole words or sentences, or key words within sentences. For more detailed information about speech audiometry tests and concepts, see Dillon and Ching (1995) and Martin (1987).

### Advantages and disadvantages of audiometric speech perception tests

The clinical advantages of the speech audiometry tests so far described lie in the precision they offer in controlling stimuli and recording responses. This is particularly useful when considering the relation between various presentation levels and the client's ability to correctly perceive the signals, and in comparing an individual client's responses to normal patterns of response. Speech audiometry techniques allow a general assessment of a client's ability to perceive speech clearly when the lack of normal volume associated with the hearing loss is compensated for by a suitable level of presentation. Additionally, audiometric speech procedures allow for: (a) each ear to be separately assessed, (b) the effects of background noise on speech perception to be systematically evaluated, (c) the client's performance to be reliably assessed across different speech materials and different modes of presentation (e.g. auditory only versus auditory/visual) and (d) assessment of the relative effectiveness of different hearing-aid settings in relation to speech perception.

However, there are associated limitations. Principally, there is the problem of generalising test results obtained in a sound-treated audiology room to the client's everyday communication situations. The speech noise used in the audiology clinic to estimate the effects of background noise on speech discrimination ability may bear little relation to the content-laden multi-babble background noise experienced by an individual working in a restaurant, for example. In contrast to the carefully calibrated recorded speech presented via headphones in the clinic, the speech of individuals important in the client's home or work life may be imprecise, accent-laden and highly variable in volume. It should be remembered that percentage correct scores obtained via speech audiometry do not indicate for all situations and all speakers the client's ability to perceive speech, because the results are specific to the material used and the context of the test setting. Additionally, as Dillon and Ching (1995) point out, audiometric speech discrimination tests may underestimate a client's potential to benefit from hearing-aid amplification. This is because the audiometer delivers the signal with a flat frequency response, in contrast to the frequency response of the individual client's hearing aid system(s), prescribed in light of that client's particular hearing thresholds and other data. Further, there are occasions when the speech-language therapist may wish to gain data about a client's speech perception ability in relation to their own spoken communication with the client, and when information is needed earlier than audiology clinic waiting lists may allow. For these and other reasons a number of live voice tests of speech perception have been developed Many of these are suitable for use by speech-language therapists, educators of the deaf and other professionals outside the audiology clinic, and they also provide complementary forms of assessment for the audiologist working primarily in rehabilitation.

## Alternative clinical approaches to assessing speech perception ability

Non-audiometric techniques of assessing speech perception ability may assess (a) phoneme detection (e.g. the Ling Five Sound Test, Ling, 1976; Ling & Ling, 1978), (b) consonant discrimination (e.g. the RNID hearing test cards for young children based on the rhyming picture test developed by Reed, 1959), (c) consonant and vowel discrimination (e.g. the Manchester Picture (MP) Vocabulary test, Watson, 1967), (d) the ability to detect speech envelope versus spectral patterns (e.g. the PLOTT Sentence test, Plant & Moore, 1992), (e) comprehension of sentences (e.g. adaptive screening of sentences, Erber, 1992), or (f) some combination of the above (e.g. the Glendonald Auditory Screening Procedure (GASP!) developed by Erber, 1982). Three of these non-audiometric, live voice approaches to speech perception will now be described briefly.

*The Ling Five Sound Test* is especially useful in checking speech sound perception abilities in hearing-impaired children who wear hearing aids. It is a very simple procedure in which the clinician says the sounds /a/, /i/, /u/, /ʃ/ and /s/, and the client is asked to close their eyes and repeat what he or she hears. The client whose audiogram shows aided residual hearing for frequencies up to and including 1000 Hz should be able to perceive the vowels /a/, /i/ and /u/. If the audiogram indicates aided hearing responses to 2000 Hz, /ʃ/ should be received, and if there is aided hearing for 4000 Hz, /s/ should be detected providing the threshold is not greater than about 80 dB HTL. If conducted carefully, and providing the child has sufficient language to cooperate, the Five Sound Test will show up any discrepancies between expected speech sound reception ability based on the audiogram, and actual ability on the day of the interaction with the clinician. If performance does not match expectations, the child may be suffering a conductive hearing loss, which adds to the existing loss and reduces the effectiveness of hearing aids (see Chapter 5 for guidelines on screening middle-ear function); the child's hearing aid(s) may not be functioning optimally (see Chapter 7 for guidelines on hearing aid checks); the child's motivation may be reduced; or some combination of these and/or other factors may exist.

*The PLOTT Sentence Test* is designed to test the auditory speech perception skills of children with profound hearing loss (thresholds on average 90 dB HTL or greater). The test stimuli are sentences, each of which is one of a closed set of four sentences. The client is asked to identify which of the four sentences was spoken by pointing to a corresponding picture. The clinician presents the sentences live voice and without visual cues, while the child is wearing their hearing aid(s) or other sound delivery system. The test items variously assess the ability to use time and intensity cues (as in the closed set 'Bob has a football' vs. 'Bob has a bike' vs. 'Bob has a baby brother' vs 'Bob has one sister and two brothers') and the ability to use spectral information (as in the closed set 'Bob saw some red fish' vs 'Bob saw some blue birds' vs 'Bob saw some red birds' vs 'Bob saw some blue fish'). As with many other live voice tests of this type the performance of individual children can vary greatly, even when audiograms are very similar.

*The Glendonald Auditory Screening Proceedure* (Erber, 1982) was developed to screen the phoneme detection, word identification and sentence comprehension abilities of hearing-impaired children aged 4 years and over. The results of the test reflect the child's ability to use audition to understand the particular speaker conducting the test. Hence it is potentially very useful for educators of the deaf and speech-language therapists. The test progresses from phoneme detection through word discrimination, to sentence comprehension. Phonemes presented are vowels (/i/ as in 'beet', /I/ as in 'bit', /e/ as in 'bet', /æ/ as in 'bat', /ɑ/ as in 'pot' /ɔ/ as in 'bought', /u/ as in 'book', /u / as in 'boot', /ʌ/ as in 'but', /ɚ/ as in 'bird'; nasals /m/, /n/; laterals /r/, /l/; voiced fricatives /z/, /ʒ/, /v/, /ð/; and unvoiced fricatives /s/ /ʃ / /f/ and /θ/. Presentation of these phonemes is interspersed with trials in which no sound is made. A response form for this phoneme detection subtest is shown in Table 4.2. Words presented are monosyllablic (e.g 'shoe'), spondaic (e.g 'tooth-brush'), trochaic (e.g. 'pencil'), or trisyllabic (e.g. 'elephant'). Sentences presented are questions (e.g. 'What colour are your shoes?'). No visual cues are given. The child is asked to point to a picture (a 'yes' or 'no' card for the phoneme detection task, and a picture of the object in word identification tasks) and to respond verbally (to the questions). The clinician may make their own materials for the test. A very helpful and full description of how to conduct and score this test is given in Erber (1982, pp. 47–71).

## Speech audiometry perception tests for languages other than English

The vast majority of methods for assessing speech perception abilities have been developed in the English and other European languages. Scandinavia, for example, has well-developed protocols for speech audiometry in Danish, Finnish, Norwegian and Swedish. In contrast, there are very few well-standardised speech audiometry tests in Asian languages, such as Cantonese, Indonesian or Malaysian, or in Aboriginal languages, such as Walpiri, one of approximately 20 Australian Aboriginal languages. However, a beginning has been made (see for example, Knight, 1987; Kei et al., 1991; Plant, 1991). When an individual with English as a second language is assessed via English speech perception tests problems of validity may arise (see for example, Danhauer, Crawford & Edgerton, 1984; Smith, Tipping & Bench, 1987; Elliot & Doyle, 1993). Countries such as Australia, the UK and the USA have increasingly multicultural populations. English speech audiometry tests are therefore not necessarily suitable for many clients attending clinics. As most of the world's population communicates in languages other than English, a great deal more work is needed in developing speech perception/audiometry tests in languages other than English.

Table 4.2: Response form for the GASP Subtest 1 (Phoneme Detection)

GLENDONALD
AUDITORY
SCREENING
PROCEDURE

Child: _____
Teacher: _____
Tester: _____
Date: _____

How was child tested?

HA
FM
AT
V

|   | L | Bin | R |
|---|---|---|---|
|   |   | • |   |
|   |   |   |   |
|   |   |   |   |

I. *PHONEME DETECTION*—Place dot(s) in the *yes/no* box(es) to indicate child's response(s).

| | beet | bit | bet | bat | pot | bought | book | boot | but | bird | no sound | nas. | lat. | voiced fricative | unvoiced fricative |
|---|---|---|---|---|---|---|---|---|---|---|---|---|---|---|---|
| | i | ɪ | ɛ | æ | ɒ | ɔ | ʊ | u | ʌ | ɜ | | m n | r l | z ʒ v ð | s ʃ f θ |
| yes | o | • | • | • | • | • | • | o | • | • | | • | • | • • o o | o • • • |
| no | • | | | | | | | • | | | • • • • • • | | | • • • • | • • • • |

● = normal intensity;  ○ = increased intensity

Reproduced with permission from Enser NP (1982). *Auditory Training*. Washington, DC: AG Bell Association for the Deaf.

# Evoked responses

The tests described under this general heading are those objective tests in which electrophysiological responses are evoked by various stimuli. These tests include:

- brainstem evoked response audiometry (BERA);
- auditory middle latency response (AMLR);
- late latency response (LLR);
- otoacoustic emissions (OAE);
- electrocochleography (ECOG);
- electronystagmography (ENG).

These will now be briefly described with emphasis on the OAE and BERA tests.

### Brainstem evoked response audiometry

Brainstem evoked response audiometry (BERA) is also known as auditory brainstem response (ABR) audiometry (Jewett & Williston, 1971). BERA (ABR) provides data about hearing in the frequency band 1000–4000 Hz, but the response is not frequency-specific.

In BERA the response of the afferent auditory system from the cochlea to the mid-brain is tested. An auditory signal comprising a series of clicks is delivered through a headphone, with masking presented to the opposite ear. If this signal is perceived, there will be very small changes in the ongoing electrical activity of the brain. These stimulus-related changes in brain activity are recorded by means of electrodes attached to the head (usually to the vertex/forehead and to the mastoid processes/ear lobes). The client is asked to relax with eyes closed. Children and infants are best tested when asleep. Sedation or anaesthesia may be necessary and do not interfere with the response. A computer averages the stimulus-related responses of the auditory system to enhance them in relation to the ongoing brain activity. The test yields a trace or waveform with a number of peaks, each peak corresponding to the response of a particular level of the auditory system. Figure 4.9 illustrates a normal ABR.

BERA has a number of applications. It may be used to:

- test for the presence of hearing loss in infants and multiply handicapped individuals;
- provide an objective indicator of auditory function in medico-legal cases and/or where NOHL is suspected;
- aid in the differential diagnosis of cochlear and retrocochlear hearing loss, being particularly useful in the detection of Schwannomas;

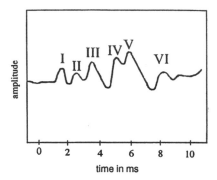

**Figure 4.9:** A normal auditory brainstem response. The peaks indicate responses from various parts of the afferent auditory system. For example, waves I and II relate to the auditory nerve and wave III to the cochlear nucleus.

- assist with detection of other neurological disorders, such as multiple sclerosis or cerebellopontine angle tumours.

The interpretation of BERA responses involves assessment of the presence or otherwise of the expected waveform peaks at various levels of stimulation, the amplitude of the response, the latency of the response, the interpeak latencies and the relative responses of the two ears.

### Middle and late latency responses

The auditory middle latency response (AMLR) and late latency response (LLR) are responses emanating from portions of the afferent auditory pathways above brainstem level. They are also called cortical responses, measured by cortical evoked response audiometry (CERA). The AMLR gives information about low-frequency hearing (not available from BERA), as well as the response from the mid-brain and auditory cortex. LLRs are made up of a number of components and can relate to the listener's alertness and auditory discrimination. Cortical responses can be usefully applied in cases of NOHL. Additionally, there are indications that aspects of the LLR may have greater than normal latencies in children with language impairment, suggesting slower processing in the central auditory pathways (Tonnquist-Uhlén, 1996). Jirsa (1992) found that aspects of the LLR appear to be sensitive to behavioural changes following therapy. Readers interested in BERA, AMLR and LLR are referred to several chapters in Katz (1994).

### Electrocochleography

Electrocochleography (ECOG) is a test of the cochlea and VIIIth nerve. As with BERA, a click stimulus is used and the response is recorded via electrodes. However, although some electrodes are placed on the forehead and mastoid/ear lobe as in BERA, the active electrode may be either placed in the external auditory meatus or inserted through the tympanic membrane to rest on the promontory of the cochlea. In the case of transtympanic electrode placement the test is done under local anaesthetic or more general sedation if necessary. A computer-averaging technique is used to generate a waveform from the responses. This may be read to estimate thresholds for frequencies 1000 Hz and above in cases where hearing loss is present. Another useful application of ECOG is in the differential diagnosis of various cochlear disorders. It is especially useful in diagnosing Ménière's disease (Coats, 1981). ECOG testing is also useful in pre-operative assessment of cochlear implant candidates (see for example, Kileny et al., 1992).

### Electronystagmography

Electronystagmography (ENG) is not a test of hearing, but a test of the vestibular system. It is mentioned here because the differential diagnosis of cochlear and retrocochlear disorders often requires vestibular assessment, and because ENG can aid in the detection of other lesions of the central nervous system (Allard & Welsh, 1990). ENG involves recording spontaneous and evoked nystagmus (involuntary, regular eye movements which indicate an attempt by the vestibular-ocular reflex (see Kileny, 1985) to stabilise images on the retina) via electrodes placed on the forehead and around each eye. Responses are evoked via caloric stimulation (application of warm and cool water or air to the tympanic membrane) and by optokinetic stimulation (watching a rotating drum with alternate black and white vertical stripes). The individual client's response is compared to expected norms and the relative response from the client's two ears is examined. ENG is useful in the diagnosis of Ménière's disease, for example, as the vestibular response from the affected ear may be significantly different in comparison to that from the other ear (Barber & Stockwell, 1980).

### Otoacoustic emissions

Otoacoustic emissions are often described as essentially an 'echo', coming from the outer hair cells of the cochlea, and occurring a few milliseconds after stimulation with incoming sound, in response to the incoming sound (Kemp, 1978; Johnson, Bagi & Elberling, 1983; Kemp, Ryan & Bray, 1990).These emissions may be detected in the external auditory meatus. If such emissions are detected, normal cochlear function can be assumed for the stimulus frequency. OAEs cannot be used to estimate threshold, but can determine whether or not a normal cochlear response is present. OAEs can occur spontaneously, but these will not be discussed here.

OAEs may be evoked by clicks and tone bursts (yielding transient OAEs), a continuous frequency sweep tone (yielding stimulus frequency OAEs) or a combination of pure tones (yielding distortion product OAEs). The stimulus is presented via a probe tip, which also contains a microphone sufficiently sensitive to detect the cochlear response. The response is analysed via a computer system. An emerging role for OAEs is to assist in the differentiation of sensorineural losses that are largely due to cochlear pathology (such as NIHL) and sensorineural losses that have a neural (e.g. VIIIth nerve) etiology. Transient OAEs can be useful in the diagnosis of non-organic hearing loss (Kværner et al., 1996). OAEs are potentially useful in screening for hearing loss, although there are problems in applying the technique to very young children and infants (see for example, Trine, Hirsch & Margolis, 1993; Dalebout, 1995b; El-Refaie, Parker & Bamford, 1996), largely because sound transfer to the cochlea is affected by the presence of middle-ear fluid and by various other changes to the function and/or structure of the external and middle ear. This characteristic of OAEs has been positively approached by McPherson and Smyth (1997), who argue that for populations in which conductive hearing loss is very common (such as Australian Aboriginals), OAEs can be an appropriate screening tool for schoolage children. It is to be hoped that in time there will be routinely available a combination OAE probe and tympanometer to allow better interpretation in such cases.

## Tests for non-organic hearing loss (NOHL)

When a client presents with inconsistencies between test results (e.g. a discrepancy between SRT and PTA), when client communication behaviour does not appear to match rest results or when responses are highly variable within or between tests, then tests for NOHL may be applied.

Tests for NOHL may be objective, such as ABR or ECOG already mentioned, or subjective, such as the Stenger test. The reader is referred to Martin (1985) or Silman and Silverman (1991) for a discussion of some other tests.

The Stenger test is applied when the client reports the hearing in one ear to be much better than the hearing in the other ear, and the clinician doubts the truth of this claim. For example, a client may give normal threshold responses in one ear and responses to unmasked tones consistent with a severe or even total hearing loss in the other ear. In reality, such a situation cannot occur, because sound delivered to an ear with even little or no measurable hearing will be perceived by the opposite, normal ear when the level of presentation is sufficient to vibrate the skull and cause cross-hearing (usually, 40 or 50 dB above the threshold in the better ear).

The Pure Tone Stenger test is based on the principle that if pure tones of the same frequency are presented to both ears simultaneously, only the tone that is louder to the listener will be perceived. If the tones are equally loud to the listener (such as would be the case if both ears had similar thresholds for that tone and the sound was delivered at the same dB HTL level to each ear) then the tone will be perceived in the mid-plane. For example, a 60 dB HTL tone of 1000 Hz presented to both ears simultaneously will be perceived in the mid-plane if both ears have thresholds of say 20 dB HTL, or 35 dB HTL, or 50 dB HTL, or some other equal level for that frequency, as long as the threshold is better than 60 dB HTL.

If the tones are not equally loud to the listener (such as would be the case if one ear had hearing much poorer than the other, or if the presentation level of the tone was greater in one ear than the other) then the tone will be perceived in only one ear, even though the tone is presented to both ears at the same time. For example, if the hearing thresholds were the same in both ears, and the 1000 Hz tone was presented to the left ear at 75 dB HTL and to the right ear at 60 dB HTL, then the tone would only be perceived in the left ear. Similarly, if the tone was presented to both left and right ears at 60 dB HTL, and the right ear had a threshold of 50 dB HTL and the left ear had a threshold of 30 dB HTL, the tone would only be perceived in the left ear because the sound would be louder to the individual on that side (presentation level of 60 dB HTL – threshold of 50 dB HTL = sensation level (SL) of 10 dB in the right ear; presentation level of 60 dB HTL – threshold of 30 dB HTL in the left ear = 30 dB SL in the left ear. Therefore the tone sounds 20 dB louder in the left ear than the right).

Figure 4.10 illustrates how these facts are used in the Pure Tone Stenger test. The tone is presented to the apparently poorer ear at a level lower than the admitted threshold in that ear (so that if the threshold is correct the individual would not be able to hear the tone), and simultaneously to the better ear at a level which is both higher than the threshold on that side (so the individual should be able to hear the tone) and at the same time lower than the level presented to the reportedly poorer ear. The individual is asked to respond when they hear a tone. If they hear the tone in the better ear (as would be the case if the admitted thresholds are genuine) they will acknowledge that they hear a tone. If they hear the tone in the apparently poorer ear (as would be the case if the admitted threshold was false) they will be unlikely to acknowledge hearing the tone.

The Stenger principle can also be used with speech material. For example, portions of a story may be delivered to alternate ears. At the conclusion of the story the individual is asked to repeat it. If portions of the story delivered to the poorer ear are recalled, then obviously that ear had sufficient hearing to perceive the signal. Additionally, a tuning fork Stenger test may be done in the medical clinic (see Ballantyne, 1990).

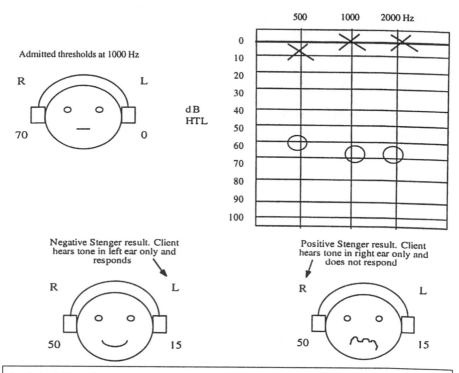

The admitted right ear thresholds appear too poor (refer discussion on cross-hearing and interaural attenuation). In the Stenger test a tone is presented at a level lower than the admitted threshold in the right ear, and simultaneously, a tone of the same frequency is presented to the left ear at a level higher than the given threshold. Since the individual will only perceive the tone which is louder to them, they will hear the tone in the left ear if the admitted thresholds are genuine and only in the right ear if they are not.

**Figure 4.10:** Example of a Pure Tone Stenger test at 1000 Hz in a case of suspected non-organic hearing loss.

# Central auditory processing tests

Central auditory processing disorders (CAPD) are essentially those problems associated with manipulation and use of sound by the central nervous system (Lasky & Katz, 1983), in which perception and cognition interact at various levels (Beasley & Rintelmann, 1979). The American Speech-Language-Hearing Association Task Force on Central Auditory Processing Consensus Development (1997) has provided a useful technical report on the nature of CAPD. CAPD is known to be associated (although certainly not invariably) with damage to the central auditory nervous system, such as can occur with tumours, vascular accidents, head injury and multiple sclerosis, and learning disorders. Persons with learning disorders may have a developmental delay in maturation of their central auditory processes, perhaps associated with myelination rate (Yakovlev & LeCours, 1967).

Methods of assessing the ability to process auditory signals have developed along two paths. First, and particularly where children are concerned, there have been various psycholinguistic approaches, such as exemplified in some subtests of the Illinois Test of Psycholinguistic Abilities (ITPA), developed by Kirk, McCarthy and Kirk (1968). These approaches are usually non-audiometric. Second, particularly in the case of adults, there has been a site-of-lesion approach, which attempts to investigate the association between various functions and known lesions of, for example, the temporal lobe. Whichever approach is employed in a given case, it is imperative to first establish the status of the peripheral auditory system, as what could be assessed as difficulty in comprehension of auditory information, for example, might simply be a difficulty in hearing what is said.

Audiological assessments for CAPD aim to test the auditory system by taxing some of the higher auditory functions, such as binaural fusion of signals reaching the brain from the two ears, and the ability to distinguish a speech signal in the presence of various competing signals. Meaningful and/or nonsense speech materials are frequently employed in CAPD assessments. The use of audiometric techniques to assesss CAPD has strong appeal because of the ability to control the signals and presentation modes used. The information gained can valuably augment audiological assessments of more peripheral auditory function, such as sound detection, and can provide useful data for the speech-language therapist whose client has difficulty dealing with auditory information.

In the case of children who appear to have hearing problems and yet have a normal audiogram, CAPD is one possible explanation. There are of course others, including language delay, reduced attention span and unwillingness to respond, although these features might in theory coexist with a CAPD problem.

CAPD assessment and treatment is a very complex topic and one in which there is a great deal yet to be understood. Bench, in Chapter 9, discusses the current status of CAPD evaluation.

## Clinical decisions for the speech-language therapist

Other than decisions involved in hearing screening, which are discussed in Chapter 5, the speech-language therapist is likely to encounter two basic decisions around hearing assessment. These are:

1. Do I need any additional information about my client's auditory function?
2. Do the test results I have received appear to match client performance?

It may be that the speech-language therapist has referred the client for diagnostic hearing assessment because a client appears to respond inconsistently to speech sounds, and the audiological report has indicated no hearing loss and no apparent middle-ear dysfunction. In this case, because the speech-language therapist continues to observe apparent hearing problems, it may be wise to refer the client for assessment of central auditory processing abilities.

If a child attending for speech therapy has a good aided sound field audiogram, indicating the ability to perceive most of the speech signal at a distance of one metre, and yet the Ling Five Sound Test reveals that the child is currently responding only to low-frequency vowel sounds, then it is wise to investigate this apparent inconsistency by referring for tympanometry to exclude current middle-ear problems, and perhaps requesting a technical check of the child's hearing aids.

In these and other ways the speech-language therapist can utilise the information contained in audiological test results to monitor the client's auditory function in relation to their performance in therapy sessions and to make appropriate referral decisions when indicated. Additionally, the information from hearing assessments can guide therapy and assist in setting realistic goals relating to the acquisition of spoken language through audition.

## Summary of key points

Routine diagnostic hearing assessment comprises: subjective tests of auditory threshold sensitivity (air- and bone-conduction pure tone audiometry via headphones with masking if necessary, and/or sound field audiometry), objective tests of middle-ear function and associated reflexes (tympanometry and acoustic reflex tests) and tests of the ability to perceive speech (speech recognition threshold, speech discrimination tests). A number of objective evoked response tests (BERA, OAE, AMLR, LLR, ECOG, ENG) may be applied in cases where routine procedures are not suitable and in the differential diagnosis of various auditory disorders. Audiometric procedures for examining cases of suspected non-organic hearing loss are available. A range of non-audiometric speech perception tests are available, which are suitable for clinicians who wish to establish how a particular client perceives that clinician's own speech using audition. Central auditory processing disorders may be assessed via audiometric techniques, but these are not available in every audiology clinic. Clinical decisions for the speech-language therapist include examination of audiometric results in comparison to client communication abilities in the speech clinic, and seeking further information and assistance if necessary.

## Further reading

Erber NP (1982) Auditory training. Washington, DC: AG Bell. (A very readable book aimed at clinicians, teachers and parents of hearing-impaired children. Gives background to and techniques for assessing and developing the child's use of audition. Lots of practical information.)

Martin M (Ed.) (1987) Speech audiometry. London: Taylor & Francis. (A review of international practices in audiometric methods of assessing speech perception abilities. Several chapters are particularly useful for speech-language therapists. These include an overview of basic properties of speech by R Wright and a discussion of speech perception tests for the profoundly deaf by AB King.)

Silman MB, Silverman CA (1991) Auditory diagnosis: principles and applications. San Diego: Academic Press. (A good reference book for those interested in more detail about the application of clinical tests in audiology. Readable and comprehensive. Also includes information relevant to the disorders described in Chapter 3.)

# Chapter 5
# Screening of hearing and middle-ear function

JANET DOYLE

The purpose of screening is to separate from among apparently asymptomatic individuals those who have a greater probability of having a hearing problem, and then to refer them for diagnostic assessment (ASHA, 1995). Screening is the most basic formal test method of detecting auditory problems. It is therefore a suitable tool for speech-language therapists and other health professionals for whom hearing status is an important item of clinical data. This chapter presents guidelines for conducting screening of hearing and middle-ear function in the clinic and other treatment locations.

The assessment of clients with multiple handicaps and of children under 3 years of age requires specialist audiological expertise (ASHA, 1994b), but the speech-language therapist can readily screen hearing in the majority of all other clients. Although speech-language therapists in Australia and the USA are trained to screen for hearing loss, it is acknowledged that screening for hearing loss by speech-language therapists in the UK is relatively rare for training and resource reasons. This chapter presents a discussion of screening from the perspective of the speech-language therapist, rather than from an epidemiological perspective. The emphasis is on the identification of hearing and/or middle-ear problems in individual clients of the speech-language therapist, rather than large-scale public health screenings, although references are provided for those readers particularly interested in the latter, and a brief summary of current approaches to population screening is presented.

## Principles

1. *Screening of hearing is an important responsibility of the speech-language therapist*. This principle is fundamental to valid assessment of communication and appropriately targeted clinical management.

Undetected hearing or middle-ear problems in any client consulting a speech-language therapist potentially compromises the effectiveness of therapy and client health care. Clients whose communication problems are associated with head injury, cerebral vascular incident, cleft palate, multiple sclerosis or genetic developmental syndromes, for example, may readily have their therapy compromised by an unacknowledged hearing loss. For all clients the following applies: if hearing assessment has not been conducted or arranged by other persons, then the speech-language therapist should arrange for audiological evaluation or conduct hearing screening.

2. *Screening yields a 'yes' or 'no' response to the question: 'Does this client appear to have hearing sensitivity and/or middle-ear function outside the normal range?'* A screening test identifies people who may have a hearing loss and/or a middle-ear dysfunction, and who therefore require further assessment. A screening test does not yield a comprehensive description of hearing or middle-ear function. Screening tests are not a casual or 'sloppy' way of assessing hearing (Doyle, 1989), but are carefully designed and applied procedures aimed at answering this basic question .

3. *Pass/fail criteria must be set* a priori *and applied consistently*. In a screening test the client's responses to a defined set of stimuli are tested. The screening stimulus (for example a 20 dB HTL pure tone at 1000 Hz in a hearing screening test) is decided before the test begins, with the understanding that individuals who do not respond to the 'screen' will be deemed to have failed the test and are therefore identified. It is not appropriate to decide that in a particular case a lack of response can be ascribed to some cause other than hearing loss, and that therefore the client may be exempted from further investigation. Only unambiguous responses are acceptable in screening. If there is any doubt about whether or not a client has responded to a particular stimulus it is best to assume no response. Possible reasons for ambiguous responses in hearing screening are discussed later in this chapter.

4. *Appropriate test specificity and sensitivity is necessary*. Every screening test has a certain chance of correctly identifying persons who have normal performance with regard to the feature of interest, for example, hearing, and this test characteristic is termed 'specificity'. Each test also has a level of 'sensitivity', the ability to correctly identify persons who have a hearing loss. The speech-language therapist is advised to choose screening tests known to have high specificity and sensitivity (for example, the pure tone procedure described in this chapter), while recognising that no single test has perfect power to make identifications correctly in all situations.

5. *The effectiveness of screening procedures must be intermittently evaluated*. Because all clinical situations are slightly different, it is

important to check the effectiveness of the screening tests used. Methods of checking specificity and sensitivity are discussed later in this chapter. Evaluation also involves determining the effectiveness of follow-up and referral procedures. These should never be assumed to be adequate.

6. *Interpretation and counselling must match the information yield.* It is important to avoid the situation of trying to explain hearing or middle-ear status beyond the limits of the information yielded by screening tests. Clients may wish to know the level and cause of an apparent hearing problem detected at screening. The most that can usually be said, on the basis of a hearing screening test, is whether one or both ears are suspected of having a loss, and at which test frequencies a loss is suspected. It is also important to remember that almost all hearing screening tests focus on detection of peripheral hearing loss. Although not a frequent occurrence, it is possible to have a perfectly normal ability to detect sound, and yet have real problems hearing. This situation is addressed in Chapter 9.

7. *All people involved should understand the screening process.* For screening to be effective, it should be understood by clinicians, clients and other relevant persons and agencies. Clients, parents and teachers need to understand that the aim of a screening test is identification of individuals who *may* have a hearing problem, and that further work is necessary to exclude or confirm that possibility. It is important to explain the process in a manner that will avoid both complacency and undue alarm among clients and their families. Agencies to which referral is made for further testing should be aware of the screening protocol used. If the screening programme involves large numbers of clients it is advisable to alert agencies to a possible flow of referrals and to discuss in advance how this will be best managed.

8. *Cost-effectiveness, liaison, personnel, follow-up, referral, resources and outcome evaluation must be considered before screening.* These considerations are as important as the expertise with which screening tests are carried out. Decisions about these issues can be assisted by asking the following questions with regard to your particular clinical environment as an individual speech-language therapist:

   (a) Which equipment is the most economical given the particular test(s) I wish to conduct? Here it is important to consider the cost of maintenance, such as calibration, in addition to the cost of buying or leasing equipment. If it is necessary to demonstrate cost-effectiveness it may be useful to devise a formula to yield a cost per client (see, for example, Bess & Humes, 1990, p. 154), although a companion formula to demonstrate the cost of not detecting hearing or middle-ear problems would also seem sensible.

(b)If there is a need to reduce costs, how can cost-effectiveness be improved? (e.g. by screening greater numbers of clients, sharing equipment among several facilities.)

(c) Which person will coordinate screening?

(d)What is the best audiological and/or medical referral route(s) for clients who have been identified by screening? Here it is important to consider waiting lists, apparent quality of service, suitability of the person or agency for your particular clientele, and possible costs to the client or your agency.

(e) What is the clinical protocol with regard to referral? For example, one protocol might have all identified clients receive a medical evaluation. Another protocol might have identified clients referred for audiological assessment, the audiologist later referring for medical opinion and management if necessary.

(f) How will I get feedback on clients who have been referred for further assessment or management?

(g)What evaluation can I make of the effectiveness of screening in terms of client outcomes?

## Managing pre-screening

There are several pre-screening steps that can inform your knowledge of the client's hearing status and augment the informational counselling that follows testing. First, for adult clients, a simple question about possible hearing difficulties can yield much information, including occasions of difficulty, family opinion of the client's hearing, ear differences, presence or absence of tinnitus, relative hearing ability of left and right ears, earache and other symptoms of aural dysfunction, and past history of medical treatment of the ears. If the client does have hearing problems, more often than not a fairly full picture is volunteered. Additionally, it is important to assess the attitude of clients to having a hearing loss, as attitude may be related to compliance with recommendations for action following screening. The literature demonstrates that compliance levels in adults can be disappointing (for a brief review see ASHA, 1992). For child clients, a parental/care giver impression of the child's hearing is valuable. Some parents can be very accurate in detecting significant hearing loss (Kankkunen, 1982; Hovind & Parving, 1987), although use of parental questionnaires as a method in large-scale screening projects is debatable in terms of effectiveness (see Haggard & Hughes, 1991, pp. 224–228 for a discussion). Parent confusion about a child's hearing status is also valuable as it can signify intermittent conductive losses. Parents of children with conductive loss may not recognise that their child has a hearing loss (Moore, 1993; Pollard & Tan, 1993), but they may report that their child's behaviour is unacceptable and that they feel annoyed or angry with their child a good deal of the time (Moore, 1993).

Second, the client's self-rating of overall hearing ability (as, for example, 'excellent', 'good', 'fair' or 'poor') is useful. Clinical experience has shown that up to 30 per cent of adult clients in some populations give a self-rating of hearing ability that appears at odds with subsequent hearing screening test results (Healey & Doyle, 1980), perhaps rating their hearing as 'good' or 'excellent' when screening detects a loss, or rating their hearing as 'fair' when the screening test fails to detect a loss of hearing sensitivity. Putting aside a discussion of the possible reasons for this apparent and interesting mismatch of client perception and screening test results, it is important to know about such inconsistencies if informational counselling and referral decisions are to be effective. For example, if the client has rated her or his hearing as 'good' and yet clearly fails the screening test, the importance of further assessment will need to be stressed without in any way devaluing the client's judgement. If the client has rated their hearing as 'fair' or 'poor' and yet passes the screening test, a decision to refer for assessment in spite of an apparently satisfactory screening test result may be wise to exclude a more central auditory disorder and to provide the client with more comprehensive information.

Third, your observation of the client's ability to use auditory information in conversation is valuable. If the client displays a heavy reliance on visual cues and/or asks for repeats, misinterprets your utterances, has a louder-than-normal voice, seems slightly vague or appears not to comprehend, hearing loss is very likely, and the client may need assistance to improve communication function. Children with hearing loss may be reluctant to tolerate distance from their parent or carer. There are of course other possible explanations for such behaviours. Similarly, clients who do not display any of these behaviours should not be assumed to have normal hearing. Many people with hearing loss naturally develop skills that allow for good communication despite some loss of auditory sensitivity. Hearing screening for these persons has the potential benefits of excluding the need for medical referral on health grounds and of providing information for the client's own use, even if no other intervention is indicated and/or agreed to by the client.

Fourth, the opinion of a range of family members about the client's hearing ability is useful. Some clients who report no hearing difficulties can have families who insist that the client does have hearing problems! As the client's communication effectiveness is related, in part, to family perceptions and communication habits, this situation needs addressing.

# Pure tone screening for detecting hearing loss

### Why pure tone screening

There are many methods of screening hearing. For infants and children these include: high risk registers, in which infants whose characteristics include presumed high risk factors (such as very low birthweight, cleft palate or family history of hearing loss) are identified for subsequent selective screening or for audiological evaluation (see Mauk et al., 1991, for a discussion of the effectiveness of risk registers); auditory brainstem response (ABR), in which the subcortical responsiveness of the afferent auditory pathway is tested objectively with an electrophysiological technique (see Fria (1985) and Bess & Humes (1990) for readable descriptions) ; sound field localisation or distraction tests, in which acoustic stimuli such as that produced by the Manchester high pitch rattle (Kettlety, 1987) are presented at a specified distance from the ear and the child's ability to localise those sounds is observed (a range of these tests is described by Ballantyne, 1990); parental and/or teacher questionnaires, in which judgements about, for example, a child's language and speech development, and presence of otological symptoms, are sought (Haggard & Hughes, 1991); and pure tone headphone tests, in which calibrated pure tones of various frequencies are delivered to each ear separately and a behavioural response from the child is sought (ASHA, 1985). There are other methods of assessing hearing in infants and children, but the examples listed above illustrate the methods most commonly used for screening. For adults, possible screening methods include pure tone headphone tests (ASHA, 1985); audioscope tests, in which a hand-held combination otoscope and pure tone generator is employed with an automatic tone presentation sequence (Lichtenstein, Bess & Logan, 1988); and client or carer questionnaires, in which questions such as 'Do you have difficulty hearing when someone speaks in a whisper?' are asked. On the whole, these questionnaires for adults (see, for example, the HHIE-S in Lichtenstein, Bess & Logan, 1988) address the question of perceived hearing handicap rather than auditory sensitivity and, there-fore, used alone, they are not really a hearing screening test. Nevertheless, the approach can have useful applications (see, for example, Ventry & Weinstein, 1983; Poltl & Hickson, 1990; Schow, 1991). In the USA there are also various telephone screening services, but these are of questionable value (ASHA, 1988).

This chapter focuses on screening with pure tone audiometry. It lists ten reasons why screening with pure tone audiometry is particularly useful for the speech-language therapist, and is the test recommended by this author.

1. Pure tone testing uses calibrated, electroacoustically generated stimuli. Provided that the audiometer used is kept in calibration, the potential problems of variable frequency and intensity that can occur with 'human-generated' stimuli, such as low-frequency voice, shaking of rattles, or speech, sounds are avoided.
2. The necessary equipment is not overly expensive and is easily mastered with appropriate training. A pure tone air-conduction

audiometer with noise-excluding headphones is not expensive in comparison to much of the other equipment used in the speech and hearing sciences. Additionally, there are now available even less expensive pure tone generators, such as the Welch Allyn audioscope, which, when used with careful attention to recommended protocols, can be very effective with many clients (Lichtenstein, Bess & Logan, 1988; Sangster, Gerace & Seewald, 1991)

3. The face validity of the test for clients is high. Although clinical artistry may allow brilliant hypotheses about the client's hearing, client confidence in clinical advice may be greater if the test has been conducted using equipment. This is not to say that clients cannot appreciate clinical expertise, but simply that the presence of scientific instrumentation may assist the client's confidence in the assessment and hence any recommendations for further investigation.

4. The information yield is in a form familiar to audiologists, audiological physicians, hearing therapists, otologists, special teachers and others likely to be interacting with speech-language therapists and their clients. Speech-language therapists share with them a knowledge of decibels, audio frequency and normal hearing. This shared knowledge should assist professional communication.

5. The specificity and sensitivity of the tests are established relatively easily with reference to diagnostic threshold audiometry. Specificity and sensitivity values are established by arranging threshold assessment for samples of clients who pass and who fail the screening test, and then determining the hit and miss rates for each of the two groups. This is discussed later in this chapter.

6. The test is fast. If the level of client cooperation is high, ambient noise remains appropriately low and clear instructions are given, it is possible to check hearing for three frequencies in each ear within 5 minutes, and in many cases in 2–3 minutes. This includes subjective equipment checks, instructions to the client and the recording of the results. The test may therefore be easily incorporated into scheduled therapy sessions, and be repeated on each occasion of therapy if indicated.

7. If accompanied by a fun play response, pure tone screening can be a way of engaging child clients in communication. In this case the test will obviously take longer than 5 minutes, but turn-taking and other communication behaviours can be observed or enhanced at the same time. When a child is reluctant to participate in screening, a turn-taking form of game, with pure tones used as the signal for turns, can help condition appropriate responses for later testing.

8. Separate information is yielded for each ear and the test gives frequency specific information. Therefore, the responses can indicate if one ear may have better hearing than the other, and if the possible loss is suspected to involve low-frequency hearing, high-frequency

hearing, or both. This information can be very useful when combined with the results of tympanometry screening, also described in this chapter.

9. Guidelines for pure tone screening have been developed by professional associations such as the American Speech-Language-Hearing Association (ASHA), the Audiological Society of Australia (ASA) and the British Society of Audiology (BSA). These guidelines reflect considerable background thinking about key issues and offer a range of detailed protocols to inform the clinical decision-making of the individual speech-language therapist.

10. Pure tone headphone screening is possibly the most valid and, at the same time, accessible hearing screening tool for the speech-language therapist, for several reasons. The validity and reliability of pure tone headphone testing is high, given satisfactory levels of tester expertise, client cooperation and ambient noise in the test environment. The concepts and expertise are not difficult to master, and the cost is relatively low compared to other equipment-based screening methods. Considerably more training and equipment is required for some of the other approaches (for example ABR). Additionally, in the view of this author, the validity and/or reliability of some other screening methods, such as distraction tests using live voice, can be very sensitive to the level of expertise of the individual persons employing them. Speech-language therapists who wish to employ live voice techniques (as used in distraction testing or cooperative play tests) are advised to seek appropriate training, use a sound level meter to ensure accurate levels during testing and to establish a good relationship with an expert in live voice techniques for purposes of consultation and refresher training.

**Room and equipment requirements for pure tone screening**

Pure tone screening may be carried out in rooms when ambient noise is sufficiently low to allow detection of the selected stimuli by listeners with normal hearing. For example, if a 20 dB HTL screening level is used, the American Speech-Language-Hearing Association recommends that ambient room noise be no greater than 41.5 dB SPL at 500 Hz, 49.5 dB SPL at 1000 Hz, 54.5 dB SPL at 2000 Hz and 62 dB SPL at 4000 Hz (ASHA, 1985). Ambient room noise per octave-band needs to be assessed by means of a sound level meter with octave-band filter. However, a general practical guide is that if a person with known normal hearing can hear the screening test tones without strain, then the room noise is likely to be of an acceptable level.

Equipment needed for pure tone screening is a audiometer or an audioscope™. An air-conduction audiometer with TDH-49 headphones on a spring steel band and MX-41 AR pads is appropriate. An audiometer that is lightweight, easily carried and has a drawer or pocket in which to carry record forms has added advantages for the speech-language therapist. If necessary, TDH-50P circumaural ('noise-excluding') headphones can be used. These contain a standard MX-41 AR pad in an external hard shell which encloses the whole ear, rather than resting on the auricle as is the case with TDH-49 headphones. The advantage of TDH-50P circumaural headphones is that they provide greater attenuation of ambient room noise. Thus they permit screening in locations that would otherwise be unsuitable and this is the case for both adult and child ears (Wright & Frank, 1992). The disadvantages of TDH-50P circumaural headphones are that they are heavier, can be more difficult to position correctly, especially on small heads, they may contribute to test-retest variability in higher frequencies and may be less comfortable for the client than the standard TDH-49 headphone. If TDH-50P headphones are considered, it should be remembered that they are not a substitute for an adequately quiet screening test environment. There are insert earphones available that provide excellent noise reduction (Wright & Frank, 1992), but these are more appropriate to diagnostic testing than screening for various reasons, including the expertise needed to use them, calibration issues and the cost of the disposable eartips.

Every audiometer used should be calibrated fully to the appropriate standards (ANSI S 3.6 1969 (ANSI, 1970), IEC 645 1979 (IEC, 1979), Australian Standard AS 2583 1986 (Standards Association of Australia, 1983)) at least annually, and be subject to electroacoustic checks of SPL output at least every 3 months. Additionally, subjective listening checks should be carried out by the speech-language therapist at the beginning of any pure tone screening test or session. This comprises a quick self-hearing test to check if the tones are audible at the expected levels, if each earphone is functioning, that there are no potentially distracting equipment noises such as dial clicks, that the headphone fit is stable and that there is no intermittency of function (see Wilber, 1985, pp.122–124 for more detailed discussion). Modern audiometers may be much less prone to these problems than their predecessors, but it is wise nevertheless to perform this check routinely. Access to a technician for calibration and repairs is vital. Under no circumstances should an audiometer be used if it is not *known* to be in calibration. Generally equipment suppliers can advise on calibration.

An alternative to a standard pure tone audiometer is the audioscope™. This is a hand-held instrument that combines a pure tone generator and an otoscope. It is a true screening device in that the user selects a screening level (20 dB HTL, 25 dB HTL or 40 dB HTL) and the unit automatically presents a sequence of pure tones (1000 Hz, 2000 Hz, 4000 Hz and 500 Hz) at that level when the start button is pressed. The three screening levels available reflect the recommendations of ASHA (1985), Schow, Smedley and Longhurst (1990) and Weinstein and Ventry

(1983), respectively. The instrument does not allow the user to present tones at intensities other than at the selected level(s) and thus is entirely appropriate for screening. The audioscope comes with a clearly written instruction book and a range of audiospec tips to enable appropriate positioning in the ear canal. The instrument is battery-operated and is stored in a recharger unit when not in use. Calibration arrangements should be made with the supplier. The audioscope is very accurate when used with adult clients (Frank & Petersen, 1987). With children, the audioscope may have less than satisfactory specificity (Gershal et al., 1985), although the current model contains features that have the potential to improve specificity levels. The maximum permissible ambient noise levels for conducting audioscope screening are 55 dB A (20 dB HTL screen) and 60 dB A (25 dB HTL and 40 dB HTL screens). The most recent audioscope (Model 23300 Audioscope 3) complies, where appropriate to the instrument, with the ANSI S3.6-1969 Standard for Audiometers (ANSI, 1970) and the IEC 645-1979 Standard for Audiometers (IEC, 1979).

### Screening levels and frequencies

The choice of screening level depends on the aim of the exercise. If the goal is to detect all hearing losses with the potential to interfere with development and/or maintenance of normal spoken communication then 20 dB HTL is an appropriate screening level (ASHA, 1985). If the aim is to detect moderate and severe hearing losses, but not mild losses, then an appropriate screening level might be 40 dB HTL (Weinstein, 1986). A two-level protocol (e.g. 20 dB HTL stimulus followed by 40 dB HTL) might be useful in some situations. The important thing is to decide on the screening level (i.e. the pass/fail fence) before conducting screening tests, and to be clear why that level was chosen. A good discussion of various pass/fail fences and suitable applications is given by Schow (1991).

Clinical decision-making around the choice of screening level involves answering the questions. (a) Who are the target individuals to detect? (b) Is it desirable to have a single protocol that is applied to all clients or a set of different protocols that may be selected for use with individual clients? (c) Is a single screening level appropriate or should I employ a multi-level screening protocol? (d) Can I act on the information yield of the test? (e) What are the environmental constraints on choice of screening level?

Although less of an issue, as multifrequency screening is almost universally accepted, the choice of screening frequencies in pure tone testing depends on answering similar questions: (a) Do I have a need for especially rapid testing with large numbers of clients, and therefore a need to limit the number of test frequencies? (b) Do I have a particular interest in detecting low-frequency or high-frequency hearing loss? (c) Is the perception of particular frequencies likely to be affected by ambient noise in the test situation? Examples of the application of various screening levels and frequencies are shown in Table 5.1. Further examples of protocols are given by ASHA (1990c).

**Table 5.1:** Examples of the application of various pure tone hearing screening levels and frequencies and the rationale for their use in different settings

---

**Speech-language therapist A**

*Client population:* entirely paediatric; most cases presenting with language development/delay; also a small specialist list of clients with cleft palate.
*Clinical environment:* one of a team of four part-time clinicians; purpose-designed treatment rooms with ambient noise below 40 dBA SPL for at least 4 hours daily; access to audiologist with 5-week wait for appointments; access to otolaryngological outpatient clinic with 3-week wait for appointments but urgent cases seen within 1 week.
*Goal of hearing screening:* detection of developmentally significant hearing loss and of intermittent and/or fluctuating conductive loss.
*Screening level and rationale:* 20 dB HTL. For this client population it is important to detect all cases in which hearing problems may contribute to the development of speech and language. Even very mild and/or intermittent hearing problems may be of significance. While there could be value in using a more sensitive screen, especially for cleft palate clients, the risk of ambient room noise invalidating response during tests at certain times of the day means that 20 dB HTL is the lowest practicable level. Therapy room set-up can be modified easily to accommodate treatment of children with questionable hearing during the wait for further investigation. Repeat screening can be carried out during weekly therapy sessions and yield a useful profile for information of audiologist and otologist. Repeat screening may reduce number of children eventually referred. A single level protocol simplifies communication among the various part-time clinicians on staff.
*Screening frequencies and rationale:* for all clients 1000 Hz, 2000 Hz and 4000 Hz (ASHA recommendation) in that order and then, subject to an ambient noise check on each occasion, 500 Hz. If a child cooperates only with responses to the first stimulus (1000 Hz) useful information about speech reception is nevertheless gained as that frequency is mid-range for English speech. Cooperation for the 1000 Hz, 2000 Hz and 4000 Hz test tones yields information about the ability to perceive both voiced and unvoiced speech sounds. If cooperation is maintained, 500 Hz is included because of the goal of detecting conductive losses, which are common in children and often effect low frequencies. The same protocol used for all clients simplifies communication among the various part-time clinicians on staff.

*Note:* for cleft palate clients and clients failing pure screening, tympanometry, including auroscopic inspection, will also be employed (see later discussion).

(contd)

**Table 5.1:** (contd)

**Speech-language therapist B**

*Client population:* residential care clients; almost all over 70 years of age; many clients have low vision and a diagnosis of dementia. Most clients have very low income.

*Clinical environment:* sole part-time speech-language therapist; no purpose-designed therapy rooms; access to day room with ambient noise of 45 dB A SPL in early morning and late afternoon and much greater levels during the rest of the day; access to quiet room with ambient noise at 35 dB A except during lunch preparation; private audiologist will visit by arrangement within 1 week; government hearing-aid audiologist will visit if client cannot be transported to the hearing-aid centre, with a 6-week wait for visits to the home.

*Goal of hearing screening:* (a) to identify clients with severe or profound hearing loss who may benefit from assistive listening device and/or hearing aid-amplification; (b) to develop a profile of clients' hearing status to assist nursing staff in their communication with residents; (c) to assist in the differential diagnosis of communication problems.

*Screening level and rationale:* for all clients 40 dB HTL, 60 dB HTL and 90 dB HTL in a multi-level screening protocol involving higher-level presentation only in the case of non-response to the preceding screen level. Ambient noise does not allow for the reliable use of lower levels. Test sensitivity will be compromised with the 40 dB HTL level, but until available resources improve, the benefit of identifying persons with hearing loss less than 40 dB, who are otherwise asymptomatic, is questionable given the need to give high priority to referrals for hearing-aid assessment. The multi-level approach, in conjunction with other clinical information, assists the development of guidelines for communication with individual clients. Clients with identified loss who are evidencing symptoms of receptive aphasia, and clients who exhibit the apparently greater levels of hearing loss, will be given first priority in referral for audiological evaluation. Pending the results of those evaluations speech-language assessments and treatment can be modified to allow for the presumed general level of hearing sensitivity loss in each case. Clients who pass the 40 dB HTL screen but whose hearing is of concern to themselves, their families or nursing staff will be given second priority in referral for audiological evaluation.

*Screening frequencies and rationale:* for all clients 1000 Hz and 2000 Hz only. These frequencies are mid-range for speech perception of English. Clients with significant hearing loss are likely to fail screening at one or both of these frequencies. Given the multi-level approach the number of frequencies needs to be limited in order not to tax clients' ability to cooperate during screening testing. Subsequent audiological evaluation will address hearing for a greater range of frequencies. Further, because of likely age-related physical changes to the auricle in these clients, ear canal collapse and other problems the validity of screening at 4000 Hz may be compromised. Ambient noise may compromise screening at 500 Hz.

*Note:* auroscopic inspection will be carried out for all clients (see later discussion).

## A suggested protocol

Notwithstanding the need to make decisions around hearing screening in individual clinical environments, the following protocol is offered as one that is likely to be appropriate to the needs of many speech-language therapists. It is stressed that this protocol is intended for use with individuals who consult speech-language therapists and is not necessarily suitable for mass hearing screening in all situations. The pure tone levels and frequencies are those recommended by the ASHA for persons up to the age of 40 years (ASHA, 1985, 1990c). The practical arrangements, such as seating, are those recommended by Osborn and Doyle (1983). The advice about hygiene is based on papers by ASHA (ASHA, 1990d) and McMillan and Willette (1988). The suggestions about instructions, client response and reinforcement are those which this author has found clinically effective over many years. Some of the suggestions are simple common clinical sense, but are worth mentioning nevertheless. The protocol assumes that matters of calibration, ambient noise, subjective equipment checks, referral mechanisms and outcome evaluation have been addressed and that pre-screening observations and questions have been carried out.

### 1. Set up room and equipment to maximise test validity and client cooperation

If working alone with the client, and using a pure tone audiometer with headphones, seat the client so that he or she is facing away from mirrors or other reflective surfaces and at an angle between about 90° relative to your own position. Position the audiometer so that the client cannot see any of the controls. This arrangement reduces the chance of the client responding to visual cues, yet gives a sense of being in touch, as you are within the client's peripheral vision. If you are working with a colleague, the client may be positioned directly opposite your position, either side-on or with their back to you, providing that they cannot see you or your equipment reflected in clinic room mirrors or windows. This arrangement frees you from worry about visual cues. Your colleague is seated facing the client and can take the role of providing instructions, and reinforcement. Your colleague can also act as a second judge of client responses. Working with a colleague is especially useful when the client is a young child or has difficulty concentrating on the task. If working alone and it is absolutely necessary to face the client to ensure cooperation, set up a small screen around the audiometer and keep your hand and arm movements to a minimum. If you wear spectacles be sure that audiometer tone indicator lights are not reflected in the lenses. If you are using an audioscope rather than an audiometer, the risk of giving visual cues is virtually non-existent.

### 2. Ensure that clinical hygiene is satisfactory

Wash your hands for 30–60 s with an appropriate soap or solution before and after all physical contact with the client. Dry your hands on paper towel or under an air dryer. Particular clinical facilities may require different and/or additional procedures for infection control.

### 3. Explain the procedure and instruct the client

A simple explanation of the purpose and scope of the test is useful as it informs the client and/or their caregiver as to what they will experience, and helps them to appreciate the meaning of the subsequent findings. Face the client when speaking. A suitable form of words is: 'This test will indicate whether or not your/your child's hearing is in the normal range. If it does not seem to be within the normal range we will arrange for further tests. I will present some simple sounds through these headphones/this audioscope and I want you to (name response) each time you hear a sound, even if the sound is very faint.' Demonstrate a pure tone and a response (this cannot be done when using an audioscope). Do this by placing the headphones on the table or holding them in your hands, about half a metre away from the ears, and producing a 1000 Hz or 2000 Hz tone at the 90 dB HTL setting on the audiometer dial, simultaneously raising your arm, tapping on the table or making some other simple and visually obvious action known to be within the clients repertoire (never introduce 90 dB HTL as a conditioning tone with headphones over the clients ears). Ask the client if they understand. If client understanding is not apparent, reinstruct.

### 4. Position the transducer correctly

If using an audiometer, ask the client to remove spectacles, earrings and anything they may be chewing. Ensure that the client's hair is behind their auricles whenever possible. Place the headphones so that the earphone is directly over the opening of the external auditory meatus. Check that the right (red) headphone is on the right ear. Adjust the headband to ensure this position is maintained. If using an audioscope, ask the client to remove anything they may be chewing. Select an audiospec appropriate to the size of the external auditory meatus. A snug fit is essential to test validity. Position the audioscope so that a clear view of the external auditory meatus and tympanic membrane is obtained.

### 5. Present a cue tone and check client response

If using an audiometer, present a cue tone of 40 dB HTL at 1000 Hz to the right ear and/or the suspected better ear, and check for client response. If the response is clear, proceed to deliver test tones as described in step 6. If there is no response, remove headphones and reinstruct. If there is again no response to the 40 dB HTL cue tone, present a cue tone of 60 dB HTL. If there is still no response in either ear, and the equipment is found to be functioning normally, abort the test and refer for further assessment. When using an audioscope a cue tone is automatically delivered at 40 dB HTL if the 20 dB HTL screen level is selected and the start button is pressed. If there is no response to the cue tone, remove the audioscope and reinstruct. If there is still no response to the cue tone after reinstruction, and the positioning of the audioscope in the external auditory meatus appears correct, simply note if there are responses to any of the subsequent test tones and use these to inform your referral.

### 6. Present the test tones and note client responses

Present the test tones immediately following a clear response to the cue tone, as follows: right (or better) ear 20 dB HTL at 1000 Hz, 20 dB HTL at 2000 Hz and 20 dB HTL at 4000 Hz, then left (or poorer ear) 20 dB HTL at 4000 Hz, 20 dB HTL at 2000 Hz and 20 dB HTL at 1000 Hz. Thus the test begins and ends with a 1000 Hz tone. For each tone note the presence or absence of client response and record the result. If the client fails to respond to any one or more of the six test tones they have failed the screen.

### 7. Rescreen clients who fail the screening.

Carry out a repeat screen on clients who fail the test, preferably on the same day, and no later than two weeks after initial screening. This will reduce the chances of false positive identification due to problems with instructions, equipment or client cooperation (Wilson & Walton, 1974).

### 8. Make the pass/fail screening decision

If the client has responded to all six test tones at either first test or rescreening on the same day they have passed the screen. If the client has not responded to each of the six test tones after rescreening they have failed the test, are identified as having a probable hearing loss and need referral.

### 9. Obtain levels of first response (this cannot be done with an audioscope)

For clients who have been identified by the screen, it is useful to obtain a level of first response (LFR) at each frequency where the client did not respond at 20 dB HTL. This is done by increasing the intensity in 5 dB steps until the client responds and noting that level (e.g. 55 dB HTL). This LFR should not be confused with hearing threshold (see the discussion of pure tone audiometry in Chapter 4). LFRs are obtained because they are useful to personnel subsequently assessing the client, and they inform the speech-language therapist as to a likely general level of hearing loss. However, LFRs are not used in counselling the client or in reaching the pass/fail decision as this is taken prior to the establishment of LFRs.

## Recording results

Record-keeping is a reflection of the quality of care given to clients (ASHA, 1994a). Increasingly, proper record-keeping is considered important, not only for reasons of quality assurance and professional standards (Paul-Brown, 1994), but also as one practical aspect of professional risk management (ASHA, 1994a). The results of pure tone screening are best recorded on a purpose-designed form, which indicates what test tones were used, the date of the test, whether rescreening was conducted and other relevant data, such as the client's opinion of their hearing. One possible model for such a form is shown in Figure 5.1. The provision of separate boxes for screening responses and LFRs in this example is to underline the fact that the pass/fail decision is made on the basis of responses to screening levels and not on LFRs.

Pure tone hearing screening record

| | | | |
|---|---|---|---|
| Client name: | | Age: | Date of test: |
| Client rates hearing as: | Excellent | Good Fair | Poor |
| Initial screening/rescreening (circle one): | | | |
| Cue tone 40 dB HTL 1000 Hz | Response | Yes | No |

Test tones

| | | | |
|---|---|---|---|
| Right ear | 1000 Hz | 2000 Hz | 4000 Hz |
| Test tones | 20 dB HTL | 20 dB HTL | 20 dB HTL |
| | Response Yes No | Response Yes No | Response Yes No |
| Left ear | 1000 Hz | 2000 Hz | 4000 Hz |
| Test tones | 20 dB HTL | 20 dB HTL | 20 dB HTL |
| | Response Yes No | Response Yes No | Response Yes No |

| | | |
|---|---|---|
| Screening test result | Pass | Fail |

Levels of first response if fail result

| | | | |
|---|---|---|---|
| Right ear | 1000 Hz | 2000 Hz | 4000 Hz |
| | 20 dB HTL (screen) | 20 dB HTL (screen) | 20 dB HTL (screen) |
| | dB HTL | dB HTL | dB HTL |
| Left ear | 1000 Hz | 2000 Hz | 4000 Hz |
| | 20 dB HTL (screen) | 20 dB HTL (screen) | 20 dB HTL (screen) |
| | dB HTL | dB HTL | dB HTL |

Screening test conducted by: _____ signature

Speech-language therapist

**Figure 5.1:** Sample pure tone screening record.

It is inappropriate to record screening results on an audiogram as audiograms are records of threshold assessment (see Chapters 4 and 6). Potential confusion can easily result if, for example, the client responds to a 20 dB HTL screening tone and this level is entered on the audiogram. The audiogram would then indicate that the client's threshold for that tone is 20 dB HTL when in fact the threshold could be 20 dB HTL, 15 dB HTL, 10 dB HTL, 5 dB HTL, 0 dB HTL, –5 dB HTL or even –10 dB HTL. Screening tests need screening forms. In particular clinical situations it might be useful to have the screening form incorporated into a general client profile form. A system of self-carbon sheets, or a computerised record might be useful. In any case, some way of retaining a record of screening test performance in a form that is clear and can be forwarded to subsequent professionals and/or retained by the client, is necessary.

### Frequency of screening

As part of a thorough communication assessment, all individual clients of the speech-language therapist require hearing screening if hearing status is not already known. Usually a pass on a single screening test (i.e. a negative screening test result) is sufficient to exclude significant hearing problems, although rescreening is recommended if there is evidence the client is not progressing as expected and/or at any expression of client, parent or teacher concern about hearing. Additionally, rescreening is recommended as part of annual progress reviews. The necessity for rescreening individuals identified by initial screening to reduce the number of false-positive identifications has already been mentioned. It is also wise to rescreen periodically if the client has shown evidence of chronic or fluctuating hearing problems, even if the client's hearing is under the management of another health professional (see example in Table 5.3).

### Common procedural problems and suggested solutions [1]

One of the most difficult problems encountered in screening is ambiguous responding by the client. Sometimes clients give responses which, because they are delayed or somehow 'half-hearted' or indecisive with regard to the requested response, are ambiguous. For example, the client asked to raise a hand when they hear a tone may offer a few arm movements that sometimes appear temporally related to the test tones and sometimes not. The tester simply doesn't know if the response is genuine. The possible reasons for these ambiguous responses include: poor instructions or modelling of the response by the tester, guessing by

[1] I wish to acknowledge the contribution of Judith Swanwick, who wrote a set of clinical teaching notes on which this and the corresponding tympanometry section are largely based.

the client, lack of understanding by the client, tinnitus or physical inability to produce the response. Although these sorts of response behaviour can be informative in some ways (see Green, 1978, for a classic description of some responses) they are an unacceptable basis on which to make the pass/fail screening decision. The remedy is to stop the test, remove headphones, reinstruct with modelling and have the client demonstrate the response. In the case of the hand-raising response, the hand should be returned to the client's lap or the table top immediately after each response, a large movement involving the whole arm, if necessary, should be encouraged and the client should receive positive reinforcement for rapid responses. Other problems that can be encountered are listed in Table 5.2, along with some possible solutions. Some of these problems would normally be detected during the pre-test subjective listening check, but they are included here nevertheless. The most important thing to remember is that the tester must arrive firmly at a pass or fail decision based on clear client responses. If this is not possible, refer for audiological assessment.

**Table 5.2:** Some problems and solutions in pure tone screening

| Problem | Possible causes | Solutions |
| --- | --- | --- |
| Ambiguous responses | 1. Poor instructions or response modelling | 1. Remove headphones, reinstruct with modelling. Have client demonstrate response to tones in free field before replacing headphones |
| | 2. Response not within client repertoire | 2. Change response, ensuring that fatigue will not compromise response clarity |
| | 3. Response continuing beyond stimulus | 3. Ask client to return hand to desktop/release button after each tone heard |
| | 4. Delay between stimulus and response | 4 Emphasise need to respond immediately. If working with a colleague have them 'race' the child client to a response. If the client is unable to respond quickly, ensure that the intervals between tone presentation are much greater than the client's response latency |
| | 5. Equipment problems | 5. Redo subjective test. If necessary use different audiometer/audioscope |

(contd)

**Table 5.2**: (contd)

| Problem | Possible causes | Solutions |
|---|---|---|
| No response at all | 1. Significant levels of hearing loss | 1. Present cue tone at greater intensity if this is in your protocol. If still no response then assign a fail decision and attempt to establish at least one level of first response. It can be distressing for the client if they have heard no tones at all during the test |
| | 2. Lack of cooperation from client | 2. Reinstruct, indicating that your previous instructions may not have been clear. Check that client can perform response to tones before resuming test |
| | 3. Audiometer or electrical supply problems | 3. Redo subjective test. If necessary use different audiometer/audioscope or power point |
| | 4. Audioscope not positioned correctly | 4. Check that best fitting audiospec is used. Check that a view of the external auditory meatus and tympanic membrane is obtained before recommencing test |
| | 5. Response not within client repertoire | 5. Change response, ensuring that fatigue will not compromise response |
| False positive responses (client responds when no tone has been presented) | 1. Client may have tinnitus | 1. Increase cue tone and check that client can respond reliably to this before decreasing to test levels. If the audiometer allows use pulsed rather than continuous pure tones. If tinnitus is limited to one ear, test the other ear first to condition the client to the stimulus |
| | 2. Audiometer has been set so that the tone is continuously on. When the tester 'presents' a tone they are in fact briefly switching the tone off | 2. Visually check audiometer settings. Redo subjective listening check. Reinstruct client |

(contd)

**Table 5.2:** (contd)

| Problem | Possible causes | Solutions |
|---|---|---|
| | 3. Client is anxious to pass the test, leading to frequent guessing | 3. Revert to cue tone and present several tones to establish a better response pattern. Reinforce client, then again present test tones |
| | 4. Clicks or other noises in audiometer dials to which the client is responding | 4. As a temporary measure only, reinstruct and condition the client to the cue tone, then vary the interval between dial movement associated with clicks and the test tone presentation |
| Poor headphone fit | 1. Headset band defective, resulting in earphones slipping | 1. As a temporary measure only, wrap rubber band or similar around headphone spike above the level of attachment to headset band |
| | 2. Failure to remove client earrings, spectacles | 2. Remove headphones, remove earrings, spectacles and start test again |
| | 3. Headset too large for the client's head | 3. Place pad of foam on top of client's head under the headset band |
| Intermittent ambient noise | 1. Unexpected noise external to the room | 1. Present test tones during periods of quiet, first explaining to the client that you are aware of the noise and are working around it. If, however, client fails to respond normally rescreen in a quiet situation before making the pass/fail decision |
| | 2. Inadequate test location and/or timing | 2. Move and/or reschedule testing |
| Colleague's reinforcement of client sometimes inappropriate | 1. Colleague's reinforcement too frequent | 1. Have a quiet word and/or refocus the colleague onto judging speed of client responses |
| | 2. Colleague's reinforcement not related to client responses | 2. Give colleague a visual signal (e.g. a raised finger) when each test tone is presented, ensuring that this cannot be seen by the client and that the colleague uses only peripheral vision to receive the signal |

Problem (contd)

**Table 5.2:** (contd)

|  | Possible causes | Solutions |
|---|---|---|
|  | 3. Colleague looks to the client or gives some other cue each time the tester presents a tone | 3. Have a quiet word with colleague to change behaviour. Check client responses to tones already presented |
|  | 4. Tester's visual signals to colleague are intermittent or not temporally related to test tone presentation | 4. Start again if necessary, perhaps changing signal to one which is easier to manage |
| Lack of cooperation from child clients | 1. Anxiety about the test | 1. Model the test and responses with colleague or parent, ensuring that the child can hear some tones, and that the experience looks like fun. Use a response mode likely to appeal to the child. If still unsuccessful reinforce for any degree of cooperation (e.g. sitting at the test table) and reschedule screening |
|  | 2. Language problems | 2. Model as above |
|  | 3. Significant hearing loss, so that the client cannot understand instructions or hear cue tones | 3. Test the other ear. If still no cooperation, remodel the test using louder tones in free field |
|  | 4. Child is distracted by an interesting toy or complex process used as a response mode | 4. Simplify the response mode, ensuring that the tester or colleague, and not the child, controls the availability of the blocks or other toys used |

## Interpreting the results

The results of pure tone screening can be interpreted alone or in combination with the results of screening tests for middle-ear function. As a stand-alone test, pure tone screening indicates: (a) whether the client's ability to detect sound is or is not within normal functional limits, (b) if the left and/or the right ear is involved in any apparent loss, and (c) what frequencies are likely to be involved in any loss. This information is communicated to the client, along with recommendations for further assessment as indicated by the particular clinical protocol. When explaining to the client that a possible hearing loss has been detected it is best not to use the word 'fail', as it may alarm clients and caregivers and upset some children.

The LFR information can indicate to the speech-language therapist the level of loss that appears to have been excluded (for example, LFRs in the 50–60 dB HTL range exclude a profound hearing loss but do not exclude mild, moderate or severe loss). The frequencies involved can indicate to the speech-language therapist if the loss is likely to involve a sensorineural component (for example, a client who responds at 1000 Hz and 2000 Hz but not 4000 Hz has a response pattern consistent with high-frequency sensorineural loss). The pattern of test results can indicate to the speech-language therapist what measures might be necessary to optimise communication in the interval between identification and subsequent audiological and/or medical assessment (for example the need to reduce the distance between speaker and listener or the need to alert classroom teachers that the child client is under suspicion of a hearing loss). Informational counselling of the client, however, should be based only on the response to the screening tones and not on LFR information. This is because (a) the LFRs are not thresholds (although they may match or closely approximate thresholds subsequently obtained in diagnostic testing), (b) the overinterpretation of responses to air-conducted sounds in absence of bone conduction information can lead to false conclusions, (c) there is, despite all care, a very small chance that the test was invalid, and (d) counselling beyond the screen-level response data invites client questions about possible causes of the apparent hearing loss. Answers to such questions must await confirmation of screening results and the further information available from diagnostic assessments. Indeed, the ASHA specifically advises that ASHA member speech-language therapists limit judgements and descriptive statements about the results of hearing screening to whether the test result was negative or positive (ASHA, 1992).

## Example of application in schoolage children

Children referred to the speech-language therapist because of concerns about speech or language development possibly provide the most widely applicable example of the need to conduct screening. Table 5.3 shows the profile of such a child. The principal features of this example are that repeated screening was necessary, that the screening test procedure was incorporated into therapy sessions as a fun start exercise, that the results allowed the speech-language therapist to maximise therapy and that the child was referred for medical management of what had been a chronic, yet previously undetected, problem.

## Example of application in adults

The example chosen to illustrate the application of hearing screening in adults is that of a person without obvious hearing problems, who has consulted the speech-language therapist because of a long-standing stutter (Table 5.4). Hearing screening in this case was conducted as a routine part of clinical assessment. The identification of an apparent high-frequency loss allowed counselling about hearing conservation and assisted in the planning of family support in an intensive fluency programme.

**Table 5.3:** Example of screening a child client

*Presenting issue*

Parental concern about language and behaviour. Child is 5 years of age and appears to be developing much more slowly than did older siblings. Occasional tantrums and aggression towards other children. Sits very close to television

*Initial assessment*

Detailed history and observation. Mouth-breathing observed. Reported to snore when he has a cold. Hearing screening yielded the following result:

| Cue tone 40 dB HTL 1000 Hz | Response | (Yes) | No |
|---|---|---|---|
| Test tones | | | |

| Right ear Test tones | 1000 Hz 20 dB HTL Response Yes (No) | 2000 Hz 20 dB HTL Response (Yes) No | 4000 Hz 20 dB HTL Response Yes (No) |
|---|---|---|---|
| Left ear Test tones | 1000 Hz 20 dB HTL Response (Yes) No | 2000 Hz 20 dB HTL Response (Yes) No | 4000 Hz 20 dB HTL Response (Yes) No |

| Screening test result | | Pass | (Fail) |
|---|---|---|---|

Levels of first response if fail result

| Right ear | 1000 Hz 20 dB HTL (screen) 25 dB HTL | 2000 Hz (20) dB HTL (screen) dB HTL | 4000 Hz 20 dB HTL (screen) 30 dB HTL |
|---|---|---|---|
| Left ear | 1000 Hz (20) dB HTL (screen) dB HTL | 2000 Hz (20) dB HTL (screen) dB HTL | 4000 Hz (20) dB HTL (screen) dB HTL |

Further questioning indicated the child had had a series of colds every winter and has always had a tendency to mouth-breathe. There has been no known earache in the last 18 months, but he suffered several ear infections before the age of 3 years. Mother is unsure about his hearing

*Action*

Rescreen confirmed screening result. Referral to family physician for medical assessment of ears. No middle-ear infection was apparent on medical examination, but large tonsils and poor nasal airway were noted. Speech-language therapist decided to monitor hearing during weekly visits for continued speech-language assessment

(contd)

**Table 5.3:** (contd)

and therapy. The following profile was obtained over a 5-week period:

| Occasion # 1: | | 1000 Hz | 2000 Hz | 4000 Hz |
|---|---|---|---|---|
| 20 dB HTL screen | Right | X (40) | ✓ | X (30) |
| (LFRs dB HTL) | Left | ✓ | ✓ | ✓ |

| Occasion # 2: | | 1000 Hz | 2000 Hz | 4000 Hz |
|---|---|---|---|---|
| 20 dB HTL screen | Right | X (25) | ✓ | ✓ |
| (LFRs dB HTL) | Left | ✓ | ✓ | ✓ |

| Occasion # 3: | | 1000 Hz | 2000 Hz | 4000 Hz |
|---|---|---|---|---|
| 20 dB HTL screen | Right | ✓ | ✓ | ✓ |
| (LFRs dB HTL) | Left | X (25) | ✓ | ✓ |

| Occasion # 4: | | 1000 Hz | 2000 Hz | 4000 Hz |
|---|---|---|---|---|
| 20 dB HTL screen | Right | X (40) | X (25) | X (30) |
| (LFRs dB HTL) | Left | X (30) | ✓ | X (25) |

| Occasion # 5: | | 1000 Hz | 2000 Hz | 4000 Hz |
|---|---|---|---|---|
| 20 dB HTL screen | Right | X (30) | ✓ | X (25) |
| (LFRs dB HTL) | Left | ✓ | ✓ | ✓ |

Given evidence of chronic mild hearing loss the client was referred to hospital Ear Nose and Throat clinic for assessment. This revealed fluid in the right middle ear and a significantly retracted left tympanic membrane due to Eustachian tube dysfunction Enlarged tonsils and adenoids were noted. Parents are considering surgery to improve middle ear ventilation. Speech-language therapist ensures therapy sessions are conducted with minimal speaker listener distance and has advised parents on tactics to optimise child's' speech reception at home

---

**Table 5.4:** Example of screening of an adult client

*Presenting issue*
Long-standing stutter, particularly with new work contacts. Client is most concerned about telephone conversations. No other communication problems reported

*Initial assessment*
Detailed history, observation, fluency rate. Voice, language and social skills all NAD.

Recent changes in work situation have caused client to seek help. Promoted from manufacturing plant of whitegoods company to their wholesale sales team. Associated stress because of greatly increased verbal communication. Routine hearing screening yielded the following result:

| Cue tone 40 dB HTL 1000 Hz | Response | (Yes) | No |
|---|---|---|---|
| Test tones | | | |

| Right ear | 1000 Hz | 2000 Hz | 4000 Hz |
|---|---|---|---|
| Test tones | 20 dB HTL | 20 dB HTL | 20 dB HTL |
| | Response (Yes) No | Response (Yes) No | Response Yes (No) |

(contd)

**Table 5.4:** (contd)

| Left ear<br>Test tones | 1000 Hz<br>20 dB HTL<br>Response (Yes) No | 2000 Hz<br>20 dB HTL<br>Response Yes (No) | 4000 Hz<br>20 dB HTL<br>Response Yes (No) |
|---|---|---|---|
| Screening test result | | Pass | (Fail) |
| Levels of first response if fail result | | | |

| Right ear | 1000 Hz<br>(20) dB HTL (screen)<br>dB HTL | 2000 Hz<br>(20) dB HTL (screen)<br>dB HTL | 4000 Hz<br>20 dB HTL (screen)<br>40 dB HTL |
|---|---|---|---|
| Left ear | 1000 Hz<br>(20) dB HTL (screen)<br>dB HTL | 2000 Hz<br>20 dB HTL (screen)<br>25 dB HTL | 4000 Hz<br>20 dB HTL (screen)<br>45 dB HTL |

Further questioning indicated a significant history of noise exposure and occasional difficulty hearing at large family gatherings and other social situations. No apparent difficulties hearing in quiet situations and/or in one to one conversations

*Action*
Rescreen confirmed screening result. Non-urgent referral to hospital audiologist for full audiogram and counselling about ear protection and further action. Speech-language therapist notes the consistency between client history of noise exposure and an apparent high frequency hearing loss in both ears. Assessment of client ability to hear work-related information over telephone reveals occasional problems with names and numbers due to apparent mishearing of voiceless consonants. Advised to discuss possibility of amplified telephone with audiologist, since anxiety about telephone fluency might be reduced by better telephone hearing. Spouse undertakes to practice telephone work with client, noting any apparent misperceptions of telephone speech. Otherwise intensive fluency programme will be conducted as usual.

# Tympanometry screening for middle-ear dysfunction

As noted in Chapter 4, the diagnostic assessment of middle-ear function involves three components: tympanometry (a dynamic measure of tympanic membrane mobility as a function of air pressure variations in the ear canal), static admittance/compliance of the ear (a measure of the resting immittance of the middle ear, which can be deduced from the tympanogram or by separate measurement depending on instrumentation) and the acoustic reflex (a dynamic measure of the integrity of the reflex arc, mediated at brainstem level, which involves stapedial muscle contraction). The first of these measures may be used easily as a screening tool and can yield information that is particularly useful for the speech-language therapist whose clients include people known to be at risk for middle-ear dysfunction. Recommended screening protocols for detecting middle-ear disorders have often included an acoustic reflex test (McCandles & Thomas, 1974; ASHA, 1979). However, this can result in unacceptably high detection rates ( Roush & Tait, 1985; Doyle & Oakes, 1993) and in the opinion of this author is susceptible to tester error, especially when non-automatic equipment is used. Some screening protocols have employed acoustic reflex testing to detect hearing losses. There are unacceptable risks of missing sensorineural losses if acoustic reflexes are used as a hearing screen (see for example, Bennett & Mowat, 1981), and this is another reason why reflex testing in screening applications is losing favour (Margolis, 1993).

## Why tympanometry?

Tympanometry is recommended as a screening tool for middle-ear function for the following reasons:

1. It is an objective procedure that does not require more than passive cooperation from the client. Although the client can offer useful observations about their experience of tympanometry, interpretation of the test is done purely from the machine dials and/or readout.
2. Tympanometry can detect the presence of abnormal middle-ear function in the absence of obvious symptoms. Clients with changes in the mobility and stiffness of the middle-ear system, such as occur with ossicular chain fixation, for example, often will not have otological symptoms other than hearing loss. Tympanometry has the potential to identify clients with such middle-ear disorders. Further, middle-ear effusion and significant negative middle-ear pressure can exist without a noticeable hearing loss. Therefore middle-ear problems in individuals who pass pure tone screening may be identified with tympanometry.

3. The overall sensitivity and specificity of tympanometry for detection of middle-ear fluid is likely to be around 90 per cent and 77–94 per cent respectively when the validators are otoscopy and myringotomy (Brooks, 1982), although the sensitivity and specificity rate depends on which particular aspects of the tympanogram are used to make the pass/fail decision (Nozza et al., 1992).

4. Tympanometry can assist in referral decisions if the results are used in combination with pure tone screening results. If a client fails both pure tone and tympanometry screening, then they are likely to have a conductive cause for at least part of their hearing loss and medical referral is indicated as a first step. If tympanometry appears to be normal and the client has been identified by pure tone screening, then a sensorineural loss is more likely. Audiological referral may be a more appropriate first referral in this case.

5. There is some evidence that some children who are referred for speech and language therapy have a greater incidence/prevalence of middle-ear problems than that in the non-referred population (Pollard & Tan, 1993; Monley, 1994; Schilder et al., 1994). Children with cleft palate or Down's syndrome are especially at risk (Schwartz & Schwartz, 1978; Hubbard et al., 1985). Additionally, children with sensorineural hearing loss requiring assistance for speech and language development can ill afford the extra handicap of undetected conductive loss as it may compromise the effectiveness of hearing-aid use, add confusion and frustration to the child's existing difficulties and, if associated with feeling unwell, reduce time in school and therapy.

6. The result of tympanometry screening is excellent information for audiologists, otologists, paediatricians, audiological physicians and others to whom the client may be referred.

7. Instrumentation for tympanometry is rapidly becoming more user-friendly and economically accessible. For example, automatic tympanometers are now commonly available. There are also various miniature tympanometers available, which helps with portability. A further development is a hand-held 'reflectometer', which assesses middle ear-function (Teele & Teele, 1984). The development of this device is analogous to the development of the audioscope for pure tone screening. The technical process is only slightly different from that which occurs during traditional tympanometry. Haggard and Hughes (1991) provide a review of the effectiveness of the reflectometer and of various versions of miniature tympanometers. They conclude that these instruments have potential as screening tools, but that further examination of their specificity and sensitivity is required. The point is that the size and cost of instruments to assess middle-ear function by tympanometry or very similar techniques is likely to continue to fall, making the devices more accessible to speech-language therapists.

8. The alternative method of otoscopy requires considerable training, is subject to large variations in judgement (Roeser et al., 1977) and hence detection rates, and it is less sensitive to some forms of middle-ear dysfunction, such as otosclerosis (Ginsberg & White, 1985).
9. With appropriate tester expertise the test is rapid. As with pure tone screening, it is possible to explain the procedure to the client, conduct tympanometry on each ear and record the result, all within 5 min.
10. The test may be conducted in situations where ambient noise excludes pure tone audiometry.

## Room and equipment requirements

Tympanometry may be carried out in almost any reasonably quiet room, as very low levels of ambient noise are not required, although the British Society of Audiology recommends that the ambient room noise be less than 50 dB A SPL if possible (BSA, 1992). The range of equipment available is considerable. A tympanometer that complies with ANSI S 3.39-1987 (ANSI, 1987) and IEC 1027 (IEC, 1991) measures acoustic admittance in either cubic centimetres ($cm^3$) or acoustic millimhos (mmho) and employs a 226 Hz probe tone is suitable. Automatic tympanometers have advantages over manual instruments as the former usually have the start sequence linked to an adequate seal and additionally may have a visual display that positions the result in relation to a 'normal result' area. Provided the 'normal result' area is consistent with the pass/fail criteria applicable to the particular clinical situation, this feature is very useful. An auroscope/otoscope is required for inspection of the external auditory meatus. Inspection via an audioscope can be an adequate alternative. A range of probe tips in different sizes is necessary. Disinfecting fluid (e.g. Sidex™, Amphel™ or Hibitane™) is necessary for cleaning probe tips. A solution of 1:10 household bleach in water is another option. ASHA also recommends the use of gloves during middle-ear testing (ASHA, 1990d). For further detailed advice regarding hygiene in test rooms see McMillan and Willette (1988)

## Available protocols

The choice of screening protocol is important because the pass/fail criteria, and thus detection rates, can vary greatly among protocols. For example, in the protocol recommended by ASHA (1990c), the pass/fail and referral criteria are based on static admittance (which is an objective measure of the height of the tympanogram peak) and tympanogram width. The British Society of Audiology recommended procedure for tympanometry (BSA, 1992), which is not directed specifically to screening applications, recommends using middle-ear pressure and admittance as indicators when interpreting tympanograms. There is no universally agreed notion as to what constitutes strictly normal values on tympanograms other than that normal middle-ear pressure is on average zero daPa/mm $H_2O$ (as discussed in Chapter 4). Normal admittance values depend on whether or not the tympanometer automatically compensates for ear-canal volume, but a mean of 0.7 $cm^3$/mmho is commonly reported. When choosing a protocol for screening with tympanometry, the speech-language therapist is strongly advised to consult their local professional association, which may have particular recommendations, and also the current clinical literature, as normative data will continue to emerge. Additionally, it may be useful to match pass/fail criteria to those used in any local public health screening programmes, provided that the criteria are not too insensitive. The protocol described in the following section is one that may be suitable to the needs of most speech-language therapists, but it is stressed that the suitability of this or any other protocol must be carefully considered in light of the particular clinical needs of the individual speech-language therapist.

### A recommended protocol

The following protocol is based in part on the ASHA guidelines for screening (ASHA, 1990c), but it retains the use of middle-ear pressure as a pass/fail criterion. The protocol is designed to be used as a companion to, or follow-on from, pure tone screening. It is not a substitute for pure tone screening. The recommendations for repeated testing in the event of detection on initial screening are seen as very necessary for clients, especially children, who do not have any obvious symptoms of middle-ear problems and who have passed pure tone screening. For clients who have other indications of aural dysfunction referral should not be delayed.

The protocol assumes that calibration and subjective equipment checks have been carried out, that referral mechanisms and outcome evaluation methods have been decided, and that pure tone screening has been conducted if the client has not otherwise had his or her hearing assessed. The background terminology, and procedures relating to tympanometry in general, are given in Chapter 4.

1. Set up the room and equipment to ensure satisfactory hygiene and client co-operation. Wash your hands and follow other hygiene protocols as appropriate.
2. Explain the test and instruct the client. It is important that the client understands that they need to be silent and still during the procedure, and that a secure fit of the probe tip in the ear canal is necessary for a valid test.

3. Inspect the pinna visually and the external auditory canal with an otoscope to determine the size and angle of the lateral portion, and to check for any contraindications to tympanometry. Contraindications include discharge from the ear, wax occlusion, tenderness of the ear, foreign bodies and obvious perforation or inflammation of the tympanic membrane (ASHA, 1990c; BSA, 1992). (Complete wax occlusion of the external auditory meatus is a contraindication to tympanometry because of the likelihood of a false result due to wax entering the probe assembly, and because of the possibility of pushing the wax further into the ear. It is, however, possible to carry out tympanometry with some wax present in the canal. If it is possible to visualise part of the tympanic membrane beyond the wax, it is usually safe to proceed with testing.) These conditions mean the client requires medical referral. Sometimes visual inspection will reveal a middle-ear ventilation tube ('grommet', 'drainage tube', 'Shepherd's tube', 'Shah tube' or other). As this indicates that the client has been under the care of a specialist ear surgeon, tympanometry need not proceed. It is important, however, to discover if the client has a medical review scheduled. If the client with ventilation tube(s) has failed pure tone screening, then referral for a current medical assessment is recommended. *Caution: Never insert a probe tip without first completing an otoscopic inspection.*

4. Select an appropriate sized probe tip. Many tips are coloured-coded and, with experience, the tester will be able to judge that a particular ear is probably a 'size green' or a 'size blue'. The common semi-rigid plastic probe tips are suitable for most clients, but foam plugs or inflatable plugs may be necessary in some cases. Be careful to place the tip firmly on the probe assembly so that it does not dislodge during later removal of the assembly from the ear.

5. Ask the client to open their mouth, and gently pull the pinna upwards and backwards. These actions will straighten the lateral, cartilaginous portion of the external auditory canal and make insertion easier. If using an automatic tympanometer, gently place the tip at the opening of the meatus. For manual tympanometers, gently but firmly insert the plug into the meatus with a twisting motion and then release the pinna. The plug should be visible at the plane of the concha but not protruding from it.

6. If using an automatic tympanometer, the instrument will indicate whether or not an airtight seal has been obtained. It will then begin the procedure either automatically or when the start button is pressed. If using a manual tympanometer, check that the manometer is still reading zero (daPa/mm H$_2$O) and, if not, use the pressure release control to release any pressure that may have been introduced during probe insertion. Introduce +200 daPa/mm H$_2$O and check that this pressure is maintained. If there is a leak present the

manometer dial will return to zero. When a seal has been obtained, gradually take pressure from $+200$ daPa/mm $H_2O$, through 0 daPa/mm $H_2O$ down to $-200$ daPa/mm $H_2O$, watching the compliance and manometer dials to observe the peak compliance and the air pressure at which that peak occurred. If the tympanometer does not have a display or printout it will be necessary to plot compliance values at 50 daPa/mm $H_2O$ intervals. If no peak is evident by $-200$ daPa/mm $H_2O$ continue to decrease pressure to $-400$ daPa/mm $H_2O$. The pressure is not reduced further because of the risk of discomfort for the client. The rate of pressure change during manual tympanometry should be gradual (the British Society of Audiology recommends about 50 daPa/mm $H_2O$/s. Automatic tympanometers generally will have faster rates). At the completion of the pressure change sweep, the following information should be available: (a) air pressure at which peak admittance/compliance occurred if a peak was discernible, (b) the value of maximum admittance/compliance at the peak, and (c) the width of the tympanogram (the pressure interval equal to a 50 per cent reduction in peak compliance).

7. Return the pressure to zero, then gently lift the pinna upwards and backwards and remove the probe tip with a twisting movement.

8. Make the pass/fail decision with reference to the suggested values in Table 5.5. Note that the suggested values for middle-ear pressure at peak compliance will pass some clients whose tympanogram may fall out of the 'normal' range suggested on some equipment, as this is a screening, rather than a diagnostic, protocol. It may be useful to make templates to which the results of individual clients can be compared (see ASHA, 1990c, for examples of width templates). The static admittance/compliance criteria are appropriate for tympanometers with a $+200$ ear-canal volume correction. If the client has values outside these ranges on one or more of these measures, then the test is positive. If the tympanometer available advises slightly different normal range values for static admittance/compliance then use those different values as they pertain to the instrument. That is, for admittance/compliance make the pass/fail decision with reference to the 'normal' area on the automatic tympanometer display, or the 'normal' areas shown on recording charts or printouts. However, for middle-ear pressure the 'normal' area shown will usually be around $\pm 50$ daPa/mm $H_2O$, which is too sensitive for screening, hence the values suggested here, which can be applied to any tympanometer.

9. If the client has also been identified by pure tone screening, and/or has symptoms of aural dysfunction, refer for audiological and/or medical opinion. If the client has no other indications of aural dysfunction, repeat tympanometry at two-weekly intervals. If the test result is positive on two successive occasions, refer for medical opinion.

**Table 5.5:** Suggested pass/fail values for screening with tympanometry

| Middle-ear pressure at peak admittance/compliance | Static admittance/compliance | Width of tympanogram |
|---|---|---|
| +50 to −150 daPa/mm H$_2$O | 0.2 to 0.9 cm$^3$/mm H$_2$O children | 60–150 daPa/mm H$_2$O children |
| | 0.3 to 1.4 cm$^3$/H$_2$O adults | 50–110 daPa/mm H$_2$O adults |

10. Inform the client of the test result, taking care not to interpret beyond the available data. A suitable form of words is: (a) for persons passing the screen: 'The test has not detected a middle-ear problem'; (b) for persons failing the screen for the first time in the absence of other evidence of aural dysfunction: 'The test shows the possibility of a middle-ear problem. If we get the same result on repeat testing in two weeks, we will recommend a medical opinion'; and (c) for persons failing the screen and who have other evidence of aural dysfunction: 'The test shows the possibility of a middle-ear problem. As you also have (cite other evidence) I recommend a medical/audio-logical (as appropriate) opinion'.

11. Keep appropriate records, ensuring that the date(s) of tympanometry screening are recorded.

**Interpreting the results**

Several cautions apply to the results of tympanometry screening. These are:

1. The results should be crossed-checked against other available information such as pure tone screening results and client history.
2. Tympanometry is not a hearing test. A normal tympanometric result does not exclude a hearing loss (although it effectively excludes otitis media and many forms of conductive loss).
3. Tympanometry is a very sensitive tool. In otherwise asymptomatic cases it is wise therefore to defer referral until rescreening has confirmed an apparently abnormal result over a period of some weeks, as recommended in the suggested protocol.

The pass/fail decision and informational counselling of the client are based on whether or not the tympanogram trace falls within the criterion limits. The speech therapist may note that the tympanogram appears flat (and is consistent therefore with the possibility of middle-ear fluid, adhesions or advanced otosclerosis, for example) or indicates negative middle-ear pressure (and is consistent therefore with Eustachian tube dysfunction and/or some degree of otitis media). These observations, however, are not used in advising the client as the diagnosis of the cause of apparent middle-ear system changes requires further specialist examination, and since there is a very small possibility that the tympanogram is invalid.

### Common procedural problems and suggested solutions

Table 5.6 lists some common problems that can be encountered in tympanometry screening. Some of these are less likely to occur when using automatic instruments. The incidence of each problem situation can be kept to a minimum with appropriate training in the technique. Performing tympanometry on oneself is a useful way of gaining confidence and expertise, of understanding what the client experiences during the test and of carrying out equipment checks.

## Evaluation of screening procedures

If screening procedures are conducted on large groups, such as, for example, the population of 5-year-old children entering school in a particular region, then evaluation is important not only from the perspective of test accuracy and cost-benefit, but also as a means of informing policy development for health and education authorities. Haggard and Hughes (1991) have provided possibly the best available review of the issues involved in screening young children's hearing, although their discussion of personnel and tester training has most relevance for the UK. Roeser and Northern (1981) have provided a good discussion of the issues involved in screening the hearing of schoolage children. Large-scale screening of adults is relatively rare, and is often part of wider aims associated with community education, the education of health professionals, research or the need to comply with workplace health and safety regulations. The evaluation of such programmes for adults has received little attention (ASHA, 1992). Richardson (1992) has provided a treatment of cost-utility analysis in health care which interested readers may find useful if they are engaged in large-scale adult screening. Turner (1991) gives examples of calculations of the relative costs in hearing screening programmes. The focus in the present discussion of evaluation is on the screening of individual clients who consult speech-therapists. The principal issues discussed are test sensitivity and specificity, follow-up of client outcomes and effectiveness vs efficiency of screening.

**Table 5.6**: Some problems and solutions in tympanometry screening

| Problem | Possible causes | Solutions |
|---|---|---|
| No seal | 1. Air leakage in system | 1. Check for leaks by occluding probe assembly tip with thumb and introducing positive air pressure (this cannot be done with automatic tympanometers). If leakage is evident check all tubing for cracks or pinholes. If the leak is near attachment to headset trim tubing back slightly and refit |
| | 2. Tip size too small | 2. Re-examine the external auditory meatus (eam) to check size and direction of lateral portion. Choose largest tip that is compatible with characteristics of the eam. |
| | 3. Tip too large, initial seal is lost as tip eases itself out of the eam. | 3. As above |
| | 4. No match of available tips and size or shape of client eam. | 4. Smear vaseline around edges of tip closest to desired size. Use a foam tip or an inflatable tip if available |
| | 5. Tympanic membrane perforation | 5. If there is a perforation and a normal Eustachian tube it may be possible to maintain a seal with negative pressure but not positive |
| Inconsistency of results with client history and/or pure tone screening results. For example, apparent failure on tympanometry with no discernible peak (type B trace consistent with middle-ear effusion) and yet client has passed pure tone screening | 1. False tympanometry result due to poor placement of probe tip and/or wax occlusion | 1. Check probe assembly for occlusion and clear with wax prick. Repeat auroscopic inspection carefully to determine angle of the eam and reinsert tip |
| | 2. Tympanic membrane perforation with blocked Eustachian tube | 2. Repeat auroscopic inspection carefully. Redo both tympanometry and pure tone screening tests. If inconsistency remains note on referral |

(contd)

**Table 5.6:** (contd)

| Problem | Possible causes | Solutions |
|---|---|---|
| | 3. Equipment problems | 3. Do a self-test to determine adequacy of equipment. Use alternative tympanometer if available |
| Erratic movement of admittance/compliance dial (on manual tympanometers) | 1. Client speaking and/or moving head during test | 1. Remove headset and reinstruct explaining the need for passive cooperation. If client is very anxious, place hand on his or her arm or shoulder during tympanometry, providing that is culturally acceptable to the client and to you. With child clients have a colleague assist |
| | 2. Client crying | 2. Model the test on yourself or a parent indicating that it is quite a fun thing to do |
| | 3. Client chewing gum | 3. Offer client a tissue and ask them to remove the gum |
| | 4. Client heart beat | 4. Find client's wrist pulse and note if it corresponds to dial movements. If so attempt tympanogram but if result is uninterpretable consider referral |
| | 5. Client breathing (occurs with patent Eustachian tube) | 5. Ask client to hold breath momentarily and note if dial movements cease. If so, ask client to hold breath while tympanometry is carried out |
| Poor headphone fit (does not apply to many newer models of tympanometers) | 1. Headset band defective, resulting in earphones slipping | 1. As a temporary measure only, wrap rubber band or similar around headphone spike above the level of attachment to headset band |
| | 2. Failure to remove client earrings, spectacles | 2. Remove headphones, remove earrings, spectacles and start test again |
| | 3. Headset too large for the client's head | 3. Place pad of foam on top of client's head under the headset band |

(contd)

**Table 5.6:** (contd)

| Problem | Possible causes | Solutions |
|---|---|---|
| Lack of cooperation from child clients | 1. Anxiety about the test | 1. Reinstruct and model the test on yourself or a parent indicating that it is quite a fun thing to do. If child remains uncooperative discontinue |
| | 2. Language problems | 2. As above |
| | 3. Hyperactivity | 3. As above |

## Test sensitivity and specificity

A measure of the usefulness of a test is how it performs with regard to the trade-off between sensitivity (the ability to identify accurately individuals with hearing and/or middle-ear problems) and specificity (the ability to identify accurately individuals who do not have hearing and/or middle-ear problems). Sensitivity and specificity are expressed as percentages, sensitivity as the percentage of valid positive test results (or the number of true positive identifications as a proportion of all persons screened who in fact have the problem) and specificity as the percentage of valid negative test results (or the number of true negative identifications as a proportion of all persons screened who in fact do not have a problem). Related concepts are positive predictive value of the test (sometimes termed the predictive validity of a positive screening test), indicated by the number of true positive identifications as a proportion of all positive identifications; and negative predictive value (sometimes termed the predictive value of a negative screening test), which is indicated by the number of true negative identifications as a proportion of all negative identifications. The overall accuracy or validity of a screening test is the sum of all correct positive and all correct negative identifications as a proportion of the total number of persons screened. Positive and negative predictive values and overall accuracy are also expressed as percentages. In combination, the values of the test attributes so far described constitute the operating characteristics of a screening test.

To establish test sensitivity and specificity it is necessary to have tested a sample of clients with both a screening and a diagnostic or 'gold standard' test (which must of course have a very high degree of accuracy). The diagnostic test must be performed on clients who pass, as well as clients who fail, the screen. This is particularly important if using a pass/fail criterion not previously assessed and/or when applying a test that may have been previously evaluated, to clients who have characteristics significantly different to those persons on whom the test was previously evaluated. An example of test evaluation is given in Table 5.7, which also shows the formulae for sensitivity, specificity, positive predictive value and negative predictive value. In this example, the screening test is more accurate in detecting persons with normal hearing than detecting persons with hearing loss. This might occur if, for example, the screen level employed was 35 dB HTL rather than 20 dB HTL. This may or may not be acceptable depending on the particular clinical situation. In general, however, greater sensitivity would be desired. Other and very readable examples of test evaluation are provided by Bess and Humes (1990).

It should be noted that in general the sensitivity of tympanometry screening tests is high and this has led to concerns about possible over-referrals (Rousch & Tait, 1985), especially when tympanometry is combined with acoustic reflex screening in children (Doyle & Oakes, 1993). The specificity of tympanometric screening has been found to be variable, but this is in part due to the nature of the diagnostic standard assessment used. One problem in assessing the accuracy of tympanometry in detecting middle-ear effusions, for example, is that tympanometry results have been judged against otoscopy in many studies, when in fact to judge otoscopy against tympanometry might be more appropriate (Haggard & Hughes, 1991) .

**Table 5.7:** Example of the evaluation of the operating characteristics of a hearing screening test. Numbers in brackets indicate numbers of clients

| | Diagnostic standard result (i.e. hearing loss actually present) | | |
| --- | --- | --- | --- |
| | Yes | No | Totals |
| Screening test | | | |
| Positive (fail) | A (32) | B (5) | A + B (37) |
| Negative (pass) | C (12) | D (50) | C + D (62) |
| Totals | A+C (44) | B+D (55) | A+B+C+D (99) |

Sensitivity = A/(A+C) = 32/44 =.7273 $\times$ 100 = 72. 73%
Specificity = D/(B+D) = 50/55 = .9090 $\times$ 100 = 90.9%
Positive predictive value = A/(A+B) = 32/37 = .8649 $\times$ 100 = 86.49%
Negative predictive value = D/(C+D) = 50/62 = .8045 $\times$ 100 = 80.45%
Overall accuracy = (A+D)/(A+B+C+D) = 82/99 = .8283 $\times$ 100 = 82.83%

## Follow-up of client outcomes

Once a client has been identified as having a probable hearing and/or a middle-ear problem, and this likelihood has been confirmed by rescreening, referral and other clinical decisions are made. One of those decisions should be to determine the nature and timing of follow-up to assess client outcome (if that decision has not been taken, as recommended, prior to screening). For example, it may be decided to make phone contact with the client 6 weeks after referral and/or to request a report from the agency to which the client was referred. The benefits of identification to the effectiveness of therapy might be measured by changes in the client's speech reception ability. Parental reports of subsequent specialist assessment or treatment might be valuable. In any case, it should not be assumed that all clients will participate in recommended actions subsequent to screening, or that further assessment or treatment occurs in a timely and satisfactory manner (Doyle & Healey, 1981; Bess & Humes, 1990; Schow, 1991). If it is not practicable to check the outcomes of screening for all clients in at least some of these ways, it should certainly be possible to have a clinic protocol that involves checking a random sample of clients screened so that a profile of representative outcomes is derived. Note that it is necessary to have decided beforehand what constitutes a satisfactory outcome.

## Effectiveness and efficiency

The particular methods chosen to evaluate screening tests and programmes will depend in part on the orientation of the evaluator. Speech-language therapists and other evaluators will be concerned to varying degrees with the efficiency and effectiveness of screening procedures. Efficiency is essentially the ratio of the work done (e.g. the number of clients screened) to the energy supplied (e.g. the number of speech therapist hours). Effectiveness is the degree to which the action (e.g. using audioscope screening) achieves the intended result (e.g. identification of persons whose communication skills may be compromised by a hearing loss). These issues will be especially important if there are large investments of staff time, equipment and other resources given to screening (as in a community hearing awareness week), but they have relevance also to the situation where speech-language therapists screen hearing and/or middle-ear function as part of their contact with individual clients. Given the current pressures on health services it seems wise for individual speech-language therapists to address the efficiency issue. Measures such as: the time taken to perform procedures; the cost of equipment and staff per client screened; and the information yield in relation to time taken to perform tests may be relevant. Effectiveness data may be gathered by client follow-up procedures as already discussed. Test specificity and sensitivity data relate to both efficiency and effectiveness. In the view of this author, it is wise to evaluate screening procedures from the perspectives of administrators and clients, as well as from the perspective of the clinical practitioner.

# Public health initiatives in hearing screening

Given the importance of early identification of children with significant hearing loss, hearing screening is very much a public health issue (see, for example, Penn & Abbott, 1997). The National Institutes of Health has supported universal neonatal screening (NIH, 1993), and ASHA has stated that it is desirable for all infants with hearing loss to be identified before 3 months of age (ASHA, 1994b). There are now large-scale neonatal screening programmes in Europe (see Grandori & Lutman, 1996). Screening at school entry occurs across the population in the UK. At-risk newborns, such as those in intensive care or special care baby units (SCBU) are a particularly important group as the prevalence rates for significant hearing loss in SCBU babies are relatively high in comparison to the general population (see, for example, Praeger, Stone & Rose, 1987). Although mass screening of pre-school and schoolage children may employ a range of techniques (such as: Toy tests, see for example, Bellman, Mahon & Triggs, 1996; otoacoustic emissions (OAE), see, for example, McPherson & Smyth, 1997; and pure tone procedures, see for example, American Speech-Language-Hearing Association Ad Hoc Committee on Screening for Hearing-impairment, Handicap and Middle-ear Disorders, 1995), recent developments in screening newborns and infants in Australia, the UK and the USA have centred on OAE and ABR (see Chapter 4) techniques.

Although there are issues related to the age of testing (see, for example, Rowe, 1991) and the effect of middle-ear disorders on test results (see, for example, El-Refaie, Parker & Bamford, 1996), it appears that OAE and ABR are emerging as powerful tools for population screening. Hunter et al. (1994) provide an example of a combined approach using both procedures. Parving and Salomon (1996) have indicated that the application of OAEs can reduce the mean age of identification of significant hearing loss. ABR techniques are popular in Australia and the USA. To pursue this topic further, the interested speech-language therapist may first find it useful to refer to information provided by the American Speech-Language-Hearing Association Ad Hoc Committee on Screening for Hearing-impairment, Handicap and Middle-ear Disorders (1995).

# Summary of key points

The speech-language therapist has a responsibility to ensure that the hearing of clients referred for speech pathology is assessed. Screening involves the application of carefully designed procedures aimed at classifying persons into two groups: those with a probable hearing loss and/or middle-ear dysfunction, and those whose hearing and/or middle-ear function is likely to be normal. The decisions facing the individual speech-language therapist in a particular clinical situation include: the choice of hearing screening procedure, the nature of client referral and follow-up mechanisms, and the method of evaluating the screening test(s) used. Test sensitivity and specificity of screening procedures must be known or established with reference to a diagnostic standard. The screening tests recommended as being particularly useful for most speech-language therapists are a modified ASHA, three-frequency 20 dB HTL pure tone test for detecting hearing loss, and a tympanometry procedure for detecting middle-ear dysfunction, in which the pass/fail decision is taken with regard to middle-ear pressure at peak admittance/compliance, static admittance/compliance and tympanogram width. Rescreening is an important aspect of maintaining acceptable test validity and containing referral rates to manageable levels.

# Further reading

American Speech-Language-Hearing Association (1985) Guidelines for identification audiometry. Asha 27: 47–52. (Details recommended procedure and includes discussion of room requirements and other practical aspects of screening for hearing loss.)

American Speech-Language-Hearing Association Joint Committee on Infant Hearing Position Statement (1994) Asha 36: 38–41. (This includes a list of high-risk factors or indicators and discusses issues around identification of hearing loss in neonates and infants up to three years of age.)

American Speech-Language Hearing Association Ad Hoc Committee on Screening for Hearing Impairment, Handicap and Middle-ear Disorders (1995) American Journal of Audiology 4: 24–40. (Provides an overview of ASHA recommendations for screening various target groups, and summarises some general principals of screening.)

Haggard M, Hughes E (1991) Screening children's hearing: a review of the literature and the implications of otitis media. London: HMSO, Medical Research Council. (A comprehensive and readable book that addresses theory and practice of screening as well as policy issues with particular reference to the identification of middle-ear problems in children. Includes a chapter on possible cognitive, linguistic and educational sequelae of otitis media. Substantial literature reviews are provided.)

Schow RL (1991) Considerations in selecting and validating an adult/elderly hearing screening protocol. Ear & Hearing 12: 337–48. (A good discussion of the pros and cons of selecting various screen levels in pure tone audiometry, and of various methods of validating screening effectiveness in adults.)

Turner RG (1990) Recommended guidelines for infant hearing screening: Analysis. Asha 32: 57–61 & 66. (An evaluation of the effectiveness of ASHA recommended procedures. Relevant for readers interested in use of public resources and in detection rates.)

# Chapter 6
# Audiograms and their interpretation

JANET DOYLE

Audiograms are probably the single most widely available formal test record of an individual's hearing. This chapter describes various forms of audiograms and gives case examples and some guidance regarding audiogram interpretation. Relatively more emphasis is given to what audiograms indicate about the speech and language of the client than to site-of-lesion considerations. This chapter builds on the information about pure tone audiometry and pure tone audiograms given in Chapter 4. The symbols used are those recommended by the American Speech-Language-Hearing Association (ASHA) and are explained in Appendix B.

## Principles

1. *Audiograms are simple two-dimensional representations of hearing sensitivity*. An audiogram is a plot of the levels at which an individual can detect the presence of sound at each of several audio frequencies. Audiograms offer no indication of how the individual responds to the temporal information available in auditory signals.
2. *Audiograms can be understood*. Even the most apparently complex audiogram can be read using the symbol code provided and a simple four-step procedure, which is described in this chapter. The procedure involves considering the level of any hearing loss and the frequency range in which the loss is present, and then making judgements about the relationship of air-and bone-conduction hearing sensitivity in each ear.
3. *Most audiograms indicate the minimum, but not the maximum, potential for oral-aural communication*. Although there is a strong general association between the degree of hearing sensitivity loss shown on an audiogram and the ability to communicate via hearing and speech, individual clients can vary greatly in this regard, particularly when hearing loss is profound (>90 dB). Hence great care must

be taken not to make limiting assumptions about an individual's ability to use residual hearing.

4. *An individual client's audiogram can change*. A particular audiogram represents the result of a particular audiometric test on a particular date, and should not be assumed to remain a true long-term representation of that individual's ability to detect sound. Young children may have variable audiograms due to fluctuating middle-ear problems. Children with sensorineural hearing loss may also develop middle-ear problems, resulting in a poorer audiogram on some occasions. Alternatively, the child with profound sensorineural hearing loss may show apparently improved audiograms over time following intensive training in using audition (see Clezy, 1984, for examples). Hence a current audiogram, especially where the client is a child and/or is known to have variable hearing, is important for the speech-language therapist.

5. *While the majority of audiograms are valid, it is useful to check for accuracy*. This may be done easily by comparing the audiometric responses of the two ears and by considering the audiometric information in light of the client's observed speech perception abilities. Examples of accuracy checks are provided in this chapter.

6. *Audiograms can inform a range of clinical decisions to assist client communication and health*. The speech-language therapist can use audiograms to plan the set-up of therapy rooms for individual sessions, to help set therapy goals and to assist referral decisions.

## Overview of audiograms

Any pure tone audiogram is a chart with decibels (indicating the level of a sound) on the Y axis and audio frequency (in Hertz) on the X axis. There are two main types of audiograms. The first and most common is the dB HTL (hearing threshold level) audiogram, also known as dB HL (hearing level) audiogram. This was briefly described in Chapter 4. The dB HTL audiogram is a record of an individual's thresholds or hearing levels for the audio frequencies tested (usually 250 Hz, 500 Hz, 1000 Hz, 2000 Hz, 4000 Hz and 8000 Hz). For each frequency the symbol indicating the threshold is placed on or near the intersection of the vertical frequency line and the horizontal dB HTL line indicating the minimum level at which the individual can reliably detect the presence of tones of that frequency.

The reference level for dB HTL audiograms is normal hearing sensitivity. Clinical audiometers are calibrated so that when the dial is set to 0 dB HTL at any frequency, the level of sound produced by the audiometer is that level required if a typical normal hearer is to just detect the tone. Hence 0 dB HTL does not mean that no sound has been produced, but that the level of sound produced is the very small amount necessary for the average, young, otologically healthy human to perceive it monaurally through headphones (for example, approx 7 dB SPL (sound pressure level) at 1000 Hz). Bess and Humes (1990, p. 77) give a clear and brief description of how this works. Hence a response at 0 dB HTL, at any frequency, can be considered to indicate no hearing loss. All dB HTL audiograms are obtained by presenting the test tones through headphones or through insert earphones placed in the ear canal. All dB HTL audiograms, therefore, usually allow for separate data from each ear to be recorded. All dB HTL audiograms are records of unaided hearing levels (aided hearing tests are discussed later in this chapter).

On dB HTL audiograms, the dB scale is presented so that the lower intensities are shown at the top of the graph, and higher intensities are visually lower down the graph. This is potentially confusing, because with other measurements (for example, percentages) greater quantities are usually visually higher up the graph, and an individual's performance is considered better when higher scores are achieved. However, audiograms are essentially an indication of the degree to which the individual's hearing sensitivity is poorer than normal (although, as will be discussed later, the result can be considered in a positive light). Thus, the lower down the graph the thresholds are visually, the poorer the hearing sensitivity, even though the dB levels have increased. On a dB HTL audiogram an individual's performance is better if the thresholds occur at lower dB levels (which are visually higher on the graph).

The second main type of audiogram is the dB SPL audiogram. This was alluded to in Chapter 4 in the discussion of sound field audiometry. The dB SPL audiogram is also a record of an individual's thresholds for the audio frequencies tested (again usually 250 Hz, 500 Hz, 1000 Hz, 2000 Hz, 4000 Hz and 8000 Hz), but the decibel scale is not referenced to normal hearing. The Y axis is therefore in dB SPL. As with dB HTL audiograms, a symbol indicating the threshold is placed on or near the intersection of the vertical frequency line and the horizontal dB SPL line to indicate the level of sound at which that particular tone is just reliably detectable to the individual.

SPL audiograms are used when the signals are delivered in a sound field, usually via loudspeakers. The test stimuli are usually warble tones (tones in which the frequency varies slightly around the frequency of a pure tone), although the SPL audiogram chart shows the same frequency scale as for dB HTL audiograms as the warble variation is very slight. SPL audiograms may indicate unaided hearing sensitivity (as, for example, with the CORA sound field assessment described in Chapter 4), or aided hearing sensitivity (as, for example, with functional hearing aid assessments). Unaided SPL audiograms are best considered an indication of binaural hearing, as in a free field situation it is not usually possible to determine which of the two ears has responded to the test tones. Aided SPL audiograms can show separate aided responses from each ear, and can allow comparisons of various hearing aids in one ear. Current hearing-aid technology and fitting techniques mean that aided SPL audiograms are not nearly as common as they once were and alternate methods of recording aided results are being developed (see, for example, Hill et al., 1996), but they remain useful to the speech-language therapist who is treating children with hearing impairment.

The decibel scale on dB SPL audiograms is usually presented so that lower intensities are shown at the top end of the graph, as with dB HTL audiograms. That convention is used in this book. However, this is not universal practice, and research publications in particular may present the scale in the other direction.

Figure 6.1 illustrates dB HTL and dB SPL audiograms, and shows in each case a threshold for 1000 Hz consistent with normal hearing. Most of the audiograms discussed in this chapter will be dB HTL or dB SPL audiograms.

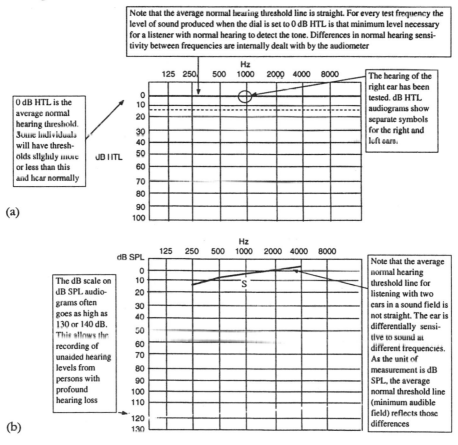

**Figure 6.1:** (a) A dB HTL audiogram with a normal threshold response recorded at 1000 Hz. The circle represents the right ear. (b) An SPL audiogram, also showing a normal response to 1000 Hz. The 'S' represents an individual's threshold when listening with both ears in a sound field, i.e. when the sound is presented via loudspeakers rather than through headphones. The 'S' symbol is not universally used.

Although it is technically possible to record the results of sound field audiometry on an HTL audiogram if a correction factor (e.g. Morgan, Dirks & Bower, 1979; Walker, Dillon & Byrne, 1984) is applied to convert the levels from dB SPL to dB HTL, this is not recommended because of possible confusion over reference levels for the dB scale. Notwithstanding the preceding comment, it is sometimes useful to have both unaided and aided results on a single graph. For example, the speech-language therapist may wish to know the amount of functional hearing aid gain to help decide whether it is necessary to reduce distance from the client or use louder-than-normal voice to enhance the client's perception of certain speech sounds during therapy. This information can be derived from a dB SPL audiogram that shows both unaided and aided responses in relation to the speech envelope for average conversational speech (see following section for a discussion of this 'speech area'). Some clinics routinely provide such audiograms. If the information is not otherwise available it may be derived by application of the minimal audible field (MAF) figures, if necessary. An example is shown in Figure 6.10 in the section on dB SPL audiograms.

## The 'speech area'

Many dB HTL and dB SPL audiograms show a shaded or outlined area designed to indicate the spectral area of conversational speech. The purpose of including this 'speech area' (also known as 'speech banana', 'spectral envelope' or, occasionally, 'speech audiogram', the last of these terms not to be confused with the speech audiogram in Chapter 4) is to allow the clinician to make a qualitative judgement about the extent to which an individual's thresholds indicate the ability to detect aspects of speech. An example of such a speech area is shown in Figure 6.2.

Although there are obvious benefits for the speech-language therapist in having such information, there are two main issues regarding speech areas on audiograms. These issues are now briefly addressed.

First, the speech area on an audiogram (which is an average spectral picture of speech imposed on a chart of response to frequency and intensity of pure tones) does not include temporal information. Hence although it may help to indicate particular phonemes difficult to perceive in the individual client's case, it is limited in regard to understanding how well the client processes running speech, especially perception of pitch. It is best thought of as 'a summary of the parts of "auditory space" involved in vowel contrasts and place/manner decisions' (Wright, 1987, p. 24.).

Second, there is no single, universally accepted speech area. The particular speech area shown on audiograms in one clinic may not exactly match that shown on audiograms from another clinic, although many clinics use the data provided by Fant (1973), Pascoe (1980) or Byrne (1977). This is because the spectral envelope differs depending on the speaker and the distance of the speaker from the microphone. Boothroyd, Erickson and Medwetsky (1994) have shown that there is substantial interspeaker variability in the speech envelope for English. The women in their study, for example, produced a higher frequency /s/ than the men, and had a stronger /m/ in relation to other speech sounds than did the male speakers. Additionally the average level of speech and the dynamic range of speech varied significantly among the speakers.

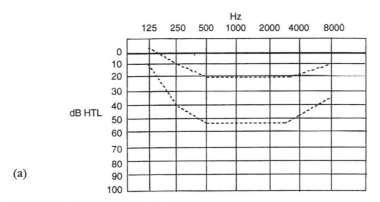

(a)

The dashed lines represent the upper and lower range of speech intensities in conversational speech (approx. 65 dB SPL) approximating the area proposed by Pascoe (1980). The speech area shown on audiograms can vary slightly between clinics because of differences in the experimental methods and subjects used to derive the reference data. The point here is that the speech area can assist in counselling clients and can be used to roughly gauge the impact of hearing loss on speech perception

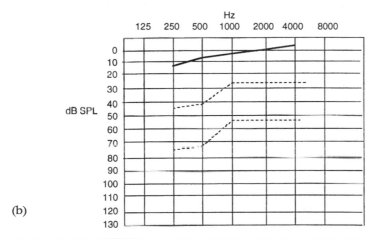

(b)

The dashed lines indicate the upper and lower ranges of speech intensities, in this case approximating the long term conversational speech spectra data proposed by Byrne (1977). The speech area shown on audiograms from various clinics can differ slightly because of the differences in experimental methods and subjects used to derive the reference data. The speech area on dB SPL audiograms has a different shape to that seen on dB HTL audiograms because of the different dB references used

**Figure 6.2:** (a) dB HTL and (b) SPL audiogram forms, showing the 'speech area'.

Despite these issues, it is generally agreed that the dynamic range for conversational speech is about 30–40 dB (Boothroyd, 1993; Pavlovic, 1993). The loudest parts of English speech (strong vowels such as /u/) are about 30–40 dB more intense than the softest parts of speech (e.g. weak consonants, such as /f/). The average intensity of conversational speech is very roughly around 65 dB SPL (which equates to about 45 dB on an HTL audiogram). Additionally, acoustic cues for the perception of intonation and nasals reside largely in low (<500 Hz) frequencies and those for vowels in middle (500–2000 Hz) frequencies, most often below 1000 Hz. The acoustic cues for consonants, particularly sibilants, fricatives and stops, reside largely in middle and high (>2000 Hz) frequencies, most often above 1000 Hz. Within these very basic and general guidelines, the audiogram can usefully inform the speech-language therapist of the likely speech perception abilities and/or potential of the client. Some examples are given later in this chapter. The interested reader is referred to Wright (1987) for a readable, but more detailed, treatment of the basic acoustic (and temporal) properties of speech.

## The articulation index (AI) audiogram

The articulation index or AI (Pavlovic, Studebaker & Sherbecoe, 1986; Pavlovic, 1988, 1989; Mueller & Killion, 1990; Humes, 1991) attempts to provide a quantitative measure of the speech-recognition difficulties experienced by persons with hearing loss. It is a development that has its base in the speech area described in the preceding section. The principal application of the AI has been in hearing-aid fitting, but the speech-language therapist may encounter the AI in some audiological reports. An AI audiogram is simply an HTL audiogram on which is shown some additional information.

The AI is reported as a figure ranging from 0 to 1.0, derived from consideration of the individual's pure tone thresholds in relation to the speech area on a HTL audiogram, which represents the proportion of conversational speech able to be perceived by the listener. An AI of 0.83 would indicate that the listener could perceive 83 per cent of the speech signal. A normal-hearing listener would have an AI of 1.0, indicating perception of 100 per cent of the speech signal. The AI does not indicate the type of errors that may be made. Humes (1991) reminds us that two individuals with the same AI might make very different types of errors in speech perception.

The more recent versions of the AI utilise a series of dots superimposed on the speech area of an HTL audiogram. For example, Humes (1991) proposed an AI audiogram in which each dot represents a 0.03 contribution to the maximum possible total AI score of 1.0. There are most dots at 2000 Hz and least at 250 Hz, reflecting the greater contribution of the former to the perception of spoken English. An AI is calculated by counting the dots above the thresholds on the audiogram, and multiplying that number by 0.03. Mueller and Killion (1990) proposed a version of the AI audiogram in which there are 100 dots, including dots at intermediate frequencies important to speech perception, and the AI is derived by simply counting the 'audible' dots in a given case. An example is given in Figure 6.3. Mueller and Killion have applied their simplified version to aspects of hearing-aid fitting.

# Reading dB HTL audiograms

## Symbols

The audiometric symbols recommended by ASHA, which were introduced in Chapter 4, are used in the audiogram examples given in this chapter. Helpfully, two symbols (O indicating air-conduction responses

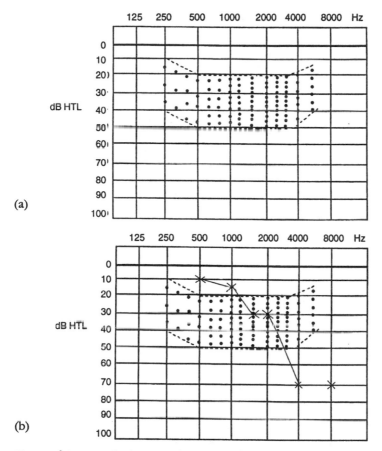

**Figure 6.3:** An articulation index (AI) audiogram, after Mueller and Killion (1990); (a) illustrates the 100 dots inside the speech area; (b) illustrates the relationship between an individual's unaided, left ear air-conduction hearing thresholds and the AI dots. Where the speech signal is above the client's threshold there are 60 dots, yielding an AI of 0.60.

of the right ear, and X indicating air-conduction responses of the left ear) are common to both the ASHA and BSA systems, which will help readers who may be exposed to both (see Appendix B).

### Audiograms obtained without masking.

In pure tone threshold audiometry, tones are presented initially by air conduction and each ear is assessed separately (see Chapter 4). If air-conduction thresholds indicate a hearing loss, bone-conduction audiometry is then carried out. For many clients this will complete the procedure, the application of masking (described in Chapter 4) being unnecessary. In such cases only two or three different symbols are used (right ear air conduction, left ear air conduction and, if necessary, a single bone-conduction symbol). Figure 6.4 illustrates two such audiograms.

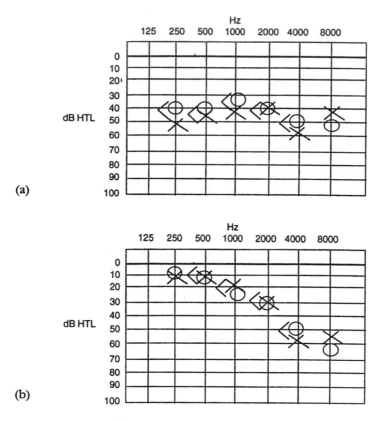

**Figure 6.4:** Two examples of unmasked dB HTL audiograms. (a) The application of masking in this case is unnecessary. There is minimal difference in the sensitivity of the two ears. Cross-hearing could not have occurred. This individual has a bilateral sensorineural loss. (b) The application of masking in this case is also unnecessary. There is minimal difference in the sensitivity of the two ears. Cross-hearing could not have occurred. This individual has a bilateral sensorineural loss in the frequency range 1000–8000 Hz.

**Audiograms obtained with masking**

In certain situations (see Chapter 4), most commonly when one ear has hearing levels much better than the other, it is necessary to apply masking to ensure a valid audiogram is derived. In these cases, the number of symbols used can reach seven (initial or unmasked air-conduction threshold of the right ear, unmasked air-conduction threshold of the left ear, masked or true air-conduction threshold of the right ear, masked response air-conduction threshold of the left ear, unmasked (initial) bone-conduction threshold, masked (true) bone-conduction threshold of the right ear and masked bone-conduction of the left ear). To read such audiograms, ignore the unmasked symbols and read the masked symbols. Figure 6.5 illustrates two audiograms which indicate that masking has been used.

# A four-step procedure for understanding dB HTL audiograms

1. *Divide the audiogram into quadrants*, so that quadrant 1 contains low frequencies and low intensities, quadrant 2 contains high frequencies and low intensities, quadrant 3 contains low frequencies and high intensities, and quadrant 4 contains high frequencies and high intensities. The audio frequency 1000 Hz forms the border between low and high frequencies. With hearing up to and including 1000 Hz we can generally expect perception of the suprasegmental aspects of speech and the first formant of all vowels. With hearing that extends beyond 1000 Hz spectral information is available to allow perception of many consonants. The dB HTL level of 50 dB HTL forms the border between low and high intensities. With hearing levels better than 50 dB HTL at least some parts of conversational speech are generally detectable at a distance of one metre. Hearing levels poorer than 50 dB HTL normally indicate significant difficulty detecting conversational speech in most situations. An audiogram divided into quadrants is shown in Figure 6.6.

2. *Consider which quadrant(s) the air conduction thresholds fall into.* This will indicate the general level of sound the client is able to receive unaided. There are six common 'quadrant patterns'. These are: (a) quadrants 1 and 2 (Q1–2); (b) quadrants 3 and 4 (Q3–4); (c) quadrants 1, 2 and 4, (Q1–2–4); (d) quadrants 1 and 4 (Q1–4); (e) quadrants 1, 3, 4 and 2 (Q1–3–4–2); and (f) quadrant 3 only (Q3). Any other patterns would be extremely unusual. Some examples of audiograms with these patterns are shown in Figure 6.7.

If all thresholds are in quadrants 1 and 2, hearing difficulty will be variable, depending on the listening situation, the speech habits of those persons with whom the individual commonly communicates

(contd)

This symbol indicates the unmasked response when the bone conductor is placed on the left mastoid. Because interaural attenuation for bone-conducted sounds is essentially 0 dB, the right cochlea (rather than the left) could be responsible for the response. It was necessary to occupy the right ear with masking and then again present bone-conducted tones to the left mastoid

This symbol, representing bone-conduction hearing of the left ear when masking is applied to the better right ear, indicates the true cochlear functioning of the left ear. With masking in the right ear responses from the left cochlea were obtained only when the tones were raised to the same level as air-conducted thresholds. This means that in the unmasked test situation, cross-hearing had been occurring

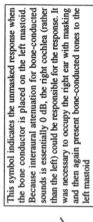
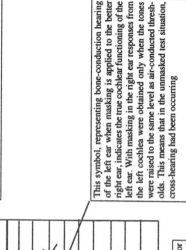

Hz

125  250  500  1000  2000  4000  8000

dB HTL

0
10
20
30
40
50
60
70
80
90
100

(a)

This audiogram is read by examining the symbols for air conduction (circles for right ear, crosses for left ear) and the masked symbol (bracket) for the bone conduction of the left ear. Bone conduction of the right ear is not shown because the right ear has normal hearing, and bone conduction cannot be poorer than air-conduction levels. This person has normal hearing in the right ear and a sensorineural loss in the left ear

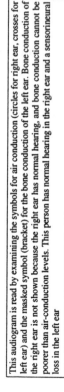

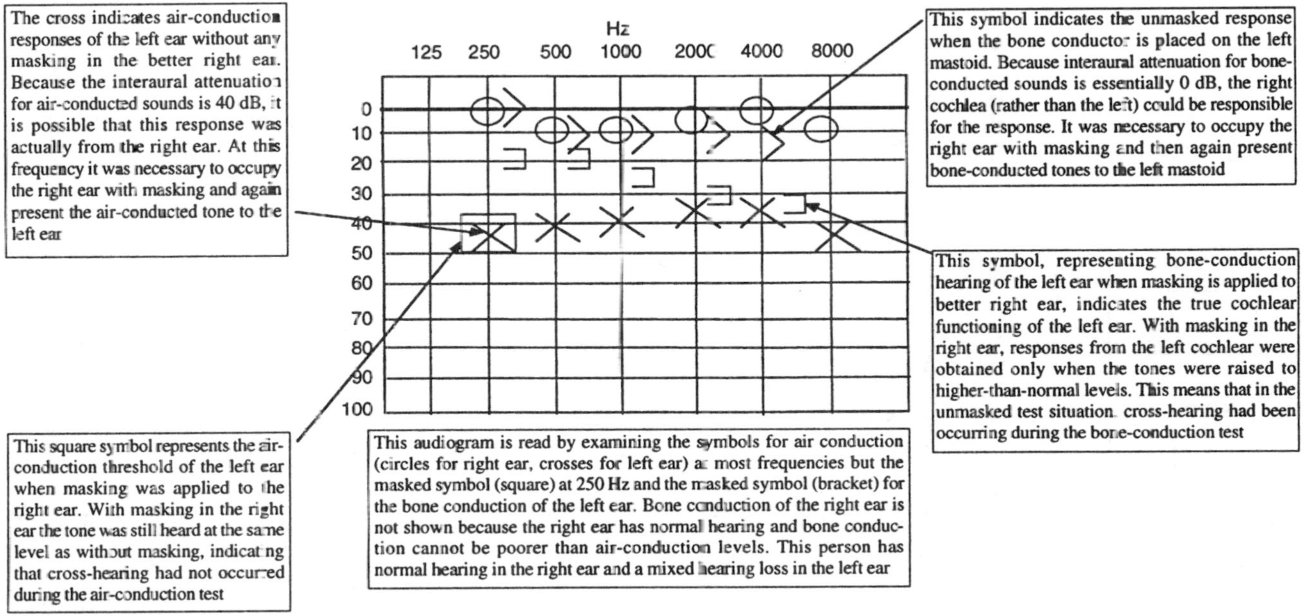
The cross indicates air-conduction responses of the left ear without any masking in the better right ear. Because the interaural attenuation for air-conducted sounds is 40 dB, it is possible that this response was actually from the right ear. At this frequency it was necessary to occupy the right ear with masking and again present the air-conducted tone to the left ear
Hz
125 250 500 1000 2000 4000 8000
0 10 20 30 40 50 60 70 80 90 100
This symbol indicates the unmasked response when the bone conductor is placed on the left mastoid. Because interaural attenuation for bone-conducted sounds is essentially 0 dB, the right cochlea (rather than the left) could be responsible for the response. It was necessary to occupy the right ear with masking and then again present bone-conducted tones to the left mastoid
This symbol, representing bone-conduction hearing of the left ear when masking is applied to better right ear, indicates the true cochlear functioning of the left ear. With masking in the right ear, responses from the left cochlear were obtained only when the tones were raised to higher-than-normal levels. This means that in the unmasked test situation cross-hearing had been occurring during the bone-conduction test
This square symbol represents the air-conduction threshold of the left ear when masking was applied to the right ear. With masking in the right ear the tone was still heard at the same level as without masking, indicating that cross-hearing had not occurred during the air-conduction test
This audiogram is read by examining the symbols for air conduction (circles for right ear, crosses for left ear) at most frequencies but the masked symbol (square) at 250 Hz and the masked symbol (bracket) for the bone conduction of the left ear. Bone conduction of the right ear is not shown because the right ear has normal hearing and bone conduction cannot be poorer than air-conduction levels. This person has normal hearing in the right ear and a mixed hearing loss in the left ear

(b)

**Figure 6.5:** Two examples of masked dB HTL audiograms.

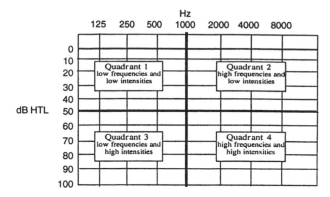

**Figure 6.6:** A dB HTL audiogram divided into quadrants.

and whether or not the loss is primarily sensorineural or conductive (see next step). If quadrant 2 thresholds approach the margin of quadrant 4 significant speech perception, difficulties may be experienced, especially in background noise. This is because quadrant 2 contains many acoustic cues for consonants important to the intelligibility of speech, and these cues are easily masked by background noise.

If the thresholds fall into quadrants 3 and/or 4, with no thresholds in quadrants 1 and/or 2, the client is unlikely to reliably perceive average intensity conversational speech via unaided audition. There is also likely to be some distortion in the signals that are received because the loss is most likely to be sensorineural (no purely conductive loss is greater than about 60 dB HTL), and because conversational partners may need to speak at much greater levels than normal, which can in turn distort normal speech patterns. Additionally, the client may not perceive warning signals, such as smoke alarms and vehicle sirens, and will usually not hear a normal telephone ring, even if in the same room.

If quadrants 1, 2 and 4 are involved, unaided hearing will usually be affected by background noise, some mishearing of consonants is likely and there may be difficulty hearing softly spoken individuals. Additionally, there may be slight difficulty perceiving some signals including the sound accompanying car indicators or wrist-watch alarms. However, in quiet listening situations, particularly if thresholds in quadrant 1 are near normal, communication may be relatively unaffected.

If thresholds are in quadrants 1 and 4, the client is likely to be able to hear much better in quiet than noisy situations, but in any case would, unless aided, have significant difficulties perceiving some English sounds important to speech perception. The impact of this on the particular individual will vary greatly, depending on the client's age and the speed of onset of loss, as well as the listening situation and the conversational habits of those with whom the individual interacts. Gradual-onset high-frequency losses are usually accommodated more easily than those of rapid onset, partly because the individual has time to adjust to augmenting audition with visual information. Fortunately, many phonemes for which acoustic cues lie in the high frequencies are also those speech elements that can be distinguished visually.

When thresholds intersect quadrants 1, 2, 3 and 4, as in the 'trough-shaped' or 'cookie bite' configuration seen in some congenital sensorineural losses, for example, the individual will usually have great difficulty perceiving and understanding speech if unaided, experiencing many of the problems encountered by the person with a Q3–4 pattern.

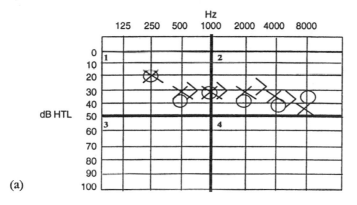

(a)

This person has a bilateral sensorineural hearing loss. The degree of difficulty in understanding speech and perceiving environmental sounds is easily influenced by attributes of the speaker and the listening situation. In quiet situations and with a good view of the speaker's face, there may be little or no difficulty. If the speaker turns away or converses from another room, hearing problems are evident. In noisy situations there may be persistent difficulty hearing speech clearly. This is because the sensorineural nature of the loss means clarity of the signal is compromised and the masking effect of background noise further reduces the ability to detect important speech sounds

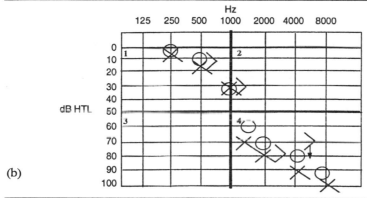

(b)

This person has a steeply sloping bilateral sensorineural hearing loss. The suprasegmental aspects of speech are easily perceived, and the first formants of vowels. However, the high frequency spectral information necessary to perceive many consonants is severely reduced in this unaided condition. Speech-reading may be of significant assistance (see Chapter 8). Ability to follow conversation will be very obviously much better in quiet situations. The impact of the loss will vary a great deal depending on the age and speed of onset of the loss, the communication abilities of conversational partners, the communication needs of the individual, and the availability of hearing aids and assistive listening devices

**Figure 6.7**: Examples of audiogram quadrant patterns: (a) illustrates a Q1–2 pattern; (b) illustrates a Q1–4 pattern.

Persons whose dB HTL audiogram displays a Q3 pattern (a 'corner' audiogram) always have sensorineural hearing loss, although they are not immune from experiencing conductive problems that will further reduce their hearing levels while the conductive loss is present. If thresholds lie only in quadrant 3 then they are likely to have very significant difficulties using audition as the primary means of speech perception, even when hearing-aid amplification or other technology is applied. However, readers should be aware that individuals with similar quadrant 3 thresholds may differ greatly in their ability to use sound. Erber and Alencewiciz (1976) have shown that among hearing-impaired children there is variation in the ability to perceive spectral information and speech envelope cues beyond what could be expected from inspection of pure tone thresholds alone. Additionally, the present discussion is about dB HTL audiograms, reflecting unaided hearing. Hearing-aid amplification or cochlear implants may very significantly augment the listener's ability to use audition for communication. Vibrotactile devices may also assist with environmental awareness and, to some extent, speech perception (see Bench, 1992a, pp. 49–54; and Chapter 7 of this book). The speech-language therapist who is treating a client with a Q3 audiogram is advised to assess speech-perception abilities rather than rely solely on the audiogram, although this can take several sessions and requires great skill. Erber (1982, 1988) provides helpful clinical protocols for this purpose. This is important because there are considerable dangers in making the wrong judgements about a client's ability to use audition.

3. *Consider the relationship of air- and bone-conduction thresholds.* This will indicate whether the loss is sensorineural (in which case some distortion of sounds is likely, in addition to a loss of volume), conductive (in which case the primary problem is lack of volume) or mixed. If bone-conduction thresholds are at approximately the same levels as air-conduction thresholds, then the loss is sensorineural. If bone-conduction thresholds are normal and air-conduction thresholds show a hearing loss, then the loss is conductive. If bone-conduction thresholds are at less-than-normal levels but are better than air-conduction thresholds, then the loss is mixed. If the loss is conductive or mixed a medical opinion about treatment and prognosis should be sought if this has not already been provided. In judging the relationship of air- and bone-conduction thresholds it is important to recognise when masking has been applied.

4. *Consider the relative levels of the left and right ears.* In the case of an asymmetrical loss, note which is the better ear, as seating arrangements and informational counselling can be improved by this information. Persons with asymmetries on average greater than 20 dB will

almost certainly experience localisation problems, such as not being able to tell which of several phones is ringing in an office. Even if the loss is confined to quadrants 1 and 2, there may be a need to consider safety issues involving localisation, such as crossing roads and judging the direction from which warning signals are coming. Persons with asymmetrical sensorineural losses should be referred for medical assessment to exclude retrocochlear lesions, if this has not already been done. When judging the relative hearing levels of the left and right ears, it is important to recognise when masking has been applied.

Together these four steps will give a fundamental indication of the challenges experienced by individuals with hearing loss, when unaided. Figure 6.8 shows two audiograms that have been read with this procedure. Additional judgements may be made if the audiogram shows a speech area (see earlier). A speech area showing individual phonemes on a transparency may be a useful tool for the speech-language therapist as it can be overlaid on a client's audiogram to indicate the nature of, for example, consonant confusions, likely with that particular hearing loss. Additional examples are given in Chapter 10.

## Reading dB SPL audiograms

### Symbols

Symbols for sound field audiograms vary among clinics. In the examples that follow the symbol 'S' is used to indicate an unaided threshold response to tones presented in a sound field, such as are obtained with behavioural assessment of hearing levels in very young children. The symbol 'A' is used to indicate a sound field threshold obtained from aided testing. These symbols indicate that the ear(s) responsible for the response is unspecified (ASHA, 1990b). Some clinics have symbols indicating aided thresholds from left and right ears, aided threshold responses using different hearing aids and even unaided thresholds from each ear when the opposite ear has been occluded during testing. For example, in Australia the symbols 'H' and 'V' have for many years been used to indicate the aided thresholds of the right and left ear respectively. These symbols will normally be explained in a key code shown next to the audiogram.

Figure 6.9 shows a dB SPL audiogram with unaided ('S') and aided ('A') threshold responses. This indicates that the functional gain of the hearing-aid amplification allows the client to perceive many speech sounds but does not permit the perception of high frequency voiceless phonemes such as /ʃ/. As with many persons who have very significant degrees of hearing loss, hearing aids and other devices do not guarantee that speech can be heard normally, or even approximately so.

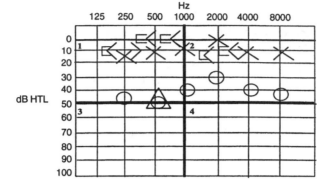

(a)

**Step 1:** The audiogram has been divided into quadrants.
**Step 2:** The left ear has a Q1–2 pattern with thresholds at or very close to average normal threshold sensitivity. The overall hearing of the right ear, indicated by the air-conduction thresholds, also has a Q1–2 pattern but at levels showing an average hearing loss of approx. 40 dB. This person will hear speech normally using the left ear, but may experience problems if the speaker is on the right side. The ability to hear in noisy situations may be affected.
**Step 3:** The bone-conduction thresholds in the right ear show essentially normal cochlear function. This, in combination with the air-conduction levels, indicates a conductive hearing loss, because when the middle ear is bypassed during bone-conduction testing, the individual can detect test tones at normal levels. Clarity of sounds perceived in the right ear would be good, provided that the signal was sufficiently loud.
**Step 4:** There is an obvious difference between ears. Masking has been applied to the normal left ear to prevent cross-hearing during checking of the air-conduction threshold in the right ear at 500 Hz, and of the bone-conduction thresholds of the right ear at 250 to 4000 Hz inclusive. Masking did not result in changes to the responses of the right ear, meaning that cross-hearing had not occurred. This individual is likely to have localisation problems. Because the loss is conductive hearing may be improved with medical and/or surgical intervention. Many causes for this type of loss are possible, but include otitis media, otosclerosis and trauma to the middle ear (see Chapter 3). Specialist medical opinion would be necessary. If hearing levels cannot be improved, the person would benefit from environmental manipulation strategies to maximise speech perception, and/or by use of a hearing aid provided there were no medical contraindications, such as infection.
**Summary:** A unilateral conductive hearing loss, which would be associated with some localisation problems. Medical/surgical treatment may improve hearing. Speech perception via hearing aid amplification would overcome the loss of volume experienced in conductive losses if medical treatment cannot improve hearing.

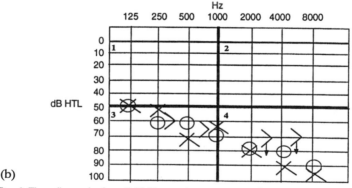

(b)

**Step 1:** The audiogram has been divided into quadrants.
**Step 2:** The quadrant pattern is a Q3–4. This person cannot reliably perceive conversational speech with these unaided thresholds. As there is measurable hearing at all test frequencies a significant improvement in speech perception should be expected with appropriate hearing-aid amplification. In the absence of hearing aids speech may be perceived if the conversational partner speaks at normal levels directly into the ear of the listener.
**Step 3:** The air- and bone-conduction thresholds are similar, indicating a sensorineural loss. Even with increased volume some clarity is likely to be missing from speech signals. At 2000 Hz and 4000 Hz the bone-conduction symbol indicates no response at the maximum level of output (70 dB HTL) for this audiometer. This is consistent with the fact that the air conduction thresholds are greater than 70 dB HTL at these frequencies.
**Step 4:** The levels of the right and left ear are very similar. The ears may differ in other ways, such as tolerance for very loud sounds (see Chapter 3), or speech discrimination ability (see Chapter 4), but the ability to detect pure tones is essentially the same in each ear. Masking has not been applied because cross-hearing does not occur in this situation.
**Summary:** A bilateral severe-to-profound sloping sensorineural hearing loss. Causes may be many. This type of audiogram may reflect congenital or acquired hearing loss. Hearing-aid amplification should be of significant benefit, and would be especially important for children developing speech and language skills. Persons living alone would also benefit from devices to enable perception of doorbells, smoke alarms and other important signals.

**Figure 6.8:** Two audiograms read with the four-step quadrant procedure.

It is worth noting that the speech area on audiograms represents an attempt to depict an 'average' speech spectrum. It may be that the speech of communication partners with louder voices and those who reduce conversational distance to less than one metre will be perceived more easily. Conversely, communication partners who have very soft voices may be understood much less well than the aided audiogram would indicate. Additionally, aspects of hearing-aid technology will influence the signal received.

Another point worth noting is that wearing hearing aids does not change the listener's thresholds, as appears to be the case from inspection of aided SPL audiograms. What is actually happening is that the hearing aid(s) amplify the speech signal to bring it within reach of the client's hearing levels. Toe (1990) gives a good explanation of this and other points about aided SPL audiograms.

The client's (unaided and/or aided) responses during sound field testing are compared with known normal threshold responses, just as with headphone (dB HTL audiogram) testing. However, the reference differs. Figure 6.9 shows two lines at the top of the graph that indicate normal thresholds in sound field for listening with one ear (line 'a') or two ears (line 'b'). These levels of dB SPL, which are just detectable by normal listeners, are the MAF values referred to earlier in this chapter. For example, the monaural MAF value at 1000 Hz is 7 dB SPL and the binaural MAF value at 1000 Hz is 4 dB SPL. The dB SPL reference for normal hearing differs according to frequency, reflecting the differential sensitivity of the human ear (see Chapter 2).

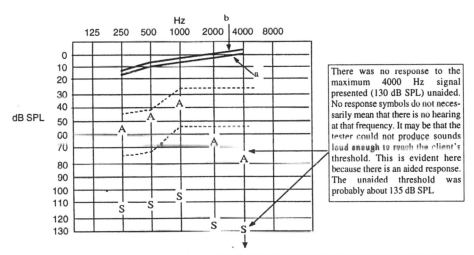

The functional gain of the hearing aids allows this client to perceive many speech sounds, but does not permit the perception of high-frequency voiceless fricatives and sibilants at normal conversational levels. The level of aided hearing for 2000 and 4000 Hz means that sounds like 't', 's', 'f' and 'sh' will be perceived only if the speaker has a loud voice or speaks closely into the hearing aid, provided that the MPO of the hearing aid (see Chapter 7) can be safely set to allow for the signal to be perceived. Many SPL audiograms will show separate symbols for each ear

**Figure 6.9:** An SPL audiogram showing unaided ('S') and aided ('A') sound field responses when both ears contribute to the response.

Figure 6.10 illustrates how information from an HTL audiogram may be translated and entered on a dB SPL audiogram by the application of MAF values. This translation may be necessary if the speech-language therapist has access to the client's unaided headphone responses (recorded on a dB HTL audiogram) and aided sound field responses (recorded on a dB SPL audiogram) and wishes to compare the two. As the reference for normal hearing is different in dB HTL and dB SPL, the MAF values need to be added to the dB HTL thresholds to convert them to dB SPL. For example, a monaural threshold of 70 dB HTL at 1000 Hz equals 77 dB SPL (HTL + MAF = SPL; i.e. 70 dB HTL + MAF of 7 dB SPL at 1000 Hz = 77 dB SPL). In similar fashion, dB SPL thresholds may be converted to dB HTL thresholds, but in this case the MAF figures would be subtracted to derive HTL values (SPL – MAF = HTL).

## Accuracy checks

The apparent accuracy of an audiogram may be checked by comparing the responses of the two ears. If the responses differ by more than 40–50 dB and there is no indication that masking has been applied, then it is wise to question the validity of the information. This is because cross-hearing (see Chapter 4) will normally occur when the level of air-conducted sound presented to the poorer ear is 40–50 dB greater than the hearing sensitivity of the better ear, as at that level, skull vibrations will occur and the stimulus will be transmitted by bone conduction (see Chapters 2 and 4) to the cochlea of the better ear. Figure 6.11 illustrates an invalid audiogram in comparison with a valid set of responses.

An additional accuracy check is to compare the client's apparent ability to respond to sound with the audiogram levels. For example, if the audiogram levels indicate the ability to perceive most of the speech signal at normal conversational levels, and yet the client appears to be having great difficulty doing so, it may be that the audiogram is no longer an accurate reflection of the client's hearing. They may for example have developed a conductive overlay to their pre-existing loss, or their cochlear hearing may have deteriorated since the time of the audiometric assessment. There are alternative explanations of course, such as hearing-aid malfunction or language problems.

## Questions to guide the use of audiograms

Table 6.1 lists ten questions that the speech-language therapist may find useful when reading audiograms. Some of these are now briefly discussed.

### Is there any indication of a need for referral for medical opinion?

Some clinics may have a protocol of medical examination for all cases of hearing loss. Where this is not the case, medical examination will usually

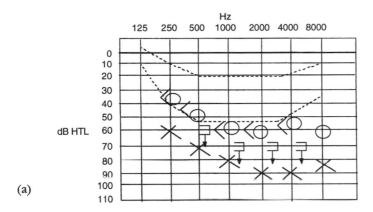

(a)

An individual's dB HTL (unaided) audiogram. There is a bilateral sensorineural loss. The right ear has better hearing levels than the left. The unaided dB HTL responses of the left ear (crosses) can be translated to dB SPL values for graphing on an SPL audiogram by the addition of monaural MAF values. These are 15 dB (250 Hz), 9 dB (500 Hz), 7 dB (1000 Hz), 3 dB (2000 Hz) and −1 dB (4000 Hz)

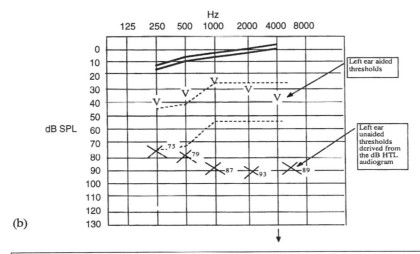

(b)

A dB SPL audiogram for the same individual showing unaided responses of the left ear (crosses) which have been derived from the dB HTL audiogram by the addition of monaural MAF values. For example, the unaided left ear air-conduction threshold at 1000 Hz was 80 dB HTL. The MAF value at 1000 Hz is 7 dB SPL. 80 dB + 7 dB = 87 dB SPL. Also shown are the aided thresholds for the left ear ('V' symbols, in Australia). It is obvious that the hearing aid gives considerable assistance to this ear, in terms of improving basic audibility. Unaided thresholds derived from headphone testing (i.e. with the dB HTL reference) are never placed on a dB SPL audiogram unless the MAF adjustment has been made

**Figure 6.10:** Translation of information between dB HTL and dB SPL audiograms: (a) shows unaided hearing thresholds on a dB HTL audiogram; (b) shows the information relating to the left ear, taken from the dB HTL audiogram and adjusted to dB SPL figures, in comparison to the aided responses in the same ear.

be organised, if necessary, by the clinician conducting the hearing tests. If, however, there is no record of medical assessment and the audiogram shows a conductive hearing loss, an asymmetrical sensorineural loss or an apparent sudden deterioration of hearing then medical examination would be a priority.

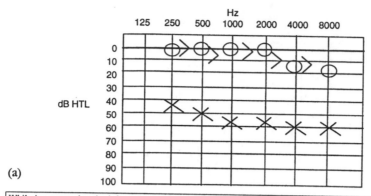

While it appears that the left ear has a hearing loss with a three-frequency (500 Hz, 1000 Hz, 2000 Hz) pure tone average of 53 dB (50 + 55+ 55 = 160/3 = 53.3 dB HTL), the difference between the ears indicates that cross-hearing may be occurring in both air-and bone-conduction testing

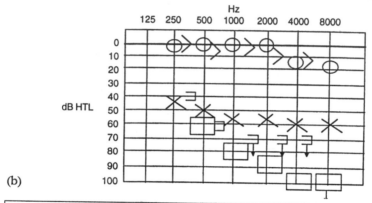

With appropriate masking it has been found that the hearing in the left ear is much poorer than the initial responses indicated. What could have been interpreted as a moderate conductive hearing loss in the left ear is in fact a severe-to-profound sensorineural hearing loss

**Figure 6.11:** Example of (a) an invalid audiogram in comparison to (b) a valid audiogram.

### Is there any indication of a need for referral for audiological opinion?

Referral for joint audiological and specialist medical opinion is often made in the cases described above. In addition, the speech-language therapist may wish further hearing assessments in cases where the audiogram information and the client's apparent hearing abilities appear to differ. In cases where the audiogram shows significant sensorineural hearing loss, referral for audiological opinion may be appropriate to assess suitability for hearing aids.

### What does the audiogram and other available audiometric data suggest is possible in assisting the client's communication in the longer term?

If the dB HTL audiogram shows a Q1–2–4, or Q1–4 pattern, for example, it may be possible to assist the client with speech-reading

**Table 6.1:** Questions to guide the use of audiograms

1. Does the audiometric information appear accurate, sufficiently current, and consistent with your observations, the client report and other clinical data?
2. Is there any indication of a need for referral for current medical opinion?
3. Is there any indication of a need for referral for current audiological opinion?
4. What does the audiogram and other available audiometric data suggest is possible in dealing with the client's presenting need?
5. What do the audiogram and other available audiometric data suggest is possible in assisting the client's communication in the longer term?
6. Is there a need to screen for middle-ear function?
7. What are the main points of information that, if necessary, I can communicate to the client?
8. In light of this information, what can I do to facilitate my own communication with the client?
9. Do I have the contact details of other professionals involved, such as audiologist, medical practitioner and teacher, and the client's permission to communicate with them?
10. What arrangements are in place for the monitoring of the client's hearing?

techniques and/or conversational management strategies to use in noisy situations, as it is in these situations that the client is least likely to be able to use their residual hearing. Referral for assessment of hearing-aid candidacy may also be appropriate especially if the thresholds in quadrant 1 approach the border of quadrant 3. Assistive listening devices (see Chapter 7) could also be judged useful, again because the lack of normal high-frequency hearing makes accurate speech perception difficult. Q3 and Q3–4 audiograms can be assessed in terms of the frequency range available to the client to make a judgement about goals for articulation therapy. Clients with Q3 and Q3–4 dB HTL audiograms will almost always be hearing-aid users and aided audiogram information is necessary.

In the case of children with significant hearing impairment, the speech-language therapist would hope to be able to rely on audiologists and other team members to provide amplification that maximises the child's audition. Putting aside concern with the dB level of the child's hearing, it is useful to consider the frequency range of sounds available to the child. Clezy (1993) reminds us that most of the components of language (prosodics, semantics and syntax) are available to the child who has aided hearing for the frequencies up to and including 1000 Hz. She gives the example of a child with hearing up to 750 Hz but no measurable hearing for higher frequencies. This child 'will have all tonal and intonational information available, most semantic and syntactic and some very important speech information (all vowels, except "i") and their transitions, diphthongs...' (Clezy, 1993, p. 26). Much can be done in therapy to help such children perceive the low-frequency elements of speech and to use that information in developing language and speech.

Appropriate attention to distance between speaker and listener, reliable hearing aids, monitoring of middle-ear function, good quality interaction and listening environment, and a developmental approach can all support such children in maximising communication skill.

### Is there a need to screen middle-ear function?

If the audiograms of the client indicate a history of intermittent conductive hearing loss, then it is wise to screen for middle-ear dysfunction with tympanometry (see Chapter 5). Two or three consecutive fails on tympanometry screening indicate the need for medical referral and the need to adjust communication behaviour during therapy in the meantime. This is important regardless of the overall level of hearing loss. A mild conductive loss could be a significant additional problem to an otherwise normally hearing language-delayed child or to the client who uses hearing aids.

## Summary of key points

Audiograms are plots of the levels at which an individual can detect the presence of sound at each of several audio frequencies. Audiograms do not show how the temporal information available in auditory signals is used. Persons with very similar audiograms can differ markedly in their ability to use aural-oral communication. Great care must be taken to assess the speech perception abilities of profoundly hearing-impaired children in particular, as audiograms provide limited information about the ability to use spectral and speech envelope cues in running speech. Using the 'quadrant' system proposed in this chapter may assist in reading audiograms. Audiograms obtained by testing with headphones (dB HTL audiograms) and audiograms obtained by testing in sound field (dB SPL audiograms) have different reference levels. However, information may be translated between them with appropriate use of minimal audible field (MAF) values. Many audiograms display a 'speech area', which can be used to assist qualitative judgements about the ability to perceive individual phonemes. The articulation index (AI) audiogram offers a quantitative method of recording the percentage of the speech signal perceived with various hearing losses.

# Chapter 7
# Hearing aids, assistive listening devices, tactile aids and cochlear implants

JANET DOYLE AND CHRISTOPHER LIND

This chapter deals with common technological approaches to assisting people with hearing loss. The aim is to provide a basic understanding of how this technology works and the ways in which it may help individual clients. Terms that are useful for the speech-language therapist to know when communicating with hearing-care professionals are explained. As technical development related to hearing loss is now very rapid, especially in the area of speech processing, the speech-language therapist is advised to maintain contact with local hearing centres who can advise on technical options as they become available.

## Principles

1. *Not all clients with hearing loss will accept or benefit from hearing-aid amplification, although many do.* There are clients whose hearing loss may be managed well with a hearing device, with communication training alone or with a combination of the two; clients who cannot manage or do not accept hearing aids; and clients whose hearing loss is of a magnitude that severely limits the applicability of hearing aids. Where hearing aids are not a workable option and yet the client has significant hearing loss, other technology may be appropriate and should be considered.
2. *The interaction between the technology and the user's real-life communication needs is a key consideration in the selection and evaluation of technology for individual clients.* Hearing aids and cochlear implants, for example, are individually prescribed so that their electroacoustic characteristics match as closely as possible aspects of the client's remaining hearing abilities. The electroacoustic characteristics of assistive listening devices are not individually prescribed, but their selection and evaluation should be carefully and individually considered, including suitability for the client's daily life

needs and compatibility with any hearing aid(s) the client may be using.

3. *Aspects of both hearing impairment and hearing handicap are considered in applying technology to hearing loss.* Hearing impairment is the loss of normal function of the auditory system due to physical changes. Hearing disability/handicap is the effect of the impairment on the client's daily communication. When using technology to address the ramifications of the hearing loss in daily communication, we need both the audiogram (a measure of impairment) and a functional assessment of the individual's daily communication needs (an indication of handicap). The speech-language therapist may be well placed to assess daily communication needs.

4. *Basic troubleshooting of hearing aids and assistive listening devices is not difficult.* As some clients who consult speech-language therapists may be regular users of such devices, it is important for the therapist to detect problems with their function or use. Some guidelines are given in this chapter.

5. *In our view the clinical service involved in the provision of technology is likely to be almost as important as the technology itself.* Clinicians advising on or providing technology for hearing-impaired or deaf individuals have technical knowledge that can be applied to the problem of living with hearing loss. The client has life knowledge about communication needs, which need to be applied to the problem if the technology is to be successful. The clinical interactions between clinicians and clients are an opportunity to marry these two forms of knowledge and support the client appropriately. It is therefore important that the client perceives the interaction as satisfactory.

## Overview of technology

Four principal forms of technology are available for the person with hearing loss. These are: hearing aids, assistive listening devices (ALDs), tactile aids and cochlear implants. A fifth type of technology, tinnitus maskers and densensitisation devices, is aimed at alleviating the distress associated with tinnitus (see Chapter 3), which may or may not be accompanied by significant hearing loss. This fifth technology is treated as a separate topic at the end of this chapter. Hearing aids, tactile aids and cochlear implants may be described as general communication devices (i.e. used in response to the individual's communication needs across many daily conversational settings). By contrast, ALDs have been designed to provide assistance for the user in specific situations. The greater emphasis on situation specificity is reflected in the assessment, selection and evaluation of ALDs. Table 7.1 compares the general characteristics of hearing aids, ALDs, tactile aids and cochlear implants.

**Table 7.1:** Characteristics of hearing aids, assistive listening devices, tactile aids and cochlear implants

| Hearing aids | Assistive listening devices | Tactile devices | Cochlear implants |
|---|---|---|---|
| • Used for general communication via audition. Very useful for speech communication. May be used to supplement speech-reading in cases of very profound hearing loss | • Used in specific situations. Used alone or with hearing aid(s) | • Used for general communication. Suitable for clients with total or profound loss who cannot benefit from hearing aids | • Used for general communication via audition, sound awareness and supplementation of speech-reading. Suitable for clients with total or profound loss who cannot benefit from hearing aids |
| • Matched to aspects of pure tone hearing impairment and speech discrimination ability | • Matched to aspects of disability, i.e. particular listening problems | • Employs vibrotactile or electro-tactile stimulation of the skin | • Matched to aspects of pure tone hearing impairment |
| • Almost all are worn external to the body, in or behind ear, occasionally on the body. Bone-conduction aids are worn on the head and mastoid process. Implantable aids have external components but surgically implanted output stages | • 'Attached' to specific signal generators, such as television | • Sound is received by an ear-level microphone, then processed and delivered to electrodes in contact with the skin, usually the hands or fingers | • Receiver implanted permanently in temporal bone. Electrode(s) positioned in or near cochlea. Other components worn externally |
| • Used when required. Individuals can differ greatly in hours of use | • Used in specific situations, e.g. noisy party, watching television, using telephone | • Use varies | • Generally used all waking hours |
| • Relatively high cost, especially dynamic speech processing hearing aids. Many clients may be eligible for government assistance | • Relatively low cost | • Cost varies with particular device | • Very high cost |

Although many people understand that a congenital hearing loss usually means very significant and ongoing challenges to successful communication, it is a widely held community perception that an acquired hearing loss is largely 'solved' by a hearing aid, implant or ALD. These technologies seldom completely solve hearing difficulties. They often do not restore to the user the functional equivalent of normal hearing. Despite this, hearing aids, ALDs, tactile aids and cochlear implants each have a place in meeting the communication needs of many people who are hearing-impaired or deaf.

Sandridge (1995) reminds us that hearing performs three functions:

- environmental awareness;
- warning or alerting;
- symbolic communication.

Environmental awareness provides access to the sounds of everyday activities, by which we orientate ourselves to the world. Warning and alerting functions direct the individual to sounds that may represent a challenge to his or her safety within a particular environment. Symbolic communication includes access to all forms of spoken language and music. Technology such as hearing aids, ALDs and cochlear implants are designed to improve the user's access to these functions within the context of the individual's daily life.

Before selection of particular technology it is important to establish the social, personal and cultural environment in which the person lives and to assess his or her sensory/perceptual and communicative skills and needs. The therapist must understand technology as a tool of intervention to be used as part of an overall therapy plan for the individual who has a hearing loss or who is deaf. For more detailed reading on the range of current aural rehabilitation techniques, including these technologies, the reader is directed to the texts by Gagné and Tye-Murray (1994), Kricos and Lesner (1995), Plant and Spens (1995) and Erber (1996).

# Hearing aids

Hearing aids are electroacoustic instruments that improve the audibility of speech and other important signals for the person with hearing loss. The aim is to increase the volume of the signal to a level that is, on average, above the individual's hearing threshold and below that individual's level of discomfort (see Chapter 3, p. 51), so that the signal is comfortably audible, and to do so in a way that maximises the intelligibility of speech signals.

## Operating features

Figure 7.1 is a schematic diagram of a basic hearing aid. The essential features are: a microphone (input transducer) to detect the signal and convert it into electrical form; an amplifier to increase the strength of the signal and shape the signal in ways that are useful given the client's particular hearing loss; a receiver (output transducer) to convert the amplified electrical signal back to an acoustic signal; and a battery (power source) to enable this process.

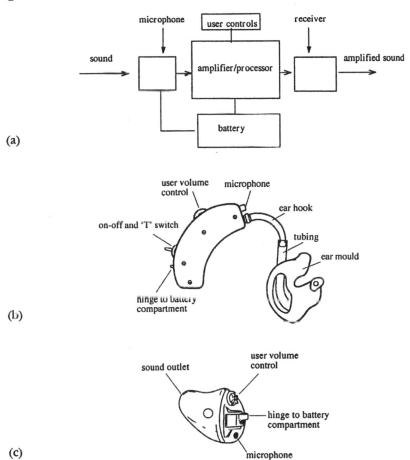

(a)

(b)

(c)

**Figure 7.1:** Schematic diagram of (a) the components of a basic hearing aid, (b) the general appearance of a behind-the-ear hearing aid and (c) the general appearance of an in-the-canal hearing aid. The size and position of the basic components varies with the style and size of the aid.

The technical characteristics and the size of these components varies considerably among hearing aids. Some modern hearing aids have additional complex speech processing abilities. Hearing aids also have some form of on-off switch and a means of varying the volume of the signal (usually a wearer-operated volume control). As well as these very basic requirements, hearing aids may have: a telecoil to allow coupling of the aid to special telephones and other listening devices (see following section); direct audio input to allow electrical signals (such as those from a hand-held microphone or some other device) to be plugged straight into the aid; tone or programme controls to allow the user to switch from one particular type of amplification to another; and remote controls, which permit the user to alter the functions of the hearing aid without having to touch the aid in the ear.

## Types of hearing aids

Hearing aids are most commonly classified by style, which is closely related to the size of the instrument. The largest and least frequently fitted aid is the body-level aid, which is worn clipped on to clothing, generally at chest level. The signal that is picked up and amplified in the body-worn aid is fed to a receiver attached to a standard earmould. Because the microphone (input transducer) and the receiver (output transducer) are a considerable distance apart, very powerful amplification may be provided with little risk of acoustic feedback. Even though powerful amplification is now available in much smaller aids, body-level aids remain appropriate for some individuals, particularly those who require very large controls because of reduced manual dexterity and/or poor vision.

In behind-the-ear (BTE) hearing aids all components are worn at ear level. The microphone, generally level with the top of the ear, is thus in a more natural position than it is in body aids. Even individuals with profound hearing losses may be fitted with BTE aids. Earmould styles and materials in BTE aids can vary greatly and are an important part of the sound-delivery system. The same hearing aid can produce very different results with different earmoulds (see, for example, Byrne, Noble & Sinclair, 1996).

In-the-ear (ITE) aids house all components in a custom-made shell, which fits into the concha and external auditory meatus. The size of ITE aids varies with the size of the individual's ear and the desired features. In-the-canal (ITC) hearing aids provide all components in a custom-made shell that occupies the ear canal and less of the concha. The smallest aids are completely-in-the-canal (CIC) aids, which are effectively not visible. There are some exciting developments in amplification with CIC aids (see, for example, Mueller & Ebinger, 1996). Deep canal hearing aids sit partly down in the bony portion of the ear canal and this appears to provide relief from the occlusion effect experienced by aid-users who complain about how they hear their own voice. Additionally it allows for greater gain than might otherwise be achieved in a canal fitting.

Many smaller hearing aids cannot provide features (such as telecoil) beyond the standard microphone, amplifier, battery and receiver because of space limitations. In addition, individuals with profound losses cannot yet be effectively fitted with many of the smallest ear-level hearing aids. However, ITE, ITC and CIC aids are very popular, presumably because of their small size and the natural position of the micro-phone. In the UK many clients who purchase hearing aids privately in preference to obtaining a free aid from the National Health Service (NHS) do so for cosmetic reasons (Rendell et al., 1992), because the smaller ITE and ITC aids are not routinely available from the NHS.

Eyeglass or spectacle aids provide amplification through hearing aids built into the frame of spectacles. The amplified signal is fed via a tube to the ear canal. Spectacle aids may or may not be worn with earmoulds, depending on amplification needs.

Spectacle aids can be particularly useful when it is necessary to provide contralateral routing of signals (a CROS fitting). A CROS fitting is indicated when, for example, the client has normal or near normal hearing in one ear and a very profound or total loss in the other ear. The localisation problems associated with such a hearing loss can be greatly assisted by placing a microphone on the side with little or no useable hearing and routing the signal to the contralateral (good hearing) ear. Although all sound is heard in the good ear, the individual can now perceive sounds arriving at both sides of the head and can soon develop the impression of binaural hearing. Other, more complex, fittings are also available using the CROS principle. CROS fittings can also be provided in BTE and ITE aids. Recently Bauman and Braemer (1996) have described an alternative method, which, in summary, is the prescription of a high-powered ITC aid for the ear with no useable hearing. The resulting ampli-fication reportedly yields a signal loud enough to transmit the signal to the better ear by bone conduction (see Chapters 2 and 4).

Radio-frequency (RF) or frequency-modulated (FM) hearing aids are instruments in which the microphone is positioned at the sound source (e.g. close to the mouth of a parent, speech-language therapist or teacher) rather than at the ear of the listener. The signal is then trans-mitted by radio-frequency technology from a transmitter worn by the speaker to a receiver worn by the hearing-impaired listener. This receiver is connected to headphones worn by the listener or to the listener's personal hearing aid(s) by means of an induction or audio input 'shoe', which plugs into the aid(s). The great advantage of this technology is that the signal reaches the listener without the loss of intensity that would normally occur over the distance between, for example, a teacher at the front of a classroom and a hearing-impaired student seated at the back of the room. The result is a much improved signal-to-noise ratio and the reception of important signals that would otherwise simply not be heard. The environmental microphone on the listener's personal hearing aid may be switched on or off depending on the situation in which the radio-frequency instrument is used. For example, if the listener is attending a formal lecture it would be useful to have the environmental microphone turned off, so that any noise occurring around the listener is not perceived. If, however, the listener needs to hear his or her own voice or the voices or others as well as that of the formal speaker, such as in a classroom or a speech therapy session, the hearing-aid microphones need to be turned on. As there are some important technical issues involved in setting the gain of RF/FM systems (Rawson & Bamford, 1995), the speech-language therapist whose clients use RF/FM units may need, on occasions, to seek the support of an appropriate hearing professional, but generally this technology is very easy to use. RF/FM units are discussed further in the section on assistive listening devices later in this chapter.

A type of hearing aid that is fitted very infrequently, is the bone-conduction hearing aid, in which the output transducer is replaced by an oscillator (similar to that used in bone-conduction audiometry) placed on the mastoid and held in place by a spring steel band over the head. This type of aid is used for persons who have chronic discharge from the ears, or who have a deformity of the external ear that prevents the use of standard hearing aids. However, bone-conduction aids are relatively inefficient and can be uncomfortable because of the necessary pressure exerted on the user. An advance on this situation is the implantable bone-conduction aid (IHA) or bone-anchored hearing aid (BAHA), in which the output stages of the aid are surgically implanted. For example Dunham and Friedman (1990) have described an implantable bone-conduction hearing aid in which the output oscillator is permanently housed in the temporal bone. Gyo, Saiki and Yanagihara (1996) have developed an implantable aid in which a vibrator is attached directly to the stapes. These aids appear to have potential for individuals with conductive or mixed losses in which bone-conduction thresholds are better than 40 dB HTL and preferably better than 20 dB HTL. However, as with some more conventional hearing aids, IHA/BAHA users can have difficulties with hearing speech in noise and listening over the telephone (see for example, Stephens et al., 1996).

### Electroacoustic data

Hearing aids can be described in terms of gain, frequency response and maximum output. Simple explanations of these concepts are provided in Table 7.2 along with other terms useful to the speech-language therapist who needs to communicate with hearing care professionals.

Gain is the output SPL minus the input SPL, i.e. the amount by which the incoming sound is increased by the aid. Gain varies with frequency, as the aid is prescribed to provide greatest gain where the client's hearing loss indicates most need (often, but not always, where the loss is greatest). Gain also varies with the position of the volume control, higher volume settings yielding greater gain. In some modern hearing aids the gain also varies in response to the level of sound reaching the microphone.

**Table 7.2:** The basic meaning of some terms commonly used in hearing technology

| Term | Meaning |
|---|---|
| Compression | A means of limiting the output of hearing aids while preserving the characteristics of the speech signal |
| Direct audio input | An attribute of some hearing aids. Allows instruments such as FM/RF (see below) receivers and some other assistive listening devices to be plugged directly into the aid |
| FM (aka RF) | Frequency-modulation (radio-frequency) systems. Use of radio waves to transmit signals across much larger areas than can be handled by hearing aids. Can be used alone or with hearing aids. Gives good signal-to-noise ratio |
| Frequency response | A curve indicating how much gain (see below) the instrument produces at various frequencies. The frequency response will differ with level of input |
| Gain | The strength of a hearing aid or other device. The difference in dB between input and output |
| Insertion gain (aka real ear gain) | Gain of hearing aid measured with a probe microphone inserted in the ear canal. Measurements are taken from the client's unaided ear and compared to measurements when the client is wearing the hearing aid. The difference is the insertion gain |
| Power (aka MPO, SSPL90) | The maximum output in dB SPL. The greatest intensity a hearing aid will produce |
| Speech processing (aka speech encoding) | Involved in cochlea implants, some hearing aids and some tactile aids. An electrical means of dynamically analysing and shaping the speech signal that has been detected by the microphone before being delivered to the user |
| Telecoil (aka 'T' coil, 'T' switch) | A coil in a hearing aid that picks up electromagnetic signals. Can be used instead of an environmental microphone when using telephones, some assistive listening devices and in areas with looped public address systems |

The frequency response is a plot of gain by frequency, usually generated with an input of 50 or 60 dB SPL. Some hearing aids may have irregular (i.e. not smooth) frequency responses. In BTE aids some of these irregularities or peaks in the frequency response are due to the effects of earmould ventings or tubing (Studebaker & Zachman, 1970; Lybarger, 1985), and others to the electronic components of the hearing aid itself. The speech perception of listeners with hearing impairment may be more adversely affected by such peaks, and to a greater degree than listeners with normal hearing (van Buunen, Feston & Houtgast, 1996). However, this danger is greatly reduced with current hearing-aid technology. In some hearing aids a number of different frequency responses may be programmed (see programmable hearing aids, below) so that the client can choose one frequency response for one type of listening situation (e.g. quiet conversation) and a different frequency response for another situation (e.g. noisy restaurant).

Maximum output, also known as maximum power output (MPO), saturation sound pressure level (SSPL) or SSPL90, is the maximum amount of sound the aid will produce with a high level input, such as 90 dB SPL or more. Hearing-aid output is limited so that very loud sounds are not amplified to the same degree as weaker sounds. In this way the danger of exceeding the client's tolerance level is eliminated or reduced. An MPO may be set, for example, at 115 dB SPL, meaning that the aid will not present the user with sounds greater than 115 dB SPL under any normal circumstances.

There are various means by which hearing-aid limiting MPO is achieved. Peak clipping, in which those parts of the amplified signal that exceed MPO are 'clipped', is the simplest approach, but because the original waveform is changed by this process some degree of distortion occurs in the output signal. Compression, in which the output signal is limited by reducing the gain as the intensity of the input signal increases, is an approach that retains the overall waveform of the input signal. There are various forms of compression (e.g. input versus output compression), but a discussion of these is beyond the scope of this book. However, it is worth noting that automatic gain control (AGC) hearing aids, which utilise compression, not only keep MPO to a desirable level but also achieve a better match between the client's hearing (which often has a reduced dynamic range, see Chapter 2) and the output signal of the hearing aid.

Digital hearing aids offer great potential for shaping the amplified signal to better suit client needs and for improving listening in difficult situations. Digital hearing aids electronically convert a continuous incoming signal such as speech into a sequence of data points or digits. This allows rapid assessment of, and changes to, the output signal in response to changes in the incoming signal. Hearing aids utilising digital technology are sometimes called speech processing hearing aids or intelligent hearing aids, because of the dynamic way they react to incoming signals. Some digital hearing aids do not require the user to make any adjustments, responding automatically to the incoming signal. Digital technology is used in programmable hearing aids in which the dispenser uses a computer to set aid characteristics. At the time of writing, digital hearing aids are still very expensive relative to more conventional hearing aids, but it is hoped that this will change somewhat as the use of the technology spreads.

As Moore (1996) has observed, the vastly increased range of prescription options in hearing aids will be a major challenge to the hearing-aid dispenser who must decide between them. Nevertheless it is true that the potential to better meet the hearing needs of aid users has improved dramatically over the last decade.

## Complexities in hearing-aid fitting

In cases of profound hearing loss, hearing-aid fitting can be problematic because of the ear's impaired ability to process amplified signals and because of the difficulties achieving a useful level of amplification that at the same time does not exceed the client's tolerance levels. The speech information received may in some cases be very limited, even with digital hearing-aid technology. Nevertheless, hearing-aid amplification can greatly support speech-reading and provide a sense of living in a world with sound, even if the amplified signal is insufficient for communication via audition.

Another problem is that amplification by very powerful hearing aids can, in some cases, cause temporary threshold shift (TTS) and permanent hearing damage in the same way as occurs with noise-induced hearing loss (Macrae, 1968, 1991). Therefore very careful attention needs to be given to the prescription of safe levels of MPO. There are some relatively simple methods of achieving this (Storey & Dillon, 1996). However, even relatively low-powered hearing aids can increase the risk of noise exposure if used in very noisy situations, such as some industrial workplaces (Dolan & Maurer, 1996), although the use of AGC can help reduce this risk.

While there are very good reasons (such as better hearing in noisy situations) for using two hearing aids if there is a loss in each ear (see, for example, McKenzie & Rice, 1990), this is not necessarily of benefit in all cases (Byrne, Noble & LePage, 1992). The question of cost may also deter some individuals from proceeding with binaural aiding. The client's attitude and particular communication needs also impact on the monaural versus binaural decision. It is therefore not automatically the case that an individual with bilateral loss should wear bilateral hearing aids, although most audiologists would agree that binaural aiding is the preferred approach if speech-perception skills in communication are to be maximised. Additionally, binaural aiding probably helps to prevent a decline in the ability to process speech sounds that might otherwise occur in an unaided ear.

If monaural aiding is selected, the aid may be fitted to the better or the poorer ear. The decision is made generally on the basis of which arrangement provides the best speech perception, in combination with a consideration of handedness and listening needs.

## Evaluation of hearing-aid outcomes

An important question is: What constitutes a good outcome? The answer is likely to be different for different individuals in the aural rehabilitation process. For example, the audiologist may characterise a good outcome as excellent real ear gain, aided thresholds in the speech banana or good aided speech discrimination ability. The client may think they have a good outcome when others do not notice their hearing aids or when they are able to hear better in church. The clinic administrator may consider that a low rate of return for aid repair is one good outcome. These, of course, are not the only possible ways a good outcome may be defined. These authors believe it is useful to ask the client what they would consider a good outcome to be prior to hearing-aid fitting, and to evaluate the success of hearing aids principally by that client criteria. A novel tool currently being developed with this in mind is the Client Measured Benefit worksheet (N. Clutterbuck & S. Clutterbuck, 1997, personal communication). Notwithstanding the need for assessment by the client, we also believe it useful to employ a combination of quantitative (e.g. number of hours of aided listening per day or per week, aided real ear performance measures or similar) and qualitative (e.g. client diaries of aided experiences, reports of communication partners) measures.

Brooks (1996), for example, reported a 10-year follow-up study of hearing-aid users. The data suggest that if clients are using their hearing aid(s) for more than 4 hours a day six months after fitting of the aid they are likely to maintain or even increase their use of the aid over the long term. If the client is over 70 years of age when they obtain their first hearing aid(s) they may be less likely to adapt to hearing-aid use and so the outcome, at least in terms of hours of use, may be less hopeful for this group. However, it could be the case that individuals who use their aids very infrequently may consider them a success on the basis of their experiences.

It may be the case that the success of the hearing-aid fitting is influenced as much by the individual's daily communication environment(s) as it is by the electroacoustic qualities of the aid itself. If the well-aided individual communicates in a range of environments that are noise-filled or distracting, and/or if their communication partners do not accommodate their communication needs, the hearing aid may be of little assistance. That is, the environment does not allow successful hearing-aid use, despite the skill with which the aid was fitted and the effort the individual makes to use it competently. Because of this possibility, practical measures of hearing-aid success should include evaluations of the environments in which the aid is used (Erber, Lamb & Lind, 1996).

Some functional outcome measures, such as the Client Oriented Scale of Improvement (COSI) (Dillon, James & Ginnis 1997) and the Abbreviated Profile of Hearing Aid Benefit (APHAB) (Cox & Alexander, 1995), acknowledge the potential influence of environment on aid use. Although the former asks open-ended questions and the latter is a forced-choice inventory, both evaluations incorporate aspects of the hearing-aid user's daily communication environment in judging the success of aid-fitting.

Another factor to consider in evaluating hearing-aid outcomes is what Gatehouse and Killion (1993) term 'HABRAT' (Hearing Aid Brain Rewiring Accommodation Time). It takes time to adjust to aided listening when parts of the auditory signal have not been heard for some time (usually at least several years) due to hearing loss. Gatehouse and Killion proposed that the brain of a person with unaided hearing loss will, over many years of no longer receiving stimulation for certain audio frequencies, 'allocate surrounding frequencies and intensities to those unstimulated regions' (p. 32). When the hearing-impaired individual is later fitted with hearing aids, the previously unheard frequencies become audible. However, the cortical areas that were initially responsive to those frequencies have been reallocated to other frequencies. It takes time for the brain to become somehow 'rewired' and for the person to make best use of the signals provided by the hearing aids. Gatehouse and Killion stress that the notion of hearing-aid accommodation time should never be used as an excuse for poor aid-fittings, but they argue that HABRAT is consistent with clinical experience and must be considered when counselling clients. The accommodation time is variable and although the adjustment can be rapid, especially when technically excellent hearing aids are provided, it may take some months or even years.

### Troubleshooting hearing aids

Table 7.3 lists some common problems that may be encountered by persons who wear hearing aids, and some ways that the speech-language therapist may assist. It is useful for the speech-language therapist who does not have immediate access to an audiologist, hearing therapist or hearing-aid technician to have some basic equipment, such as a battery tester, spare batteries and a stetoclip for listening to hearing aids (Table 7.4). This will permit basic troubleshooting and appropriate referral. *Caution: Never use a stetoclip without first turning the hearing aid volume to the lowest setting.*

The speech-language therapist whose client has hearing aid(s) is advised to know (a) where the aid was obtained, (b) the recommended volume and tone settings (in cases where the aid is not programmable or automatic), (c) the client's ability to use and care for the aid, and (d) the degree to which the aid benefits the client (as indicated by client report,

**Table 7.3:** Troubleshooting hearing aids

| Problem | Possible causes and what to do |
|---|---|
| 1. Aid whistles | (a) Aid or earmould may not be inserted correctly. Check fit |
| | (b) Wax in ear canal. Check visually and refer for wax removal if necessary |
| | (c) Break in casing, tubing or earmould. Check visually and then test for acoustic leakage by placing thumb over sound outlet and any vent while aid switched on. If feedback ceases leakage is not the cause |
| | (d) Aid worn at or near full volume. More likely to cause feedback in severely hearing-impaired children where frequent changes of earmould are needed as child grows. Check fit of earmould. All hearing-aid users periodically need new earmoulds (for BTE and body-level aids) |
| 2. Aid seems dead | (a) Flat battery. Test and change |
| | (b) Battery inserted incorrectly. Check and reverse if necessary |
| | (c) Sound outlet blocked with wax. Wipe sound outlet and if necessary inspect and remove with wax tool (ITC and BTE aids) or a pipe cleaner. With ITE/ITC/CIC aids take great care |
| | (d) Aid switched to 'T' rather than 'M' |
| | (e) Corroded battery terminals. Common if the battery has been left in an unused aid. Remove battery and clean terminals with emery board or the eraser from the end of a pencil |
| | (f) Microphone/amplifier/receiver damaged. Refer back to hearing-aid dispenser for repair and loan aid |
| 3. Signal distorted or weak | (a) Battery run down. Check and replace. Check that client is using recommended battery type |
| | (b) Incorrect tone setting. Check recommended setting |
| | (c) Blockage in sound outlet. Check and clear as necessary |
| | (d) Internal fault. Listen to aid with stetoclip. If distorted and there is no other cause evident, refer to audiologist |
| | (e) Dirty controls or switching. 'Dry', clean controls with air blower, or 'wet' clean with a purpose preparation |
| | (f) Volume turned too high. Check ear for wax occlusion. If occluded refer for removal. If not occluded refer for evaluation of client's current hearing levels and hearing-aid prescription |
| 4. Client not happy with amplified sound | (a) Many possible technical and non-technical causes. Refer back to dispenser and if necessary for audiological opinion |

**Table 7.4:** Things to have handy when working with clients who wear hearing aids

| Item | Description |
|---|---|
| 1. Batteries | • Selection of zinc-oxide (air) and mercury batteries in sizes 675, 13, 312 and 10 or 230<br>• Zinc-oxide batteries last longer on the shelf and in the aid, but some clients still use mercury batteries |
| 2. Battery tester | • A single tester that can handle all battery sizes |
| 3. Stetoclip (aka stethoscope) | • For listening to hearing aids to subjectively judge quality of signal<br>• When listening to BTE aids detach hearing aid from earmould and attach end of stetoclip to aid ear hook<br>• When listening to ITE, ITC and CIC aids insert ITE adapter into end of stetoclip and then insert that into sound outlet of aid. When listening to body-level aids, remove earmould from output receiver, remove flexible tube from stetoclip and clip output receiver into neck of stetoclip. *Caution:* Never use a stetoclip without first turning the hearing aid volume to the lowest setting. The volume may then be carefully increased for the listening check |
| 4. Eraser or emery board | • Small eraser from end of pencil or emery board nailfile are useful for cleaning corroded battery terminals in aids where size permits |
| 5. Air blower | • For blowing moisture from earmoulds and earmould tubing after cleaning or in case of perspiration |
| 6. Devices list | • List of assistive listening devices and their compatibility with hearing aids, including current sources and costs |
| 7. Auroscope (aka otoscope) | • To examine the client's ear canal to detect the presence of wax. Need a supply of batteries, disposable speculae and appropriate hygiene protocol |
| 8. Telephone contacts | • The telephone numbers of a local hearing-care professional who can advise in case of difficulty |

report of client's family and friends, clinic tests such as aided thresholds and speech discrimination tests, and clinical observation). He or she should also have readily available the telephone number of the audiologist or hearing-aid dispenser who provided the hearing aid(s) so that advice may be sought quickly if necessary.

The volume control on most non-automatic and programmable BTE aids is numbered, commonly from 1 (softest) to 4 (loudest). A suitable volume setting is often about halfway (i.e. 2–3), although with severe and profound losses, especially those with a conductive component, the client may wear the aid at higher volume settings.

The volume control on many ITE/ITC aids is not numbered. The hearing-aid dispenser may place a dot of coloured nail polish on the control to allow easy checking that the volume control is set at an appropriate level.

Many clients will need to alter the volume control to positions slightly above or below the recommended setting for particular listening situations. Many new hearing-aid users like less volume. If the client reports needing more volume than usual, and no obvious reason can be found on troubleshooting the aid(s) (see Table 7.3) it is wise to refer back to the dispenser because the client's hearing may have deteriorated, the aid may be malfunctioning or there may be wax occlusion of the ear canals.

**Clinical decisions for the speech-language therapist**

1. One important role of the speech-language therapist is to help the client obtain hearing-aid evaluation and fitting. In the UK there is now a system of Direct Referral Hearing Aid Clinics, which means that individuals can be referred direct to audiology centres by their general practitioner without the need for an assessment by an otolaryngologist, as was previously the case for NHS clients. In some clinics, the non-attendance rate has dropped considerably since the introduction of the Direct Referral system (Zeitoun et al., 1995), and waiting times for a hearing aid are shorter (Reeves et al., 1994). The system is thought to work best for clients aged 60 years or over, as younger clients with significant hearing loss are more likely to have conditions requiring specialist medical treatment (Koay & Sutton, 1996).

   In Australia the federal government supports the provision of hearing-aid services to eligible older adults via a system of accredited audiologists and audiometrists. Children receive free government funded hearing aids via the Australian Hearing Services (AHS) hearing centres. The particular details of these systems may vary over time, but referral is often made by general medical practitioners. The speech-language therapist can assist by having a supply of the appropriate forms. Persons wishing to obtain hearing aids privately may be referred directly to the audiologist by the speech-language therapist or may arrange appointments directly.

In Canada and the USA methods of arranging hearing-aid fitting vary according to the particular legislation and practices in various states and provinces. In Asia practices also vary between and within countries.

2. Deciding when the client may need referral for review of their amplification is an important responsibility. It is sometimes very obvious when a hearing aid is not working and therefore referral back to the dispenser or to another professional is necessary. However, even if the aid appears to be functioning well any suggestion that aided functioning has declined or seems inadequate should be taken as an indication that audiological review or further assessment is indicated. It may be that the client's hearing has changed or that the hearing aid has an intermittent or subtle fault that compromises the signal. Additionally, the client may have wax occlusion or a middle-ear disorder (see Chapter 3). Simple live voice checks of hearing function, such as the Ling Five Sound Test (see Chapter 4) can assist with the referral decision.

3. The decision to explore options other than, or in addition to, hearing-aid amplification is more complex. However, the speech-language therapist can greatly assist the client by completing a communication-needs assessment. This may highlight aspects of daily functioning that need priority treatment. For example, it may become apparent that reliable telephone communication is vital to the client's work and home life. As a result the client may be advised to consider various assistive listening devices for the telephone.

## Assistive listening devices

Three groups of people are potentially assisted by ALDs. First, ALDs can assist adults with acquired hearing loss whose access to daily verbal communication is compromised by their hearing loss. Second, ALDs provide technology to assist the deaf community. People who are deaf (who may communicate either by spoken or signed language) require telecommunications that are appropriate to their communication needs and to cultural and linguistic aspects of their community. The final group of people to be assisted by ALDs are the family and friends of individuals who have hearing impairment or are deaf. Often the impetus for the purchase of an ALD comes from the frequent communication partner rather than the individual with the hearing loss. Thus ALDs are chosen in response to the nature of the individual's communication milieu.

ALDs may be classified by their major purpose. The four major categories of ALDs are:

- telephone devices;
- television and radio devices;
- alarms;
- general communication devices.

These are described briefly below. For more detailed reviews of current ALD technology the reader is referred to Compton (1991), Garstecki (1994), Ross (1994) and Sandridge (1995).

## Telephone devices

Telephone devices fall into two broad categories: devices that alert the individual to the telephone ring; and devices that increase the individual's access to speech transmitted over the telephone.

Alerting devices for the telephone are usually auditory (such as a high-intensity, low-frequency signal in place of the usual telephone ring) or visual (such as a lamp, which, when connected to the telephone, will flash when the telephone rings), although vibratory devices (e.g. vibrating personal pagers) may also be used. The auditory and visual devices may be permanently installed or portable. In general, the greater the distance between an auditory or visual telephone alarm and the individual relying on it, the less its effectiveness.

Increasing access to the spoken signal depends on both increasing the volume of that signal and minimising the effects of background noise. Permanently installed or portable volume controls are available for the telephone. The possible benefits of portable devices to increase volume of the speech signal depend on the pattern of telephone use. Frequently used telephones may benefit from permanent installation of a volume control for the voice.

Hearing-aid wearers who have a 'T' switch built into their aid(s) may take advantage of electromagnetic signals. Most electrical devices use the energy or power that they draw inefficiently. The wasted energy 'leaks' from the electrical device as electromagnetic energy. This wasted energy can be picked up and converted to acoustic energy by a hearing aid with a built-in telecoil. Normal domestic telephones do not usually have sufficient electromagnetic leakage to allow successful telecoil use without modification. However, the telephone can be made compatible with the telecoil by inserting a small resistor or induction coil into the telephone handset. This resistor increases the electromagnetic leakage to a level sufficient for the telecoil in a hearing aid positioned near the handset to receive the telephone signal. The hearing aid then converts this to an acoustic signal, amplifies it and presents it to the listener's ear. The telecoil in the hearing aid is activated by the 'T' switch. In most (but not all) cases, once the telecoil has been turned on, the microphone in the hearing aid is automatically turned off. On this setting, the hearing aid will pick up the electromagnetic signal but will not pick up environmental sounds, hence reducing or eliminating possible interference from background noise in the vicinity of the telephone user. Many, but not all, public telephones have induction coils installed. The traveller who uses more than one telephone regularly may benefit from a portable induction coil that is fitted over the telephone receiver and converts the acoustic signal into an electromagnetic signal. For a more detailed and technical review of telecoil and induction loop function see Ross (1994).

The use of telephone amplifiers and induction devices presume the user has access to spoken communication, which is not the case for many people who are deaf or who have a severe or profound hearing loss. These people may choose to use telephone typewriters (TTYs), also known as telecommunication devices for the deaf (TDDs). The most common form of contact between TTYs involves the sending and receiving of a typed message. A typed message from a keyboard at one end of the telephone connection is transmitted to a visual display at the other end. To achieve this, a typewriter keyboard is linked to an acoustic transmitter (i.e. a speaker) and receiver (i.e. a microphone). As each different keystroke is made on the TTY transmitting the message, a distinct tone is transmitted via a speaker, through the handset of the telephone and down the telephone line to the TTY at the other end of that line. The TTY receiving the acoustic signal converts it back into orthographic symbols, presented on the electronic display. Some TTYs have built-in printers that will allow a permanent record of the conversation.

Commercially available TTYs do not convert a typed message into spoken language. To achieve this, a relay service must be used. A TTY relay service allows people who do not have the same communication modes to communicate over the telephone via an intermediary who has access to both spoken and written communication. Contact via a relay service is a crucial aspect of independence for people who cannot access spoken telephone messages, but it is limited both by the indirect nature of the conversation (i.e. being passed on by a third party) and the subsequent effect on the speed of the conversation.

The time involved in direct or relayed TTY calls is of concern for many users, particularly when long-distance or international timed calls are involved, and this could be seen to discriminate against TTY users. Recent developments, such as voice carry-over and hearing carry-over (based on the development of combined TTY and voice telephones), help ameliorate this problem as well as providing assistance to people with a range of problems relevant to communication via the telephone.

Voice carry-over and hearing carry-over allow two people who have either expressive or receptive communication difficulties, but not both, to communicate more efficiently and more directly with each other. For example, voice and hearing carry-over are useful when one person has (a) good hearing but unintelligible speech (e.g. a person with a neurologically based expressive communication difficulty) or (b) adequate speech skills but insufficient hearing (e.g. an adult with severe acquired hearing loss). In both of these cases, the benefit of the TTY as a visual communication device is only for communication in one direction. In example (a), the person with the expressive difficulty can hear the other person's spoken message but needs to type his/her response. In example (b) the person with the auditory receptive communication difficulty can speak their message but needs to receive a typed message in response.

As many members of the deaf community have both insufficient hearing to perceive the spoken message on the telephone and insufficient oral speech skills to have their spoken message understood, typewritten TTY to TTY communication and TTY/oral communication via the relay service remain the most effective methods of telecommunication. Members of the deaf community who primarily use sign language will ultimately be better served by video telephones.

**Television and radio devices**

Television and radio devices fall into three broad categories: those that provide suitable volume for an individual watching/listening alone; those that provide suitable volume for an individual while maintaining suitable volume levels for other people; and those that provide a visual representation of the spoken message on the television screen.

The technology used to access the television depends on whether the individual is wearing a hearing aid with a 'T' switch. If a 'T' switch is available, the television signal can be passed to the hearing aid via an electromagnetic induction signal, in a similar manner to that described in relation to telephone use. In this case, the listener uses a neckloop, which plugs in to the headphone socket on the television and carries the electrical signal to wire around the user's neck and thus to the vicinity of the hearing aid. One of the disadvantages reported by users of neckloops is that they are 'hard-wired' to the television by the neckloop and must remove the neckloop each time they get up and move away from their seat. Alternative induction loop devices, such as an induction cushion on which the user sits or an induction antimaccassar hanging on the back of the chair, overcome this. Induction signals are the lowest cost form of electroacoustic access to the television signal.

For persons who do not wear hearing aids or prefer an alternative to induction, the more expensive frequency-modulation (FM) and infrared (IR) devices provide wireless reception of the television signal at a comfortable volume to some form of receiver or headphone worn by the listener. In some cases the receiver can be coupled to a hearing aid. FM and IR systems also provide a higher-quality signal in comparison to induction systems.

An additional television device includes a radio that picks up the acoustic signal from the television. This allows the user to listen via headphones with fully independent volume control, while others can set the volume on the television at a desirable level. The drawback of these devices is their inability to work with video-recorded programmes, which do not rely on the signal transmitted directly from the television station.

Another alternative is visual display of the speech signal. Subtitled (also known as captioned) television programmes may be accessed via a decoder, which presents on the screen an abridged typewritten version of the spoken content. A distinction can be drawn between open captions, which are available without special equipment and are often seen on foreign language films, and closed captions, which are accessed only via a decoder. Although decoders are easily connected to the television, they are not always easily tuned or operated. Ease of operation should be considered before purchase.

## Alarm devices

In the home situation the three most common reasons for requiring an alarm are: (a) hearing the doorbell, (b) awaking to bedside alarms and (c) perceiving cries from babies and very young children (telephone alarms are discussed earlier in this chapter). The alerting signal may be auditory, visual, vibratory or some combination of these. The benefit of alarm devices is that they alert the individual at a distance from the source of the alarm signal and can present the signal via a sensory modality other than hearing.

Alarms are also required in the work environment for safety and other purposes. Flashing-light emergency alarms placed in the individual's field of vision can replace the auditory alarm commonly used as a warning signal for groups of people. A second option is the use of vibrating personal pagers, preferably directly connected to the alarm system.

## General communication devices

Aside from hearing aids, which have already been discussed, general communication devices include individual and group amplification devices, and those designed for specific environments (for example, amplified stethoscopes for doctors, nurses and other health practitioners). General communication devices are chosen for their ability to provide more effective communication in a range of frequently encountered situations. Briefly, these devices provide assistance in:

- amplifying many voices at once (e.g. in meetings, seminars, etc.);
- amplifying one voice for many listeners (e.g. a teacher's voice in a classroom of children with hearing impairment);

- amplifying a voice over substantial background noise (e.g. in a car or other vehicle).

Many of these devices require hearing aids, usually aids with a 'T' switch. The devices amplifying to many listeners commonly rely on IR or radio-frequency (particularly FM) signal transmission because of the freedom to have many receivers for the one signal source. However, in some circumstances (especially when FM systems are being used in class-rooms) it is necessary to limit the range of signal transmission to prevent systems being used in the vicinity of each other, causing interference. Ross (1994) gives a very detailed description of FM systems in class-rooms and other educational settings.

## Criteria for selecting ALDs

Unlike hearing aids, most ALDs are not designed to provide frequency-specific amplification. However, the amplification characteristics of ALDs are thought by some experts to be an important criterion for choosing ALDs. Palmer (1992), and Lesner and Klingler (1995), for example, advocate a detailed acoustical assessment of ALDs prior to supply. The rationale given for such an assessment is that the match between the acoustic characteristics of the ALD and the client's hearing levels should be as close as possible with respect to frequency response and maximum power output. The latter is especially important if we do not wish to exceed the individual's discomfort level or induce further hearing loss because of very high-intensity output. Given a thorough analysis of acoustical characteristics, the device can be recommended without the client having prior hands-on experience of it. This is useful, because in many clinics it is not always possible to have a full range of demonstration devices.

An alternative view is that as ALDs are situation-specific devices, the preferred method of selection is trial and comparison in the relevant situations. Given this approach, the clinician needs only a general sense of the amplification characteristics of the device prior to a carefully conducted clinical trial. This view assumes that the clinician has a range of devices to demonstrate, can advise of another facility with a devices display or has a sufficient knowledge of device characteristics to recommend one or two particular ALDs for purchase and trial.

In addition to the acoustic characteristics of ALDs and the client's clinical trial of them, other factors to be considered when selecting particular devices include:

- the clients' manual dexterity, alertness and vision levels;
- cost of the device, its installation and maintenance;
- client preference;

- portability of the device;
- manner of signal transmission.

Alongside these factors it is important to consider the regular communication partners' communication skills, needs, understanding and ability to use the devices. In much aural rehabilitation therapy there is increasing emphasis on communication partners and the role they play in successful interaction.

A further important consideration in selecting a particular ALD is its compatibility with hearing aid(s). The two common methods by which ALDs can pass signals from the environment to hearing aids are induction (i.e. via a telecoil) and direct audio input (i.e. via direct electric connection with the hearing aid). There are benefits and limitations associated with each method.

Induction is included in most BTE hearing aids but usually has to be specifically ordered for ITE aids. ITC and CIC hearing aids are often too small to contain an induction coil. The advantages of induction are that it does not usually require a direct connection with the hearing aid and is relatively inexpensive. The disadvantages of induction are its poor high-frequency response characteristics and the fact that the induction/electromagnetic signal has to compete with other random electromagnetic 'noise'. Direct audio input has the great advantage that no other unwanted signal competes with the input signal coming from the ALD. However, direct audio input is limited by the relatively small range of hearing aids in which it is available.

Many clients obtain their hearing aid(s) and their ALD(s) at different times and thus compatibility of the two technologies may not have been considered. Additionally, many people who enquire about ALDs have not had detailed hearing assessments or, having had them, do not present with their audiogram. Hence it may be necessary to arrange an audiological review of the client's current situation to achieve the best balance between further expenditure and the ability to meet communication needs.

In our experience, once close scrutiny is made of the environment in which the person wishes to use an ALD, the range of devices that may be appropriate commonly narrows to a choice of two or maybe three devices, which are then trialed.

It is not always possible to collect, store and maintain a selection of ALDs, because of space, staffing, financial and other constraints. To overcome these difficulties, Dr Catherine Palmer and colleagues at the University of Pittsburgh have developed a computer-generated Assistive Listening Devices Selection Process. The program uses the application 'Hypercard' and a personal computer. A series of questions about various listening situations is presented to the client on the computer screen. These questions assess the degree of communicative difficulty in those situations, and the answers provided indicate the general class of devices required (e.g. television or telephone amplifiers or door alarms) and the specific devices and models that may be suitable. In situations where it is difficult to arrange a hands-on trial for clients this method has much merit.

## Measuring outcomes of ALD use

We suggest that ALD use is successful when (a) the client is comfortable with and able to use the device independently or with support, (b) the client perceives that it is of assistance, and (c) some numerical measure of change in listening experience has been documented. Importantly, successful device use depends on the client's ability to use the device well *in the situation for which it is intended*.

Indicators of client comfort and ability to use the device are generally available from client report and/or the reports of frequent communication partners. The user's perception of the success of the device may be accessed by using some of the many self-assessment of hearing-handicap scales, either in their original form or adapted to reflect the specific nature of ALDs. Of particular interest is the Client Orientated Scale of Improvement (COSI) (Dillon, James & Ginnis, 1997). This scale is simple to administer. It is based on the client's perception of his/her needs and the benefit derived from intervention in meeting those needs.

A numerical measure of the client's daily listening routine before and after device purchase may be indicated by, for example, the number of times a day that the client initiates telephone calls. A well-chosen television device may increase the number of hours of viewing or increase the number of hours of viewing with other people. A successfully used conference microphone may allow greater participation in/attendance at meetings or social events. The disadvantage of such numerical assessments is that they are time-consuming. However, they have a place in informing both client and clinician of the results of using an ALD.

## Training in the use of ALDs

Some devices can be used with little or no supportive training, whereas others require intensive education in their use. Those clients who require significant clinical support are most likely to be those who also need to apply communication tactics (the use of situational context, manipulation of the physical environment, choice of appropriate seating positions, use of questions designed to give most information, and so on) and to enlist the help of their communication partners in developing clear conversational behaviours. An example is the client who has a severe or profound hearing loss and uses telephone devices. One of the most well-developed training systems for ALD support is Erber's (1985) telephone training method. The telephone is particularly difficult for persons with significant hearing loss because of the absence of visual cues and the limited frequency-range of the speech signal received over the telephone line (usually reported to be between 300 Hz and 3000 Hz). The amount of perceptual information available to the hearing-impaired listener is therefore reduced over and above that imposed by the hearing loss.

## Tactile aids

Tactile aids are devices that provide some speech information through stimulation of the kinaesthetic system. Tactile aids capture auditory speech signals, process them and deliver a signal to the individual's skin surface, most commonly on the wrist or hands. There are other, more natural, means of using the sense of touch to gain speech information, such as the Tadoma method (Alcorn, 1932; Reed, 1995) and Tactiling (Soderlund, 1995), but these are not discussed in the present chapter.

Tactile aids utilise either vibrotactile or electrotactile stimulation. Vibrotactile devices stimulate the sense receptors in the dermis by pressure vibration. There are a number of different receptor systems that mediate these tactile sensations (Bolanowski et al., 1988; Verrillo & Gescheider, 1992). Electrotactile devices aim to stimulate the nerve fibres rather than the sense receptors. Electrical stimulation of the nerve fibres under the skin seems to be more comfortable than stimulation of nerve fibres in the skin (Blamey & Clark, 1987; Alcantara et al., 1990).

Tactile aids may be single channel or multichannel, and may employ various speech-encoding strategies. The simplest wearable tactile aids utilise the amplitude envelope of the speech signal and thus provide time and intensity cues to a single transducer. Others may provide speech envelope information to two transducers, one dealing with low frequencies and one with high frequencies. The most promising approach now seems to be with multichannel electrotactile aids, such as the Tickle Talker developed at the University of Melbourne (Blamey & Clark, 1985). The Tickle Talker obtains acoustic information from an ear-level microphone. This signal is fed to an integrated speech processor/stimulator, and then to a wrist-mounted handset with leads to electrodes mounted in rings worn on the fingers. Although it appears that cochlear implants provide superior speech perception performance where post-lingually deafened individuals are concerned, the Tickle Talker may provide benefits similar to cochlear implants in individuals who are prelingually deaf (Blamey & Cowan, 1992). Devices such as the Tickle Talker also cost much less than cochlear implants.

Proctor (1995) provides a useful table summarising 30 studies, from 1926 to 1993, of deaf children's speech perception and production using various tactile devices. Proctor concludes that 'there is consensus, internationally, that a tactile device can improve lipreading and speech perception as well as improve voice quality and selected features of speech production for profoundly deaf children' (Proctor, 1995, p. 133). Of particular interest to the speech-language therapist are the findings that the use of tactile aids can increase vocalisation (Neate, 1972; Goldstein & Stark, 1976), improve production of stress patterns in speech (Stratton, 1974; Shelly & Hansen, 1983), help children produce closer approximations of correct consonant production (Oller et al., 1986) and reduce the incidence of abnormal articulation habits, such as intrusive schwa and bilabial clicks. Bench (1992a) asserts that vibrotactile devices 'can compete with cochlear implants if they are developed as wearable communication devices' (p. 50). His review concluded that tactile aids are useful in distinguishing speech feature contrasts, especially at the segmental level. In general, multichannel devices are clearly superior to single-channel devices. For more detail about tactile devices, see Summers (1992) and Weisenberger (1995).

## Cochlear implants

'The cochlear implant is an electronic device, part of which is surgically implanted in the ear and part of which is worn externally like a hearing aid. It produces an electrical stimulus that bypasses the damaged or missing hair cells in profound sensorineural hearing loss and directly stimulates the remaining auditory neural elements' (House & Berliner (1991, p. 9). Cochlear implant systems have an external microphone to pick up sound, an external speech processor to deal with the signal electronically and an external transmitter coil that sends the processed signal through the skin to an internal receiver and electrode(s).

Cochlear implants vary in the type and position of electrodes, the number of channels used to deliver the signal, the ways in which the speech signal is treated and the method of stimulation. Figure 7.2 illustrates a multichannel cochlear implant system. New developments mean that the external speech processor will soon be available housed in the same behind-the-ear case as the microphone, further reducing the size of the system.

Cochlear implants require major surgery, extensive pre-operative assessment and lengthy postoperative adjustments and rehabilitation support.

### Candidates for cochlear implants

Persons with bilateral profound or total hearing loss who cannot benefit from hearing-aid amplification or tactile devices and who wish to receive speech information via a sense of audition, are potential candidates for cochlear implants. Recently it has been suggested that persons with severe hearing losses (rather than profound or total) may also be appropriate candidates for cochlear implants. Persons who have benefited from cochlear implants include both postlingually and prelingually deafened adults and children.

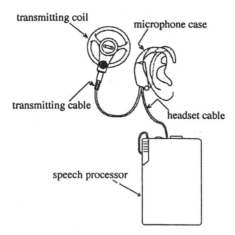

transmitting coil

microphone case

transmitting cable

headset cable

speech processor

**Figure 7.2:** Schematic diagram of external components of a multichannel cochlear implant system. Reproduced and adapted with permission from Cochlear Ltd.

The cochlear implant procedure is not reversible and hearing aids cannot be used in an implanted ear. Therefore selection for cochlear implant surgery is an extremely important decision. A basic discussion of the medical criteria for cochlear implant eligibility is provided by Gray (1991) and a detailed discussion of some assessment procedures is given by Abbas and Brown (1991). Essentially, the client must have a clear cochlear duct to permit insertion of the electrode array, an auditory pathway that is responsive to electrical stimulation and a state of health sufficient to cope with a major operation. Additionally, it is important that the client's motivation and expectations are assessed, and that a well-developed rehabilitation programme is available to assess and support the potential implantee.

Many persons who have been accepted into implant programmes have been deafened by progressive hearing loss, trauma or disease, such as meningitis. Therefore speech-language therapists whose caseloads include clients with profound or total hearing loss from these causes may usefully refer to a cochlear implant centre for evaluation. It has recently been suggested that some persons who have become deaf through surgical removal of bilateral acoustic Schwannoma (see Chapter 3) may prove to be candidates for cochlear implants provided that the auditory nerve has been preserved (Vrabec et al., 1995).

The majority of cochlear implants have involved postlingually deafened adults, but implants have now been provided for many children with post- and prelingual deafness. The age at implant is an important consideration in cases of prelingual deafness. Ramsden and Graham (1995) suggest that this should be as soon as the child can be reliably diagnosed as being totally deaf, which is generally around the age of 2 years. Beyond the age of 7 years the auditory pathways tend to lose plasticity and hence learning to use sound after that age can be assumed to be much more difficult.

Post-implant improvement on some speech perception tests (such as closed and open set word recognition tasks) may be evident in children who are postlingually deafened after about 6 months of cochlear implant use, while children who are prelingually deaf may require a longer period of implant use before significant improvements are seen (Fryauf-Bertschy et al., 1992).

Individuals whose residual hearing fluctuates may require special monitoring after implantation to optimise the result (Skinner et al., 1995).

Implantation of elderly adults can reportedly yield successful results (Kelsall, Shallop & Burnelli, 1995). When cochlear implantation is not a suitable option in elderly people, tactile aids may be effective (Soderlund, 1995), provided the kinaesthetic system remains sufficiently receptive (skin sensitivity can decline with increasing age; Verrillo, 1979, 1982).

The degree of benefit from a cochlear implant is not easily predicted. A range of physical and other variables appear to contribute to the outcome (Cooper, 1991). However, individuals with postlingual deafness tend to progress more rapidly than those with prelingual deafness. The assessment for, design of and rehabilitation after cochlear implantation are developing very rapidly. It is anticipated that in future the range of people who can benefit from this technology will significantly increase.

The speech-language therapist has an important role in the cochlear implant team (Dornan & Del Dot, 1996; Moore, 1996). Voice and articulation therapy, and assistance in the development of speech-reading (see Chapter 8) and auditory skills are key contributions of the speech-language therapist. For excellent descriptions of the clinical role played by speech-language therapists with cochlear implantees, including case descriptions, see Everingham (1996) and Moore (1996)

# Tinnitus maskers and desensitisation devices

Persons who have tinnitus or noises in the head (see Chapter 3) may also have hearing loss of a level that requires the use of hearing aids. In such cases use of hearing aid(s) may alleviate the tinnitus problem because the hearing aids provide amplified speech and environmental sounds, which then occupy the user's attention. In cases where a tinnitus sufferer does not require hearing aids for communication, tinnitus maskers or desensitisation devices may help.

Tinnitus maskers and densensitisation devices look very much like hearing aids, and are available in ITC, ITE or BTE styles. Maskers produce a broad band noise (white noise), the level of which is controlled by the user. The aim is to 'mask' or overwhelm the tinnitus with the white noise. For some people this technique appears to provide relief, although the proportion of cases for whom successful relief is achieved appears relatively small, and there is discussion as to whether the effect is due to the masker itself, the process of counselling and support that accompanies fitting of a masker, or the sense of control the user develops.

Tinnitus maskers may work because: the white noise is a more pleasant sound than the tinnitus; the white noise is a fairly monotonous external sound and therefore more easily ignored than the tinnitus; the user can control what they are perceiving; or some combination of these factors (Tyler & Baker, 1983; Vernon, 1987; Vernon, Greist, & Press, 1990). They may be combined with hearing-aid functions, so that the user is wearing a combined hearing aid-masker.

Tinnitus desensitisation devices also produce white noise, but the noise is at a very low level. The aim is not to overwhelm the tinnitus, but to subject the cochlea to a constant low level of stimulation. It is proposed that this low-level stimulation will have a neurophysiological effect that will eventually reduce the awareness of the tinnitus (Jastreboff & Hazell, 1993).

The degree to which tinnitus maskers and/or desensitisation devices assist and the mechanisms involved in achieving client improvement by these and other therapeutic means are complex areas that are the subject of much ongoing research (see for example, Dineen, Doyle & Bench, 1997b).

## Summary of key points

The choice of technology for individual clients ideally follows an examination of the client's real-life communication needs and a discussion of the client's preferences and resources. Appropriately fitted hearing aids can assist even profoundly hearing-impaired clients. The range of options in modern hearing aids is very large. Programmable and digital aids provide great flexibility and precision in hearing-aid fitting, but are more expensive than conventional hearing aids. The speech-language therapist can benefit by a knowledge of basic hearing-aid terminology. Assistive listening devices (ALDs) are available to help with hearing telephone rings, conversation, television, radio and alarms. ALDs may be used independent of, or in conjunction with, hearing aids. The compatibility of various ALDs with the individual client's hearing aids is important. Telephone typewriters (TTYs) allow direct or relayed telephone communication for persons who have receptive and/or expressive problems that preclude the use of the telephone via hearing aids or via other ALDs. Expert assistance in the selection of devices and training in their use are important to successful outcomes in ALD therapy. Tactile aids provide stimulation of the kinaesthetic system. Multichannel electrotactile aids appear particularly useful in delivering aspects of the speech signal to individuals who cannot benefit from hearing aids. Cochlear implants provide direct electrical stimulation of the auditory nerve for individuals with profound or total bilateral hearing loss who are unable to benefit from hearing aids. Selection for cochlear implant surgery follows intensive assessment of the individual's auditory system, general health, motivation and expectations. Tinnitus maskers or desensitisation devices may assist some people with distressing tinnitus. Given the rapid advances in technology related to hearing loss, the speech-language therapist is advised to establish contacts with appropriate centres who may advise on technical options as they become available.

## Further reading

Garstecki DC (1994) Assistive devices for the hearing-impaired. In Gagné J-P, Tye-Murray N (Eds) Research in audiological rehabilitation: current trends and future directions. Journal of the Academy of Rehabilitative Audiology (Monograph Supplement) 27: 113–32. (Reviews practice in evaluating for and dispensing of devices, and discusses the need for research addressing the performance characteristics of devices.)

Lesner SA, Klingler MS (1995) Considerations in establishing an optimum assistive listening devices center. Journal of the Academy of Rehabilitative Audiology 28: 60–7. (Describes the key features of a dedicated ALD room, including furnishings as well as technical features, with special reference to the devices room at the University of Akron, Ohio.)

Plant G, Spens K-E (Eds) (1995) Profound deafness and speech communication. London: Whurr Publishers. (About a quarter of this book deals with cochlear implants, detailing in a readable fashion the research into speech perception and production in cochlear implantees. Very good for readers who want a reasonable degree of detail. Other major sections deal with tactile aids, speech perception testing, speech production and computer-based training.)

Ross M (Ed.) (1994) Communication access for persons with hearing loss: compliance with the Americans with Disabilities Act. Baltimore: York Press. (Excellent descriptions of a range of large-space listening systems, personal listening systems and telecommunication devices. Also provides information on appropriate technology and communication approaches for persons with both vision and hearing loss. Especially relevant for US clinicians but widely applicable.)

Summers IR (Ed.) (1992) Tactile aids for the hearing impaired. London: Whurr Publishers. (A comprehensive coverage of tactile aids, their development, operation and function as providers of speech information. Includes some assessment of commercially available devices.)

# Chapter 8
# Speech-reading

JOHN BENCH, NICOLA DALY, CHRISTOPHER LIND AND
JANET DOYLE

This chapter considers some of the basic issues in speech-reading, including sociolinguistic aspects in relation to English language and Western culture. The place of speech-reading in child and adult aural rehabilitation is also outlined. The term 'speech-reading' is used in preference to the commonly used 'lip-reading', because there is more to the processing of visual speech than simply watching the talker's lips. For example, the talker's face, gestures and body posture may be monitored as well as the lips. Additionally, this chapter uses the term speech-reading to indicate a listener's understanding for speech through a combination of visual and auditory inputs, even when auditory imput is reduced, as in hearing loss. The term can also be used to refer to purely visual monitoring of the talker with the listener's use of residual hearing considered separately. This second definition is not used in this chapter.

## Principles

1. *Virtually every sighted person uses speech-reading at times to help in understanding speech.* Speech-reading is not the sole preserve of severely hearing-impaired or profoundly deaf people. For example, sighted children use visual cues in their development of speech perception (Dodd, 1987). Adults with normal hearing also find it easier to follow someone's speech if they can see the person's face. This becomes particularly obvious in a noisy environment. Hence to some extent the teaching of speech-reading may actually be a matter of helping people develop an awareness of an existing skill, rather than training in a new one.
2. *Less than half of speech sounds can be seen on the lips.* Therefore it is not possible to follow everything a person says by simply recognising sounds on the lips. Speech-reading by visual cues alone is an imperfect means of communication.

3. *Speech-reading and (residual) hearing are, to a degree, complementary*. Those speech sounds that cannot be seen on the lips tend to be the easiest speech sounds to hear. Speech-readers will usually benefit by using all of the visual and auditory cues available to them.
4. *Knowledge of the language, a willingness to guess when unsure, good general knowledge and awareness of context help to make for good speech-reading*. These attributes compensate in part for the deficiencies noted in principle 2. Knowledge about the possible sounds, words and sentences in a language can help combat the fact that many sounds cannot be seen, and a good general knowledge makes guessing more likely to be correct. This knowledge is only useful, however, when the speech-reader is willing to risk guessing. Contextual information, which provides much of the basis for this guessing, is available also from non-linguistic sources, including the physical and social environment, the talker's face, gestures and body language.

## Introduction

'Why can I hear better when I'm wearing my glasses?', asked a nearsighted woman in our clinic. What she did not realise was that, besides her myopia, she also had a mild hearing impairment, which impaired her hearing for speech except in quiet conditions. Her glasses allowed her to see her conversational partners' faces more clearly, and hence to speech-read them, although she was not aware that she was doing so.

This anecdote illustrates an important point. When it is difficult to understand speech because of hearing problems, whether caused by internal factors such as hearing impairment or external factors such as background noise, or both, we tend to monitor the talker's face to augment our hearing. Even people whose hearing is within normal limits generally use speech-reading in noisy situations (Summerfield, 1983). Their speech-reading may not be very sophisticated. It may amount to little more than picking up gross speech-timing cues from the talker's lip movements, but even such crude information helps in following speech when hearing alone is insufficient. To consider this situation in another way, the presence of background noise produces a virtual hearing loss in normally hearing people. As a result, they become as though hearing impaired and can then follow a talker better by combining speech-reading with their situationally reduced hearing. Sumby and Pollack (1954) estimated this benefit to speech reception with speech-reading is equivalent to improving the signal-to-noise ratio by 15 dB. There are at least four possible explanations for this effect (Bench, 1992a, p. 68). First, at the phonemic level, some acoustic cues (especially for place of articulation, e.g. /p/, /b/, see below) are transient and of low amplitude (volume), while the accompanying visual cues are relatively easily perceived. (When seen, speech sounds are commonly referred to as 'visemes', by analogy with 'phonemes'.) Second, speech-reading assists in reinforcing the perception of segmental information. Third, speech-reading directs the attention of the hearer to the talker rather than the noise. Finally, speech-reading enables the hearer to assimilate visual contextual information from talker characteristics and the surroundings.

Speech-reading obviously involves at least two participants, a talker who speaks the message and a speech-reader who receives it. That there are these two types of participant 'subjects' considerably increases the complexities of experimental design in research in speech-reading, because there will be one set of possible variables associated with the talker (e.g. Berger, 1972, pp. 141–150; Lesner & Kricos, 1981; Kricos & Lesner, 1982; Lesner, 1988; Demorest & Bernstein, 1992) and another set of possible variables associated with the speech-reader (e.g. Berger, 1972, pp. 109–139; Conrad, 1979, pp 176–203; Fletcher, 1987; Gailey, 1987, pp. 115–137; Demorest & Bernstein, 1992). To facilitate the speech-reading of a message, the talker and speech-reader may need to share some of these variables, such as a common language and familiarity with the topic of the message, but not necessarily others, such as visual acuity or use of facial expression. Also, variables associated with the talker may interact with variables associated with the receiver, because different talker characteristics are likely to interact differently with different speech-reader characteristics. Given these natural complexities in speech-reading in everyday spoken interaction, and the fact that many research studies reported in the literature may not have addressed the issue of representativeness of the talker(s) selected (Daly, Bench & Chappell, 1996a), the results of some studies must be considered indicative rather than representative (see section below on talker effects in speech-reading).

## Hearing speech by eye

It is often said that speech-reading is like hearing speech by eye rather than by ear (Bench, 1992, p. 66). In the clinic, hearing-impaired clients may report having 'heard' a successfully perceived sentence presented to them visually, without auditory cues. In the research laboratory the 'McGurk effect' illustrates this correspondence in a dramatic way. McGurk and MacDonald (1976) found that hearing 'ba' while seeing a videorecorded 'ga' produced by the talker's lips produced the illusory percept 'da'. There was thus a fusion, where what was perceived shared the phonological features of the phoneme (heard) and viseme (seen), producing a new consonant. The subject's perception is that of hearing, not seeing, the illusory syllable. This illusion provides strong evidence that the same perceptual system processes both auditory and visual aspects of spoken syllables.

Further, speech-reading is analogous to reading. Thus, hearing by eye when speech-reading resembles hearing written material by eye when reading (Williams, 1982). The common feature shared by speech-reading, reading and hearing is inner speech or subvocal speech, the language we use for thought (Conrad, 1979). Whether material is speech-read, read or heard, it is processed by an auditory or articulatory code into inner speech. Failure to acquire inner speech results in poor speech-reading performance. This conclusion explains why people who become deafened after acquiring speech and language via hearing are usually better speech-readers than those people who have been deaf from birth (Conrad, 1979), although the former do not generally compensate for their adventitious hearing loss by becoming better speech-readers (Lyxell & Rönnberg, 1989; Rönnberg, 1990). Persons born deaf (i.e. unable to use audition as a primary means of communication, which includes many persons with hearing losses in excess of 90 dB), despite modern treatments and the provision of sophisticated hearing aids, are at a severe disadvantage in acquiring oral language and, consequently, inner speech. Clinical experience shows that some of the best speech-readers seem to be those people who have developed a hearing loss during their language-learning years and whose degree of loss is sufficient to cause reliance on visual information to assist development of language skills, yet not so severe as to render them unable to use audition as a significant part of communication.

## Visibility of speech

Speech is produced by moving or articulating the vocal folds, jaw, soft palate, tongue and lips to modulate an airstream from the lungs. Such movements or articulations may be visible, permitting speech-reading. Often, however, they are not visible and cannot be speech-read. Speech-reading alone is a weak means of understanding speech, because speech elements vary in their visibility. Rather more than half of the speech sounds are not visible on the lips. Thus, although speech elements may be seen fairly readily if their perception relies on movements of the lips, jaw and teeth, and tongue, it is all but impossible to perceive the many features that depend on voicing and intonation. Other speech elements can easily be detected on the lips but are virtually impossible to distinguish from the articulatory movements of other elements (for example, /b/, /m/ and /p/). A similar problem occurs with words, sentences or other connected speech because more words look similar when speech-read (e.g. 'do' versus 'to'; 'give' versus 'gave') than sound alike when heard. It is therefore fortunate that auditory information often supplies what cannot be seen on the lips, thus complementing speech-reading. For example, most vowels are difficult to distinguish when speech-read in running speech, but the distinctions are relatively easy to hear. Hence, a combination of speech-reading and residual hearing usually proves better than either one alone.

Speech sounds are conventionally separated into vowels and consonants, both of which can be grouped in various ways (e.g. Jeffers &
Barley, 1971; Markides, 1983; Kaplan, Bally & Garretson, 1987; Jackson,
1988). Although speech-reading is not simply a matter of recognising
particular speech sounds, a brief discussion of individual speech sounds
follows for reference.

Vowels involve an unimpeded flow of air from the vocal chords
through the vocal tract. They tend to be higher in intensity, lower in
pitch and longer in duration than consonants. Overall, they are easier to
hear than consonants, but are less easy to see. Besides differences in
modulating the frequency of vibration of the vocal folds, differences in
tongue and lip position are mainly responsible for the differences
between vowels. Thus the tongue may be elevated in the front of the
mouth (e.g. /i/ as in 'see') or in the rear of the mouth (e.g. /u/ as in
'shoe'). A central tongue position produces the vowel in 'curve' or 'bus'.
The mouth opening can be wide (as in 'cat') or narrow (as in 'tea').

In contrast to vowels, consonants involve some impediment to the
flow of air through the vocal tract using the teeth, tongue and/or lips.
Many consonants are weaker in intensity, higher in pitch and shorter in
duration than vowels. They are therefore usually more difficult to hear
than the vowels, but tend to be more important for conveying meaning.
Consonants are conventionally classified in groups by place of articulation, manner of articulation and voicing.

Place is the region of the mouth where the consonant is produced.
Thus, /b/, /p/, /m/ and /w/ are produced at the front of the mouth and are
easily seen (but the first three are not easily distinguished). Also
produced at the front are /f/ and /v/, involving the lips and teeth. Many
consonants are made in the centre of the mouth and are partly visible.
They mainly involve the tongue and soft palate, as in /t/, /d/, /l/ and /s/. A
smaller number of speech sounds, such as /g/ and /h/, are produced at
the back of the mouth and are virtually impossible to see.

Manner, refers to the way in which the air flow is impeded to produce
a consonant. For example, the consonants that involve stopping the
airflow momentarily (/p/, /b/, /t/, /d/, /k/, /g/) are known as stops. Those
consonants that send the airflow through the nasal passage (/m/, /n/,
/ng/) are known as nasals. Other commonly used labels to describe
manner are fricatives, affricates, laterals and glides.

Voicing distinguishes consonants according to whether vibrations of
the vocal folds are involved or not. Thus /v/ is voiced whereas /f/ is
unvoiced. All vowels in English are voiced. The voiced/unvoiced distinction in consonants cannot be seen.

In addition to the fact that a large proportion of visemes cannot be
seen, or are only imperfectly seen, some visemes are characterised by
such small differences that, for practical purposes and especially in the
fast flow of running speech, they are identical. For example, 'bay' looks

the same as 'may'. Such viseme pairs are known as homophenes. Knowledge of which visemes are homophenous is of value in speech-reading, because mistaken perception of, for example, 'bay' as 'may' can be subsequently corrected if the mistake is realised from the ensuing context of the message, as often it can be.

From the 'bay' versus 'may' examples, it will be appreciated that homophony can occur at the word level and at the visemic level. Unfortunately for speech-readers, a large proportion of English words are homophenous. Estimates vary, but probably around 50 per cent of English words in everyday conversations are homophenous (Nitchie, 1915; Berger, 1972).

## What makes for good speech-reading?

Success in speech-reading is not mainly a matter of correctly detecting and recognising such visemic structure of visible speech as can be seen; there is much more to good speech-reading than the accurate processing of visemes. Apart from a few exclamations and interjections (e.g. 'Oh!'; 'Eh?'), speech sounds rarely occur in isolation. In natural, connected speech, the sounds that make up words are run into one another, so that the end of one word is run into the start of the next word. The result is that, even as a speech sound is being made, it is being shaped to produce the next speech sound in sequence. This anticipatory shaping means that 'o' as part of the word 'open' is articulated differently from 'Oh!' produced in isolation. This phenomenon is known as coarticulation. It affects speech-reading as well as hearing, so that teaching people to improve their speech-reading by working only on individual visemes is to take a limited and misleading view of what is involved in speech-reading. Indeed, it is very unlikely that segment-by-segment perception of continuous speech occurs (Berger, 1970). Further, speech-reading is time-pressured. Natural speech is so fast and complex that the eye cannot follow all the lip, mouth-opening, tongue and jaw movements as they are produced, even though vision has a wide dynamic range and can resolve time differences as fine as 20 ms (Geldard, 1972). So some speech movements will necessarily be missed (Kaplan, Bally & Garretson, 1987).

Other aspects of speech affect speech-readability, such as speech rate, lip movement and degree of mouth opening, talker age and gender, visibility of the talker, familiarity with the talker's speech style, and so on. These aspects are considered later in this chapter.

Although the information carried by visible speech is poor, a speech-reader with sufficient vision, a good knowledge of the language, a good appreciation of the context of the message and a good general knowledge can usually augment most of the partial information received by speech-reading alone. A good speech-reader will also make use of further clues from the physical background and from the personal characteristics of the talker, such as gender, age, body movement, posture and facial expression. For example, a frown, nodding or shaking of the head, or a raised hand in a classroom (Markides, 1983, p. 167) convey clear information. The talker's dress may provide helpful context cues, as when the talker wears a recognised uniform or other 'dress for the job'. Thus any non-verbal and social cues may be used by the speech-reader to provide additional information about the message from the talker. Rönnberg (1995) expressed the situation as involving abilities in the cognitive architecture underlying speech-reading skill and the effectiveness of the speech-reader in capitalising on social and contextual constraints, as well as the effectiveness of the cognitive system in receiving and processing the speech signal.

Drawing on the results of several experiments, Rönnberg went on to specify three direct and three indirect predictors of (sentence-based) speech-reading ability, common to hearing-impaired and normally hearing speech-readers. Direct predictors are: decoding ability when the speech signal initiates lexical activity via a phonological access route (cf. inner speech); information-processing speed (e.g. speed of lexical access); and guessing (verbal inference-making) in situations where the contextual information is relatively low. Indirect predictors are: visual-evoked potential measures; working memory (reading span); and the ability to solve antonyms and synonyms (related to guessing). Speech-reading is therefore a multicomponent activity. Phonology was thought to play an important, if low-level, role in speech-reading because, unless the speech-read information is phonologically coded in working memory, it does not obtain access to the lexicon or other implicit knowledge of likely speech content. On the other hand, high speech-reading ability was found to depend on higher-order cognitive functions, such as complex verbal working memory, rather than such lower-order functions as decoding and processing speed. A high-capacity working memory was thought to assist in speech-reading by freeing capacity for predicting the parts of the message to come next, and by maintaining previous stimuli in an active condition to allow for their re-interpretation in the light of new information.

## Talker effects in speech-reading

It has already been noted that two parties are involved in the process of speech-reading: the speech-reader and the talker. In aural rehabilitation the emphasis is often on helping the speech-reader to improve their speech-reading skills. However, it is important for the speech-language therapist to be aware that the talker also has an effect on the 'success' of the speech-reading interaction. Of course the therapist cannot work with every talker that a speech-reader may encounter, but it may at least be possible to work with the frequent communication partner(s) of the speech-reader. The therapist may also wish to discuss with the speech-reader, the idea that talkers vary in how easy they are to speech-read. It is important for the speech-reader to realise that responsibility for the success of any interaction does not rest with them alone. This section deals with the effect of the talker on the speech-reading process. In particular the visual intelligibility of talkers (how easy or difficult a talker is to speech-read) will be considered.

Many speech-reading texts have discussed the contribution made by the talker to speech-reading efficiency (Jeffers & Barley, 1971; Berger, 1972; Kaplan, Bally, & Garretson, 1987). These texts generally advise that a talker may improve their visual intelligibility by speaking more slowly than normal and by using clear articulation and facial expression. However, when these three speech behaviours have been investigated in research studies, results have not consistently supported the advice given by speech-reading texts. It has been suggested that one of the main reasons for this is the fact that most of these studies based their results on only one talker (Daly, Bench, & Chappell, 1996a).

Because individual talkers vary in visual intelligibility, the extent to which increased lip movement, facial expression or decreased speed of speech improves visual intelligibility is likely to vary between talkers. For example, if a talker uses little lip movement, instruction to increase lip movement may well result in increased visual intelligibility. By contrast, if a talker already uses clear lip movement, using more may make their speaking style unnaturally exaggerated and thus decrease visual intelligibility.

Studies by Kricos and Lesner (1982, 1985) have shown that the visual intelligibility of talkers varies considerably. In both studies, the visual intelligibility of female talkers was shown to be related to the number and nature of consonant visemes used by the talkers. The larger the number of distinct consonant visemes used by talkers, the higher the speech-reading scores attained by speech-readers.

Daly, Bench and Chappell (1996a) conducted a study of what constituted visual intelligibility in talkers presenting sentences on videotape. They found that two factors influenced the visual intelligibility of the 24 talkers: a 'speed' factor and a 'tongue' factor. As speed of speech decreased, teeth visibility, lip rounding and mouth opening increased, and the visual intelligibility of the talkers also increased. Thus it appears that slow speech affects speech in such a way as to make it more visually intelligible. Visible tongue movement was not affected by speed of speech. However, it was shown that visible tongue movement was strongly correlated with visual intelligibility: as visible tongue movement increased, the visual intelligibility of talkers increased. Therefore the speech-language therapist attempting to improve the visual intelligibility of a talker may have success by concentrating on slowing the speed of speech and increasing the visibility of tongue movements. Work has yet to be done to establish the useful limits of these behaviours.

Gagné et al. (1994) investigated the effect of 'clear' speech on the auditory, visual and audiovisual perception of individual words presented by ten Caucasian female adults. Results suggested that talkers' speech intelligibility in each of the three modes were not related, i.e. a talker whose auditory speech was clear did not necessarily have clear visual speech. Several talkers produced a negative clear speech effect in the visual mode (i.e. the speech-reading score for their 'clear' recording was worse than the speech-reading score for their 'normal' recording). This phenomenon suggested that some talkers did not know how to improve the intelligibility of their speech. It is possible that talkers interpreted the instruction to speak clearly in auditory terms only, and in the process of emphasising articulation for auditory clarity, visual clarity was distorted. Apparently, although it is sufficient simply to ask some talkers to speak clearly, for other talkers it may be necessary to make specific suggestions to improve the clarity of their visual speech. In summary, the hearing impaired speech-reader may: (a) rely on the talker's awareness of the communicative environment and the ability to make the necessary changes to his/her speech or (b) direct the talker to alter his/her speech characteristics in response to the environmental conditions. Either way, the person with an acquired hearing loss should recognise the role the talker has to play in tailoring their message to particular communicative circumstances.

Another study has pointed to variation in the visual intelligibility of talkers based on gender. Female talkers on videotape received higher speech-reading scores on average than male talkers on videotape (Daly, Bench, & Chappell, 1996b). This finding fits in with sociolinguistic research showing that English-speaking women in Western cultures tend to use language in a way that encourages interaction and is more cooperative than the speech of men (see, for example, Fishman, 1983; Coates, 1993; Holmes, 1993).

There is a large body of research showing that people use language to form interpersonal impressions of others (see Bradac, 1990, for a review of the area). This research largely involves subjects listening to audio-tapes of a number of people talking, and then indicating their impressions of the talkers on scales for such items as friendliness, successfulness, trustworthiness and educatedness. A recent study has investigated interpersonal impressions formed after speech-reading without sound (Daly, Bench & Chappell, 1996c). Results showed a relationship between the visual intelligibility of talkers and how they were scored on the impression scales. The easier a talker was to speech-read, the more favourably they were scored on the impression scales. This relationship was significantly stronger for female talkers. These results illustrate the complexity of communication, which is so intimately connected with interpersonal relationships. Thus when there is a communication difficulty, much more than the transmission of messages may be affected. This is part of the complex situation encountered by the speech-language therapist in many cases.

In summary, it is clear that the talker contributes significantly to the process of speech-reading. The speech of the talker can make speech-reading more easy or more difficult, and this can affect interpersonal relations between the talker and speech-reader. It may be possible to improve the visual intelligibility of talkers by working with them to slow their speech, and use more visible tongue movement.

## Context effects in speech-reading

So far we have considered the visual (and audiovisual) perceptual cues of spoken language. Emphasis has been placed on the variability of speech patterns of different talkers, and the ability of the talker to modify his/her speech patterns in response to both background noise and to message complexity. These issues influence the success with which a message is understood in a particular conversational environment. Other factors have been found to influence message intelligibility also, including: (a) the facial expressions and gestures of the talker; (b) information about the environment or situation in which the message is being uttered; and(c) the linguistic context in the form of the immediately preceding utterance(s) spoken in the interaction. All of these cues have the potential to enhance the intelligibility of a spoken message.

Hearing-impaired adults speech-read sentences accompanied by a relevant gesture better than sentences without gesture and better than sentences accompanied by an unrelated gesture (Berger & Popelka, 1971; Popelka & Berger, 1971). Speech-readers also benefit from sentences presented with related facial expressions, by contrast with those presented with neutral facial expressions (Dudich & Duff, 1977; Miller, 1977). Similar effects have been noted when adults speech-read sentences with prior linguistic cues (De Filippo, 1982; Gagné, Tugby & Michaud, 1991). Comparison of the influence of related, neutral and unrelated linguistic context cues on the speech-reading of adults with hearing impairment indicated a significant decrement in performance as relatedness of the context lessened (C. Lind, N.P. Erber & J. Doyle, in preparation). In concert, these studies indicate that context provided from outside the confines of the sentence, can have a beneficial effect, no effect or a detrimental effect on speech-reading of the sentence.

The influence of situational cues on speech-reading performance is more equivocal. Garstecki and colleagues (Garstecki, 1976; Garstecki & O'Neill, 1980) found that related and unrelated auditory and visual cues were inconsistent in their influence on speech-reading of sentences presented without voice.

Although unrelated gestural and linguistic cues were found to be distracting, and to result in poorer speech-reading than when stimuli were presented in the absence of context or with neutral context, no such consistent difference was noted when people were presented with situational cues. This suggests that although the former can both enhance and detract from the person's understanding of the spoken message, the latter cues can provide confirmation for related stimuli but do not detract from stimuli unrelated to the scene. Together, these studies suggest that the salience of talker-generated cues (e.g. language, gesture and facial expressions) seems to be greater than that of situational cues. Perhaps this is not surprising given that: (a) the interrelationship between verbal and non-verbal cues in conversation; and (b) the equally frequent occurrence of conversations that bear little relationship to the physical environment in which they take place. In summary, it would seem that talker-related contextual cues can detract from identification of the spoken message (i.e. unrelatedness cannot be equated with irrelevance). This does not seem to be the case for situational cues and in this sense the latter cues are less powerful indicators of the verbal message. However, the strength of the relationship between the spoken message and the situation in which it occurs (i.e. the 'typicality' of the message) may influence these findings (Samuelsson & Rönnberg, 1991).

It remains to be seen whether increases in the amount of relevant contextual information available will be accompanied by further improvements in speech-reading performance or whether the law of diminishing returns will apply. In any case, this research direction is laudable as an attempt to more closely imitate daily-life audiovisual speech reception. The clinical implications of this approach are outlined later in this chapter.

## Speech-reading training

Much useful information on the training of speech-reading is given in the texts by, for example, Sanders (1971); Oyer and Franckman (1975, pp. 125–126); Berg (1976, pp. 112–164); Ling (1984) and Kaplan, Bally & Garretson (1987). Although somewhat dated, these sources contain a fund of precepts and detail in easily readable form. More recent developments are conveniently described in Gagné (1994) and in Section V, 'Teaching and learning speech-reading', of De Filippo and Sims (1988, pp. 193–313).

Training in speech-reading has been traditionally developed from two basic positions, from which most later training methods have been derived: the analytic position and the synthetic position. It needs to be pointed out, however, that in practice, speech-reading schools do not adopt one of these positions exclusively. The distinction is conceptual rather than real.

Analytic models of speech-reading training assume that audiovisual speech perception may be learned without reference to the linguistic structure(s) or context the articulatory events represent. The analytic position assumes that the flow of speech can be differentiated into separate articulatory movements, which are characterised by recognisable patterns, though to different degrees. The analytic position also requires an ability for fast and accurate recognition of these movements as individual speech elements (visemes), and assumes that this recognition will transfer to the related speech elements as they occur in natural, connected speech. This position thus relies on the ability to recognise the individual visemes fast enough and accurately enough to identify what is being said and, consequently, emphasises training in the recognition of individual speech elements and syllable stresses rather than the recognition of words or longer strings. As the Jena method, it was popularised by Bunger (1961); as the Mueller-Waller method, it was promulgated by Bruhn (1960). Both methods use drills requiring the client to develop visual recognition of rhythmically presented groups of speech elements with increasing speed.

Bunger, whose approach was the more analytical of the two, began with the recognition of individual vowels and consonants, with the vowels considered to represent differences in mouth opening (as affected by lips, tongue and jaw), and consonants to form fast closings of the vocal channel (by the lips, tongue, hard palate, teeth, back of the tongue and the velum). Bunger then progressed to drills with syllables containing the vowels or consonants in question. These syllable drills were followed in turn by word drills based on the syllables, and thence by sentences. Bruhn placed more of an initial focus on syllables, arguing that such a focus on syllables rather than words helped the client to concentrate on the articulatory movements, instead of the meaning of the material.

There is clearly a place in the training of speech-reading for the analytic methods, as an adjunct to more real-life audiovisual communication training. They help to answer the 'Where do I start?' question, especially with the child client who has little speech-reading ability. However, the focus on articulatory movements places insufficient emphasis on higher-level abilities (e.g. language and general knowledge) that are important for good speech-reading. It is useful to have available a large mirror and good lighting, so that clients may compare their own articulatory movements with those of the clinician. It is also helpful to use tactile speech clues, with the client sensing the type and presence or absence of vibrations in the throat for the voiced/unvoiced distinction and in the nose for nasal speech elements, and so on. Such tactile stimulation, when combined with visual speech-reading inputs, is best-suited to analytic methods at the start of speech-reading training. The client will find that tactile discrimination of speech elements is a demanding task, and concentration on both the visual and the tactile channels is tiring. A list of helpful tactile speech cues for use in speech-reading was presented by Berg (1976, pp. 134–138).

The synthetic position was expounded by Nitchie (1912) and later taken up for children by Kinzie and Kinzie (1936). Whereas the analytic position may be described as a 'bottom-up' approach, which emphasises speech elements, the synthetic position is a 'top-down' approach, which focuses on meaning. Thus, the synthetic position is that the recognition of meaning is the main aim in the training of speech-reading, rather than the recognition of speech elements. The focus of the synthetic approach is on linguistic and higher-level cognitive factors, and on situational variables. Whole words are used for training, not visemes or syllables. Although a speech element may be the target of such training, clients are taught to speech-read words and sentences that contain that element. The client is presented with words that have a given articulatory movement in a beginning and/or a final position. Each new articulatory movement is connected and contrasted with previously learned articulatory movements so that a word containing the new speech element is paired with a word containing a speech element taught in a previous session. Thus training, which is assisted by mirror practice, develops as a progression.

The speech-reading training method advocated by Jeffers and Barley (1971) directs that speech-reading needs training in: (a) quick recognition of visemes; (b) use of context and non-verbal cues; and (c) flexibility to reinterpret a percept if the original does not make sense. The Jeffers and Barley method uses a variant of the synthetic approach for its quick recognition exercises, which make use of contrast words. For example, the clinician presents three words that differ in one speech element, such as 'by', 'my', 'pic'. These words are presented in different sequences, when the client has to report them in the correct sequence.

An alternative, conversational analytic approach, has been proposed by Erber and Lind (1994), who suggest that the multifaceted nature of spoken interaction be recognised in speech-reading training. The analytic and the synthetic models focus on speech materials that range from the nonsense syllable up to and including the sentence, spoken in isolation. However, in the same way that phonemes are seldom spoken in isolation from other phonemes, words and sentences are seldom spoken in isolation either from other words or sentences or from the broader non-linguistic context that accompanies the conversational interaction. The conversational analytic approach endeavours to incorporate contextual cues that are relevant to the client's stated daily communication environments and needs.

The studies reporting on the audiovisual perception of the sentence-in-context have been discussed in the preceding section on context effects. Erber and Lind's conversational analytic model of speech-reading intervention draws on that work and reflects an emphasis on aspects of interaction in audiovisual speech perception, yet recognises the current limitations of our understanding of context cues. It is hoped that ultimately speech-reading could be learned via, what we may label in anticipation, a 'conversational synthetic' approach, which will incorporate all aspects of daily interaction in clinical intervention.

The principles of this model are that speech-reading training should be conducted in ways that reflect as much of the individual's real-life communication milieu as possible. Briefly, this manifests itself in the clinic as practice with: (a) both frequent communication partners and strangers; (b) text-level language materials (as opposed to syllables, words or sentences in isolation) covering a wide range of topics and levels of complexity; and (c) across a range of environmental conditions (e.g. altered lighting, distance, background noise). Speech-reading assessment and training methods of use in this approach include Tracking (De Filippo & Scott, 1978), and QUEST?AR, Sent-Ident and TOPICON (Erber, 1996).

Although cognitive, linguistic and speech development improve ability in speech-reading (Markides, 1983, p. 168), it is sadly the case that firm evidence for success in direct speech-reading training, which produces fluent conversational interaction, is hard to find (De Filippo, 1990; Bench, 1992a, p. 75; Rönnberg, 1995, p. 408). In view of the above discussion, this situation is perhaps only to be expected. First, speech-reading has available only a poor source of information in the visual speech signal. Second, it is a complex multicomponent activity and depends on complex underlying processes, which are not well-developed in many hearing-impaired children. If speech-reading is to improve, these underlying processes must be developed, as their development sets a limit to what can otherwise be achieved. Although a narrow approach, focusing on particulars such as individual visemic patterns, can be successful in training recognition of these particulars (Walden et al., 1977, 1981), that recognition is unlikely to generalise well to connected speech. Third, there is ample evidence from several studies that, for subjects with a good command of language, untrained practice permits a noticeable improvement in speech-reading scores (see below), implying that the unwary therapist or teacher may misinterpret such practice effects as successful training.

However, this is not to say that certain techniques and insights are not viable therapeutic tools. The methods for the training of speech-reading outlined above focus the client's attention on some basics of the speech-reading task and allow distinct progress to be made. Also, the use of contextual cues in speech-reading can be drawn to a client's attention, and the client's own speech can be used to illustrate some speech-reading activities. It is relatively rare, however, for training in such speech-reading methods alone to lead to the degree of speech-reading expertise required for even partial success in monitoring everyday connected speech.

## Cued speech

As many English speech sounds are not visible on the lips or look the same as other speech sounds, the speech-reader has to depend on knowledge of language or context to make good the deficiencies. This situation is, of course, problematical for the hearing-impaired child, and especially the younger hearing-impaired child, whose knowledge of both is sketchy. A possible solution to this predicament, namely, cued speech, was proposed by Cornett (1972, 1985). In cued speech, the hands are used to signify those speech elements that cannot be seen on the lips, while allowing dependence on speech-reading of the lips for the information that they can thereby provide. Thus the hand signals of cued speech are incomplete by themselves, which forces the child to speech-read the talker's lips, with the hand signals as a supplement. Cued speech has distinct advantages. It can keep up with the natural flow of speech because it works with syllables rather than phonemes, and therefore it does not disrupt speech as happens with simultaneous fingerspelling. Yet, despite such advantages, cued speech has not become widely used (Calvert, 1986). Possibly its demands on the visual speech-processing systems are too great, or perhaps the hand signals interfere too much with the natural gestures made during speech (Mohay, 1983).

## Speech-reading tests

When considering clients for speech-reading, the therapist or teacher will be interested to know about the clients' natural speech-reading ability, their individual strengths and weaknesses, which training methods are most suitable, how much speech-reading adds to clients' communication abilities and how to demonstrate changes in speech-reading with training. Tests of speech-reading ability are useful for such purposes, but the implications of test results need careful evaluation, for the following reasons.

Different tests measure different aspects of speech-reading ability, so that a client who performs well on one speech-reading test may perform less well on another, because the tests assess different aspects of speech-reading ability or because one test is easier than the other. Also, good performance on a speech-reading test is good in relation to some standard known to be typical of the related population of speech-readers. Good performance on a test is not good performance if most of the relevant population score better on the test than the speech-reader in question. Further, unless a test reflects at least some characteristics of everyday communication, good performance on the test may bear little relation to communication in daily conversations. Such a test has weak validity.

In addition, there are serial effects that may confound the interpretation of speech-reading tests, especially when assessing the results of training in speech-reading by means of tests before and after training. For example, there is clear evidence that practice on speech-reading materials tends to increase speech-reading scores for both normally hearing and hearing-impaired subjects (Rosen & Corcoran, 1982; Squires & Dancer, 1986; Lesner, Sandridge & Kricos, 1987; Warren et al., 1989; Bench et al., 1994). Such practice generally results in an increase in speech-reading scores of some 3 to 10 per cent in early trials. Performance then levels off or increases more slowly towards an asymptote. Such increases are similar to those attributed to training, so that, before the effects of training can be accepted as valid, checks for practice need to be made. Sufficient pretest trials need to be presented to avoid this occurrence. C. Lind, N.P. Erber and J. Doyle (in preparation) found that as many as 15 or 16 trials were required before learning effects were reduced in sentence-based speech-reading assessment.

Besides the relatively short-term effects of practice, longer-term serial effects may be at work to confound the unwary therapist, especially when working with children. For instance, the therapist may wish to attribute increases in speech-reading scores to a programme of training in speech-reading over many weeks or months. However, before such claims can be accepted, it is important to be able to rule out the influence of maturational or developmental changes in cognition and language. Thus, Conrad (1979) observed that extended training may appear to produce an improvement in speech-reading, whereas the improvement may be due to increased ability in language skills.

What is it that makes for a good speech-reading test? Berger (1972) argued for:

- test validity, with the test resembling natural conversations;
- vocabulary and grammar appropriate to the speech-reading ability of the client;
- careful choice of a range of talkers varying in speech-readability;
- test items gauged to be neither too easy nor too difficult;
- test conditions varying from easy to difficult (e.g. a well-lit to a poorly-lit test environment).

Ijsseldijk (1988) reviewed 18 speech-reading tests, mostly sentence-based but sometimes based on consonants in CV form, isolated words or short stories. Four major differences were found in test presentation:

- live versus video mode;
- audio signals present or absent;
- number and gender of talkers, and their familiarity with deaf communication;
- the number of times test items were presented.

Rosen and Corcoran (1982) and Bench et al. (1993, 1994, 1995) prescribed:

- consistent test administration, requiring a filmed or videorecorded test for reliability, and hence ruling out live testing;
- a large number of equivalent forms of the test (e.g. a large number of word lists or sentence lists) to avoid learning due to repeated use of the same items;
- material appropriate for the task, with vocabulary, grammar and semantics known to be familiar to the client, so as not to confound speech-reading ability with language ability;
- careful selection of talkers.

It is difficult to include all such desirable properties in just one speech-reading test, and compromises may need to be made unless the test is designed to assess only specific aspects of speech-reading under conditions where other variables can be at set levels.

Of these prescriptions, perhaps the greatest difficulty has occurred with talker selection. The authors of most published speech-reading tests have made rather arbitrary and poorly described selections of a single talker (Ijsseldijk, 1988; Bench et al., 1994).

An important aspect of talker selection for speech-reading tests is that the accent of the talkers (i.e. the phonetics and phonology) should either match the accent used by the speech-reader, or at least represent an accent with which the speech reader is familiar. If speech-reading tests employing unfamiliar accents are used, it is likely that speech-reading scores will confound difficulty with accent with speech-reading ability. Given this caution, and aiming to fulfill as many of the other prescriptions as possible, three speech-reading tests are recommended: The Utley Lipreading Test (Utley, 1946); the BKB/A Speechreading Test (Bench et al., 1993); and the Video-recorded BKB Sentence Lists (Rosen & Corcoran, 1982). These are described in Table 8.1.

It must be remembered that speech-reading tests do not measure all aspects of communicative ability. It is possible to improve on measures of communicative ability (e.g. the Denver Communication Scale) but to show no improvement in speech-reading scores (Kaplan, Bally & Garretson, 1987)

## Clinical decisions for the speech-language therapist

The principal decisions likely to be encountered by the speech-language therapist are (a) when to suggest therapy to improve speech reading communication and (b) what clinical tests and approaches might assist. The following comments are offered to assist those decisions.

1. The speech-language therapist may decide to work towards improving the hearing-impaired client's speech-reading skills when

**Table 8.1:** Recommended speech-reading tests

*For speakers of American English: The Utley Lipreading Test*

Utley J (1946) A test of lipreading ability. Journal of Speech and Hearing 11: 109–16.

A female talker presents 62 sentences and then 72 words on silent film. The number of correct words reported is scored. Six stories are presented with no more than two interactants (from a pool of four more talkers: one boy, one man and two women) for each story. After each story there are five questions based on the content of the interactions. Scores are given for correct answers to the questions.

Strengths and weaknesses: Use of a number of talkers. Use of connected discourse. Use of black and white film. No option to include sound in testing conditions. Dated. However the Utley test remains popular with American audiologists.

*For speakers of Australian English: The BKB/A Speechreading Test*

Bench RJ, Doyle J, Daly N & Lind C (1993) The BKB/A Speechreading Test. La Trobe University, Melbourne, Australia.

Two male and two female talkers present 21 lists of 16 sentences on videotape. Each sentence list contains 50 key words which may be used for scoring. The test may be administered without sound, and with sound against background speech babble.

Strengths and weaknesses: Videorecording allows for consistent test administration; there are 21 lists of 16 sentences, thus providing a large number of equivalent forms; the vocabulary, grammar and semantics are known to be familiar to hearing-impaired children of age 8 years and above, and normally hearing children of age 6 years and above; the four talkers were selected to be of good but not exceptional visual intelligibility. A weakness is that the sentences do not represent everyday inter-actional material.

*For speakers of British English: Video-recorded BKB Sentence Lists*

Rosen S & Corcoran T (1982) A video-recorded test of lipreading for British English. British Journal of Audiology 16: 245–54.

A female talker presents 21 lists of 16 sentences on videotape. Each sentence contains 50 key words which may be used for scoring.

Strengths and weaknesses: Videorecording allows for consistent test administration; there are 21 lists of 16 sentences, thus providing a large number of equivalent forms; the vocabulary, grammar and semantics are known to be familiar to hearing-impaired children of age 8 years and above, and normally hearing children of age 6 years and above. However, there is only one talker and she is described as a female phonetician of southern British origin. Thus she may have exceptionally distinct articulation.

any of the following apply:

(a) the client has had recent changes in hearing levels that have led to communication difficulties in some or all of the individual's daily activities;

(b) the client reports communication difficulties across a broad range of communication settings, regardless of his or her hearing levels;

(c) recent changes in the client's communication environment (e.g. a change of job) have increased the pressure on communication success.

2. The speech-language therapist may decide to work with the visual intelligibility of a talker when:

(a) there are one or more people with whom the speech-reader communicates frequently and whom the speech-reader has difficulty understanding;

(b) the frequent communication partner displays a lack of understanding of the communication needs of the person with the hearing impairment;

(c) the talker has unusual speech/articulation patterns or habits. Of course it is necessary that the talkers concerned be amenable to such intervention.

3. If it is possible to have some sessions with both talker(s) and speech-reader, the speech-language therapist may be able to encourage the speech-reader to develop awareness of the constituents of visual intelligibility during normal conversations. It may also be possible to encourage the speech-reader to make appropriate requests to improve the visual intelligibility of the talker. The talker could benefit from a knowledge of specific ways in which they may contribute to better communication. Such therapy has the potential to address the needs of the client and their communication partners in a naturalistic and practical way, which has high face validity for the participants.

4. Measurement of the client's pre- and post-therapy speech-reading skills is useful. The Utley Lipreading Test, the BKB/A Speechreading Test and the Video-recorded BKB Sentence Lists fulfill many of the requirements of good speech-reading tests as discussed earlier in this chapter. Pre- and post-therapy client reports are also useful as a functional indicator of progress in the development of better speech-reading. This is important, as improvement measured in the clinic on a specific speech-reading task does not necessarily indicate improvement in speech-reading in real-life spoken interaction.

## Summary of key points

Speech-reading is used by all sighted people, whether hearing impaired or normally hearing. Speech-reading and hearing are both mediated by inner, or subvocal speech, the language we use for thinking, so that speech-reading is like hearing speech by eye. Speech-reading is difficult because less than half of speech sounds can be seen though, fortunately, the speech sounds which are the most difficult to see tend to be the easiest to hear. It helps greatly if the speech-reader knows the talker and the context of the message to be speech-read, is familiar with the language used, has a good general knowledge and is prepared to guess at the meaning when unsure. The talker can greatly influence the success of a speech-reading interaction. Talkers may also be judged interpersonally by the speech-reader in terms of how easy they are to speech-read. Therapists may find it useful to have the client practice speech-reading under a range of different environmental, linguistic and interactional settings that mimic the client's daily-life conversational settings. The therapist who attempts to improve a client's speech-reading skills needs to bear in mind that speech-reading can improve significantly with practice alone. In selecting therapy techniques the speech-language therapist may utilise aspects of the analytic, synthetic and conversational-analytic approaches. It may be particularly useful to include in the intervention programme the talkers with whom the client frequently communicates.

# Further reading

Erber NP (1996) Communication therapy for adults with sensory loss, 2nd edn. Clifton Hill: Clavis. (Readable conceptualisation of therapy for adults with hearing loss. Guidelines for conversational therapy are especially good.)

Gagné J-P (1994) Visual and audiovisual speech perception training: basic and applied research needs. In Gagné J-P, Tye-Murray N (Eds) Research in audiological rehabilitation: current trends and future directions (Monograph). Journal of the Academy of Rehabilitative Audiology 27: 133–59. (A summary of the current theory and research underlying clinical practice in speech-reading assessment, training and outcome measurement.)

Jeffers J, Barley M (1971) Speechreading (lipreading). Springfield, IL: Charles C. Thomas. (An introduction to analytic and synthetic models of speech-reading training.)

Kaplan H, Bally SJ, Garretson C (1987) Speechreading: a way to improve understanding, 2nd edn. Washington, DC: Gallaudet University Press. (A readable introduction to clinical procedures in speech-reading, environmental and hearing tactics, and communication strategies for the therapist or teacher.)

Rönnberg J (1995) What makes a skilled speechreader? In Plant G, Spens K-E (Eds) Profound deafness and speech communication. London: Whurr Publishers, pp. 393–416. (A summary of research into aspects of cognitive and linguistic processing of audiovisual speech materials.)

# Chapter 9
# Central auditory processing disorder

JOHN BENCH

This chapter describes, in outline, abnormal responses to sounds, especially speech sounds, beyond any difficulties attributable to malfunction in peripheral hearing. The chapter is thus concerned with those retrocochlear hearing problems, which give rise to what is commonly referred to as central auditory processing disorder (CAPD), alternatively known as central auditory dysfunction, central deafness, auditory agnosia, auditory imperception or sometimes as obscure auditory dysfunction. Some consequences of CAPD for other aspects of behaviour are also considered.

## Principles

1. *Central auditory processing disorder (CAPD) refers to impaired ability, or inability, to attend to, discriminate, recognise, remember or comprehend information presented through the auditory channel* (Keith, 1986; Keith & Pensak, 1991).
2. *CAPD is an 'umbrella' concept, not a unitary concept.* CAPD covers a range of individual disorders, so that different CAPD tests tend to produce different response patterns with different test subjects.
3. *CAPD is concerned with hearing problems beyond the peripheral hearing mechanism, at the brainstem or cortical levels.* CAPD may be present when (a) peripheral hearing is within normal limits and (b) in addition to peripheral hearing problems. Thus, CAPD may occur where there are no measurable hearing problems associated with the outer, middle or inner ear. It may also occur in addition to such problems.
4. *A high proportion of children with language learning disabilities have CAPD.* Several studies have found that many children experiencing learning disabilities, particularly language learning disabilities associated with difficulties in reading, writing and spelling, have central auditory processing problems.

5. *Clients with certain known neurological problems show reduced performance on tests for CAPD, but the converse is not necessarily true.* Some neurological disorders with confirmed sites of lesion have been associated with poor scores on specified CAPD tests. However, in the absence of a confirmed site of lesion, it cannot be assumed that poor results on such CAPD tests uniquely indicate a specific neurological locus. In other words, CAPD tests alone can rarely, if ever, be used to determine site of lesion, they indicate some probabilities only.

## Overview of the development of CAPD tests

Serious clinical and research interest in the area of central auditory processing is conventionally dated from the work of Bocca and co-workers (e.g. Bocca, Calearo & Cassinari, 1954; Calearo & Lazzaroni, 1957; Bocca & Calearo, 1963). Bocca et al. (1954), for example, described ways of assessing hearing in cases with temporal lobe tumours. Speech was used as the test stimulus on the assumption that the perception and recognition of speech were needed for testing higher cortical functions. The speech stimuli used in such tests, however, are not natural, free speech. Such speech contains too many cues about its message content, namely, too much redundancy, to tax the auditory pathways sufficiently for dysfunction to be identified readily. Instead, the speech is distorted by electroacoustic manipulations, including filtering, interruption and time-compression. These manipulations reduce the redundancy in the speech signal, limiting the auditory system to the processing of fewer cues, which are more readily affected by the 'central masking' effects of CAPD (Ferre & Wilber, 1986). The result is reduced speech perception, weakened according to the degree of the dysfunction. The extent to which the distortions are imposed on the speech is largely an empirical matter at the present state of knowledge. The degree of distortion is gauged so that a normally functioning person can just report all, or nearly all, of the speech material correctly, whereas a client with higher auditory dysfunction will experience significant difficulty.

Since the early work mentioned above, further tests using ingeniously manipulated speech stimuli have been developed (see for example Willeford, 1977; Lasky & Katz, 1983a). Clinical work with such stimuli continues to be used at the present time, though not without some difficulties of test interpretation, as we shall see. These tests with speech stimuli have been augmented by other tests, which use tonal, noise-band or other non-speech signals for specific purposes.

The newcomer to the area is confronted by a plethora of tests and procedures, far too numerous to describe or even to list here, which developed in a somewhat *ad hoc* fashion without much by way of protocol for their application (Spitzer, 1983). This situation arose because: (a) CAPD represents a constellation, rather than a small group, of disorders; (b) the disorders may be relatively discrete or may overlap one another; (c) the underlying neurology and physiology are imperfectly known; (d) intervening variables, such as intelligence, linguistic features, short-term memory, attention, metacognition, metalinguistics and motivation affect the test results; and (e) some of the effects are subtle, requiring special care and skill in their assessment. The central auditory system is complex and its assessment can be affected by many influences. The reader will find useful synopses of test materials and their applications presented in relevant chapters of Keith (1977, 1981a), Lasky and Katz (1983b), Willeford and Burleigh (1985), Pinheiro and Musiek (1985), Bamford and Saunders (1991), Katz, Stecker and Henderson (1992), among others.

However, it is useful to indicate here how this otherwise complex, voluminous and sometimes confusing material can be organised. In a published tutorial, Spitzer (1983) courageously undertook to impose some clinical order on this situation. Her protocol, designed to promote development and refinement of CAPD testing systematically, consisted of the following:

1. Prerequisite knowledge to conduct central auditory evaluations. Deeper than usual knowledge (for an audiologist) is needed of neuroanatomy and neurophysiology, knowledge of current research on speech perception and information processing, theories of language development and its disorders, and information about available CAPD assessment techniques and their application to special groups.
2. The role of case-history taking and basic audiological evaluation: where case-history taking, sensitised for possible central auditory pathology, is particularly concerned with noting attributes and abilities that can directly or indirectly affect CAPD test performance, such as motivation, gross motor and linguistic abilities, unusual headaches, vomiting, nausea, visual field defects, etc.; and where basic audiological evaluation includes pure tone air- and bone-conduction thresholds, speech discrimination performance, acoustic immittance, acoustic reflex thresholds and acoustic reflex decay (see Chapter 4 for description of these procedures).
3. Hypothesis formation, which is a fundamental step in reaching a diagnosis. Hypothesis formation is complex in central auditory evaluations, because of the complexity of the problems. It is probably best attempted as a staged progression from a broad level (e.g. cortical dysfunction) to a narrow level (left temporo-parietal region of the cortex).
4. First-level diagnosis, consisting of a rapid survey of several CAPD functions, and including such tests as the SSW test (see following section), performance-intensity functions and tone decay tests.

5. Second-level diagnosis, involving the use of more specialised tests, including pure tone measures (e.g. masking), level difference tests, speech measures (e.g. alternating speech, filtered speech), electro-physiological tests (e.g. electrocochleography, auditory brainstem responses) and tests of vestibular function.

Spitzer's tutorial ended with some caveats concerning CAPD test interpretation, enjoining: (a) economy of interpretation of test results; (b) recognising that multiple lesions may coexist in the auditory system; (c) understanding that medication can affect test results; (d) caution in assessing clients with peripheral hearing loss; and (e) recognising that results may be contaminated by variable client cooperation.

Spitzer's work met with general approval from her reviewers (Beasley, Keith and Musiek; see Spitzer, 1983, pp. 229–30). They did, however, raise several queries, some of which were answered briefly by Spitzer in the same article. It is informative to mention some of these queries. For example, Beasley queried whether (a) the measures from the first-level diagnosis would necessarily lead to an appropriate choice of tests at the second-level diagnosis, and (b) whether there was sufficient validity for tests designed to measure the integrity of function of specific cortical areas. Keith asked (a) if it was appropriate to administer CAPD tests in the presence of significant peripheral hearing loss, given the difficulties in partialling out the test results between the effects of the peripheral hearing loss and CAPD (even allowing for the hearing loss itself), and (b) if it was appropriate to rely on the SSW test at first-level diagnosis to evaluate site of lesion. Musiek inquired whether (a) some of the listed brainstem tests could be contaminated by involvement of the cortex, and (b) whether there was a risk of confounding some effects of high frequency cochlear hearing loss with mild CAPD.

This author points out that Spitzer's protocols were directed mainly to the assessment of site of lesion, presumably in adult clients, with some emphasis on neuroanatomical and neurophysiological features. Reference to cognitive and maturational aspects was weak or missing, perhaps because most of the work on children with learning disabilities, which has to deal with such aspects, came after the emphasis on site of lesion in adults.

The remainder of this chapter will focus mainly on issues concerned with the test battery approach, some well-known tests with which this author has clinical experience, aspects of CAPD in children and some criticisms of work in the area.

## The test battery approach

Momentum for assessing CAPD increased in the 1960s and 1970s. During this period systematic investigations of central auditory processing also began to depart from single standardised tests to a test battery approach. One of the main reasons for this was that the performance of clients on CAPD tests often differs considerably from test to test. These differences are not surprising. Rather they are to be expected because of dependency on the site of the lesion, or on sets of interacting functions each of which is predicated on specific operations of the brain (Ferre, 1987), by mechanisms as yet only dimly understood. The test battery approach uses several different, but complementary, tests to assess the full complexity of speech-processing measures needed to examine a range of clients who might suffer from a variety of auditory processing problems. Well-known test batteries were designed by Flowers and Costello (1970), Goldman, Fristoe and Woodcock (1974) and Willeford (1977), who aimed to provide multiple opportunities to assay the nature of a client's auditory processing problem through several different test procedures. Most of the currently available test batteries had been developed by the early 1980s, although further assessment protocols, often comprising a mix of established individual tests in new combinations or with new additions have been published from time to time (e.g. Ferre & Wilber, 1986; Smoski, Brunt & Tannahill, 1992).

The test battery has found widespread use in North America (e.g. Musiek, Geurink & Kietel, 1982). However, the use of test batteries elsewhere has been much more limited. The reason is largely that, although most Western clients are familiar with North American accents from the broadcast media, the tests from the USA contain some unfamiliar semantic associations and, where pre-recorded, less familiar pronunciations, especially at the word level. Where there are no semantic or syntactic cues to guide the non-American listener, this relatively unfamiliar pronunciation of words, often presented under designedly less than optimal listening conditions, causes misperceptions even in clients without CAPD problems (e.g. 'pass' pronounced to rhyme with 'lass' rather than with 'farce'). Our own observations suggest that some 10 to 20 per cent of stimulus words are so affected. It follows that the North American recordings and test norms are of dubious validity for use elsewhere. The solution is, of course, for non-North American countries to record their own test batteries, using native talkers, and to standardise them with native listeners. Until this work is done, there will be no satisfactory speech-test batteries for the assessment of central auditory processing outside North America. To date, however, such work has generally been limited to just a few tests (rather than a full test battery), and/or has been of an *ad hoc* nature in response to local, one-off clinical needs with little by way of published test norms. A notable exception has been the test battery for obscure auditory dysfunction, as described by Saunders, Field and Haggard (1992).

# Drawbacks of the test battery approach

A major drawback to the use of the test battery approach is that it is time-consuming (typically involving about one hour of testing or more), which makes it unattractive to the busy clinician. This problem can be readily compounded by client fatigue, because clients, especially children, with CAPD often have difficulty in concentrating on listening tasks over long periods. Consequently, they tire easily. Some more recent work (see below) has led to the development of auditory processing test batteries that can produce useful, though not necessarily full, information in a relatively short time (around 20 to 30 minutes). With child clients, such tests tend to focus on areas relevant to complaints about unexpectedly poor auditory performance in relation to the developmental stage of the child, and to specific aspects of the child's auditory environment (as in teacher's reports of unusually depressed listening ability in the presence of classroom noise).

# The SCAN test

An example of the shortened approach is the Screening Test for Auditory Processing Disorders (SCAN) of Keith (1986). The SCAN test was designed for assessing children between 3 and 11 years of age who have language disorders or problems with academic progress. Such children will include those whose learning is affected by short attention span, difficulty in following spoken instructions and difficulty in understanding speech in background noise. This test is also available as the SCAN-A test for screening for CAPD problems in adolescents and adults.

It was Keith's intention that the SCAN test be used to identify children with possible (language) learning problems together with central auditory processing problems. Should the test indicate the likely presence of auditory processing problems, detailed evaluation could then be undertaken to explore the problems in depth with further procedures. It is thus emphasised that the use of the SCAN test is as a screening procedure. It is useful, first, for screening numbers of children in school, where it can identify children at risk for learning and language disabilities who could gain advantage from further, detailed evaluation of auditory processing skills or language assessment. Second, it may also be used for screening children who present with behaviour suggesting auditory processing problems, such as weak auditory comprehension, difficulty in understanding speech in noisy classrooms and/or poor auditory memory. Third, it can be used to assist in the identification of an auditory processing problem in children who experience academic difficulties in spite of average-to-high intelligence, hearing within normal limits and reasonable opportunities for learning.

The SCAN test features Filtered Words, Auditory Figure-Ground and Competing Words subtests for presentation via a stereo cassette player and headphones in a quiet room. It takes about 20 minutes to complete. The test is presented in a convenient book-sized test kit, which includes an audiocassette (with prerecorded test instructions and auditory stimuli), examiner's manual and record forms. The examiner's manual contains comprehensive information on test administration, scoring and test norms, although Keith cautions that the norms for 3- and 4-year-old children are based on small samples. The results of each subtest can be considered separately or summed to form a composite score.

The Filtered Words subtest consists of two lists of monosyllabic words, low-pass filtered at 1000 Hz with a 32 dB/octave roll-off. This filtering removes the high-frequency components, making the words more difficult to perceive but still intelligible to normal listeners. Following a few practice words, 20 test words are presented to the right, and 20 to the left, ear. The child is asked to repeat each word, with responses scored correct for accurate repetition of the whole word. Keith (1986) argued that as some of the acoustic spectrum is missing in low-pass filtered speech, so that the child has to supply the absent high-frequency information, the Filtered Words subtest is a kind of auditory closure task. Hence, poor performance on Filtered Words may suggest a receptive language disorder. At any rate, poor performance should reflect problems in understanding words in certain auditory environments, such as difficulty in following low-quality audio recordings or following a teacher who is talking with his/her back to the class while writing on a board.

The Auditory Figure Ground (speech-in-noise) subtest contains similar lists of words to the Filtered Words subtest for the speech signal, and the words are presented and responses scored in a similar way to the Filtered Words subtest. The words are spoken against a multitalker speech babble as background noise, at a signal-to-noise ratio of 8 dB (i.e. the speech is 8 dB above the background babble). This background babble contains the voices of many speakers, with the acoustic peaks removed by electronic compression. Hence, it is rather more like broad-spectrum noise (as from an audiometer) than the natural speech babble of a smaller number of speakers. Natural speech babble would tend to make the client's task more difficult, and possibly offer a more discriminating test. However, it is important to appreciate that the purpose of the subtest is that of screening, rather than verisimilitude. Notwithstanding such comments, the Auditory Figure Ground subtest does provide a measure of poor listening behaviour when background noise is present, a common complaint of teachers and parents.

The Competing Words subtest contains two lists each of 25 monosyllable word pairs presented with simultaneous onset times to the right and left ears. The words in each pair are matched for duration and are semantically unrelated (e.g. 'drop', 'hen'). The child has to repeat both words of each pair, starting with what was heard in the right ear for the first 25 pairs. The child then reports what was heard, starting with the left ear, for the second 25 pairs. Competing Words is a dichotic listening task, as different words are presented to each ear at the same time. Keith states that a depressed score on Competing Words may indicate that the child's auditory processing system is functioning in a similar way to that of a younger child, and that repetition of the test can indicate developments in maturation of the central auditory pathways. Few would contest such a statement, which also holds for performance on the Filtered Words and Auditory Figure Ground subtests, and for the SCAN test as a whole.

Informal reports from clinical colleagues suggest that the SCAN test goes a long way towards meeting the need for a quick-to-administer screening test for CAPD. For such purposes it has been adopted with alacrity.

# The Katz (1992) Category System and test battery

## Some problems with the test battery approach

We remarked earlier that the test battery approach, although comprehensive, has its drawbacks. It requires considerable testing time, which places a load on the busy clinician. It is also tiring for the client, who is asked to listen to and report auditory stimuli presented in several tests under purposefully difficult listening conditions. A further problem is that of the plethora of tests that might be included in a test battery, which, at the present state of knowledge, reflects the lack of a comprehensive theoretical base on which to ground test development and test-battery compilation. There is a related conceptualisation difficulty. It is often difficult for practitioners to match the findings derived from CAPD test batteries directly with the many puzzles that arise from the client's disordered communication, as in such problems as short memory span, poor comprehension of complex spoken messages or slow progress in reading and writing.

Katz (1992) attempted to address these issues. Although by no means pretending that it answers all the questions presented by CAPD cases, this author has found Katz's work, with some variations, to be both theoretically informative and practically useful. Hence a brief account (taken largely from Katz (1992) to which the reader is directed) is now given of Katz's approach. His test battery, as explored in our clinical laboratory, is also described.

### The Staggered Spondaic Word (SSW) Test

Katz used his extensive experience with his well-known Staggered Spondaic Word (SSW) test (Katz, 1968; Arnst & Katz, 1982) as a basis from which to develop a Category System. A brief account is now given of the SSW test, but the reader is encouraged to seek a demonstration of the test from an audiologist, if possible, as experiencing the test will help greatly in understanding how the test items are sequenced.

In the SSW test the client is asked to repeat 40 pairs of familiar, different spondees (bisyllabic words, e.g 'upstairs'), presented to alternate ears through headphones. The presentation is arranged so that the first syllable of the first spondee is presented to one ear, then the second syllable of the first spondee is presented to the same ear while simultaneously the first syllable of the second spondee is presented to the second ear, and finally the second syllable of the second spondee is presented to the second ear. Thus the second syllable of the first spondee (heard in one ear) overlaps (competes with) the first syllable of the second spondee (heard in the other ear). Figure 9.1 shows, for example, the first test item.

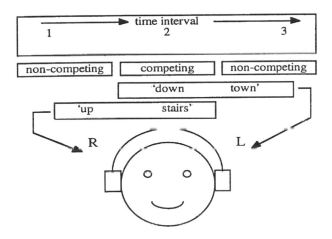

In the SSW test the timing of the presentation of test words is arranged so that each ear receives part of each word without competition and part of the same word with a competing message delivered to the other ear. In this example, the first syllable ('up') of the word 'upstairs' is delivered to the right ear alone and the second syllable ('stairs') is presented to the right ear at the same time as the first syllable of a word presented to the left ear. The client's responses and the types of errors made can describe central auditory processing problems.

**Figure 9.1:** Example of the Staggered Spondaic Word (SSW) test.

The first item containing the two spondees ('upstairs/downtown') may start in the right ear (right ear first, REF) in time interval 1 with 'up', and end in the left ear in time interval 3 with 'town', as shown. The second item of another two spondees (not shown) then begins in the left ear (left ear first, LEF), and ends in the right ear. For each item, the first ('up') and last ('town') word is non-competing (no word in the opposite ear), while the second ('stairs') and third ('down') words are competing (word present in the opposite ear). Analysis of the results begins with error counts. Errors are counted from the four conditions:

1. right non-competing (RNC);
2. right competing (RC);
3. left competing (LC);
4. left non-competing (LNC).

The error scores can be analysed in different ways, and hence may inform the clinician as to site of lesion or type of CAPD problem. For example, when the error count on the second halves of test items (the second spondees) is five errors or more greater than on the first halves (the first spondees), this outcome is considered to show a significant Order Effect (in adults). This type of Order Effect (referred to as 'low/high') has been linked with lesions in the area of Heschl's gyrus and the auditory cortex, the posterior temporal region (Katz, 1978), and with phonemic decoding (Luria, 1966, pp. 103–13). When the error count is greater for the first halves than the second halves of test items (the opposite type of Order Effect, 'high/low'), a problem linked to the anterior part of the brain, and speech-in-noise difficulties, may be suspected.

As another example, clients with marked difficulties in reading and spelling (dyslexia) often produce a 'Type A' SSW pattern, where the errors in the LC condition outnumber the errors in each of the remaining three conditions (RC, RNC and LNC). Such cases are thought to implicate the temporal-parietal-occipital region (the angular gyrus) or the posterior corpus callosum (Damasio & Damasio, 1983).

A further example is the instance of Reversals, where the client responds to at least five items with the words reported in an incorrect order (e.g. 'downtown/upstairs' reported in place of 'upstairs/downtown'), provided that there is not more than one word error. These sequencing problems are thought to be associated with the frontal-temporal-parietal and premotor regions, and the rolandic area of the frontoparietal region (Katz & Pack, 1975).

**Evaluation of the SSW test**

It will be clear to the reader that the SSW test presents many opportunities for obtaining insights into CAPD problems. It is reasonably reliable, and can be administered easily in about 10 minutes, given access to a modern two-channel audiometer and a two-channel audiotape or cassette recorder. Scoring takes some time to master, but is not difficult.

The SSW test was designed to identify lesions, mainly in adults, affecting the auditory reception areas of the cerebral cortex. As indicated by Keith (1983), much of the work on how well the SSW meets this aim was not easily gleaned from the early literature on the test. More recently, however, accessible information has become available (e.g. Arnst & Katz, 1982), together with a body of clinical experience, to create an established place for the test in helping to identify the locus of brain lesions affecting the auditory reception areas. Also, the SSW test has found a place in the assessment of CAPD in children with learning, especially language learning, disabilities. Katz himself was instrumental in this development, tending to focus on his original aim of identifying brain lesions, although it is problematical to identify site of lesion in children, if indeed localised sites exist in many instances.

Additional approaches are needed to interpreting the results of SSW in children. In particular, there are maturational or developmental effects in children, suggesting that an approach based on developmental neurology would be of great advantage. For example, performance on the SSW test improves, and the standard deviations of test scores decrease, from age 6 to age 11 or 12 years, when performance becomes similar to that of adults. There is also a strong right-ear advantage in younger children, which reduces as the central auditory pathways develop. This strong advantage disappears by age 11 years (Keith, 1983). Hence, unless specific neuroanatomical damage is at issue, the 'site of lesion' concept is rather less useful in the management of child clients than a rationale based on maturational concepts and which emphasises the cognitive and psycholinguistic implications for treatment. Following Keith (1983), such implications have become increasingly recognised, with increasing emphasis on the child client's functional abilities as these affect academic progress.

## The Category System

Drawing on findings and observations from the two Order Effects, the Type A pattern, and the Reversals of the SSW test Katz (1992) described a Category System containing four categories:

- Decoding;
- Tolerance-Fading Memory;
- Integration;
- Organisation.

The aim of this Category System was to facilitate interpretation of CAPD test results and to assist in explaining the results in the context of the client's speech, language and academic problems. Katz noted that the categories were not mutually exclusive, as dysfunction in more than one category was observed in half or more of clients with CAPD.

The Decoding Category is concerned with breakdown at the phonemic level, which may occur because the phonemes are weakly imprinted on the brain, presumably in the posterior temporal region (cf. Order Effect low/high). If so, it would be expected that clients will be unsure about the auditory stimulus presented, and will take a relatively long time to process it. Their phonemic awareness will be weak. Thus, these clients will have problems with abilities or tasks that require remembering and manipulating phonemes, such as auditory memory, phonemic analysis and synthesis/phonics, reading, spelling and most receptive language tests. The remediation of these clients is probably best directed to improving their phonemic awareness and related abilities. For example, a relatively slow speech rate might be used to begin remediation, gradually increasing the rate to normal as phonemic awareness increases.

Tolerance-Fading Memory (TFM) is typified by problems in receiving speech-in-noise and in short-term memory. In TFM, memory for the early parts of an auditory stimulus is weaker than for subsequent parts (cf. Order Effect high/low). TFM is possibly associated with the anterior temporal region and is characterised in around 75 per cent of cases by breakdowns in auditory memory and in perceiving speech-in-noise. Clients with TFM experience difficulties in reading, expressive language and writing, and are readily distracted. Reading comprehension may be a particular problem because, although they can usually pronounce individual printed words and understand word meanings, their recollection and comprehension of a body of text is weak. Distractiblity (low speech-in-noise results) and poor auditory memory would be expected to produce just such an outcome. Therapy for such cases can be approached by speech-in-noise desensitisation and auditory memory exercises. Alternative therapies may involve tactics that do not rely heavily on auditory processing, such as compensatory or augmentative therapy via the visual modality.

Description of the Integration Category is less well-developed than the two preceding categories, and includes cases that are not as homogeneous. As the title suggests, clients with integration difficulties have problems in putting information together, but the form of the difficulty varies. For example, some cases have auditory-visual integration problems, whereas others seem to need extended periods of time in which to respond to questions. All cases produce the Type A pattern in the SSW test (a high proportion of errors in the LC condition), but can be considered as forming two types (Integration Types 1 and 2).

Clients with Integration Type 1 disorders produce similar test scores and have similar classroom problems to cases in the Decoding Category. Clients with Integration Type 2 behaviour are similar to the TFM group. Integration Type 1 cases have severe reading and spelling problems (dyslexia), and often very poor handwriting and drawing abilities. They perform poorly on phonemic synthesis tasks, but do not necessarily produce severely depressed scores on speech-in-noise tests. Their difficulties may be associated with the corpus callosum and the parietal-occipital region of the brain. Appropriate therapy may include phonemic awareness and sound–symbol training, to match and integrate the visual and auditory inputs.

Clients with Integration Type 2 difficulties differ from those with Integration Type 1 characteristics insofar as they may not have auditory-visual integration problems, and have less difficulty with academic subjects. They do, however, have rather poor handwriting, as found with TFM cases. Their speech-in-noise performance is relatively weak, but they perform well on tests of phonemic synthesis. Integration Type 2 cases are relatively few in number, so that Type 2 characteristics are less well-defined than for Type 1 cases. Type 2 clients may have problems associated with the anterior region of the brain.

Clients in the Organisation Category are also relatively uncommon, and hence this category is not well characterised. However, clients with Organisation problems can be typified as producing Reversals on the SSW test and speech sound reversals in phonemic synthesis tasks. They tend to have difficulty in organising information and to be disorganised in their general behaviour, especially when carrying out sequential tasks. Remedial work may emphasise sequencing tasks and the use of (written) lists. There may be an anatomical association with the fronto-temporal-parietal and premotor regions of the brain.

## A test of the Category System

How well does this Category System work in practice? Considerably more research needs to be done, but Katz (1992) has described one study of learning-disabled children with CAPD in which there was complete agreement among three investigators in classifying a large proportion of cases. Of 94 clients assessed, 50 per cent showed a primary Decoding disorder, 20 per cent had a primary TFM problem, 17 per cent had an Integration problem (13 per cent Type 1 and 4 per cent Type 2) and 4 per cent had an Organisation difficulty. Thus almost all the cases could be categorised. The remaining 8 per cent, who had normal or few abnormal CAPD test outcomes, could not be categorised. A secondary category was chosen for 52 per cent of the children because of problems in two or more CAPD areas. The most common secondary area was TFM (26 per cent of total cases), followed by Decoding (16 per cent) and Organisation (10 per cent). Few clients (5 per cent of the total sample) had a tertiary problem (4 per cent Organisation and 1 per cent TFM). As the majority of cases could be categorised on the basis of three tests for CAPD, the Category System appears to have gone some way towards meeting the puzzles arising from the CAPD test battery approach, which we outlined at the beginning of this section.

## The test battery

Katz (1992) suggested a test battery of just three tests to provide the information on which categorisations can be made in his Category

System. Thus, tests of phonemic synthesis and speech-in-noise are added to the SSW test. These three tests take about 30–40 minutes to administer in total. We have adopted this test battery, with minor variation, for use in our own clinical laboratory. The test materials were rerecorded with a female second generation Australian speaker who has a cultivated Australian speech style (Horvath, 1985) and presented via headphones at 50 dB sensation level.

The SSW test has already been described above. We have changed some of the SSW spondee pairs because some North American spondees, (e.g. cornstarch) have little meaning for Australians. (Recently, Golding, Lilly and Lay (1996) have described a further Australian version of the SSW Test.)

Speech-in-noise is a useful test, as Downs and Crum (1978) showed that, even when a speech signal is highly intelligible, processing demands during auditory learning are significantly greater than in a quiet environment. Various speech signals and noise backgrounds can be used for the speech-in-noise test. The common preference is to use monosyllabic words for the speech signals and broad-spectrum noise ('white noise' or 'pink noise') or multitalker babble as the noise background. The words are typically presented 5–10 dB above the noise. We use the BKB/A everyday word lists (Bench, 1992b) presented 10 dB above a four-talker speech babble, scored by whole words correct. The BKB/A words are taken from the key words in the BKB/A sentences (Bench, Doyle & Greenwood, 1987), so that performance on the words may be compared with performance on the sentences, where such comparison is of interest. We use four-talker speech babble as the background noise, rather than broad-spectrum noise or speech babble with more than four talkers, because four-talker babble seems to discriminate more clearly between those clients who have speech-in-noise problems and those who do not. It appears that, with four-talker babble, it is more difficult to employ selective attention to resolve the auditory figure ground distinction.

In the Phonemic Synthesis test (Katz, 1983, pp. 269–95), the client is required to synthesise whole words from auditory presentation of their constituent phonemes at a rate of about one phoneme per second (e.g. /d-o-g/ = dog). The test consists of 25 items increasing in difficulty from the first to the last item. Phonemic synthesis, sometimes referred to as sound-blending, is a metalinguistic skill ,which depends on phonemic awareness. It requires the client to detect and recognise the phonemes, retain them in memory and combine them into words in the given phoneme sequence.

We have also added a test of auditory memory span, the Digit Span subtest of the Weschler Intelligence Scale for Children – Revised (Weschler, 1980). This test is presented with live voice (taking care not to offer speech-reading cues), rather than from a recording, for the following reason. Because the digits are presented without falling intonation for the final digit (which conventionally would signal the end), the client has no cue as to when the sequence of digits has finished. However, if the digits are presented with live voice, the client can be instructed to observe the tester for a signal (e.g. nodding the head) to determine the end of the sequence.

We have conducted a factor analysis (not reported in detail here because the study is ongoing and incomplete at the time of writing) of data from the use of these four tests on a group of 36 children. These children were aged 8 to 12 years and had diagnosed language learning disabilities, varying in severity from little or none, to severe. The factor analysis to date suggests that, for three factors isolated: the Total SSW score loads mainly on Factor 1; SSW Reversals load mainly on Factor 2; speech-in-noise loads mainly on Factor 3; Phonemic Synthesis, like speech-in-noise, loads mainly on Factor 3, perhaps suggesting that speech-in-noise impairs phoneme perception; and the Auditory Digit Span test loads on Factors 1 and 3. Because of the small size of the sample and the varying severity of language learning disability, it would not be reasonable to conclude too much from this outcome. It is nonetheless reassuring that the four tests cannot be said to be measuring the same things and, in some instances, are clearly measuring different things. It is particularly interesting that Reversals appear to form a condition of their own, as Katz noted some question as to whether Reversals could form a separate category in his System.

## Test battery for obscure auditory dysfunction

Before leaving this section, we make passing comment about the test battery for obscure auditory dysfunction (OAD) by Saunders, Field and Haggard (1992). The concept of OAD has been used specifically to refer to people aged 15 to 55 years who have normal peripheral hearing and no known (other) central audiological problem, but who have difficulty with perceiving speech in all types of noise background or with understanding speech in the presence of other speech. A battery which characterised this population consisted of tests for: (a) poor speech perception threshold in noise; (b) the individual's view of, or confidence in, his/her ability to discriminate speech in noise; (c) dichotic listening as a measure of attention; and (d) masked thresholds for 2000 Hz tones in notch-noise (broadband noise with a 1000 Hz-wide notch centred at 2000 Hz). This test battery was presented as part of a package, in which other components were a special clinical interview and a brief questionnaire, taking 37 minutes to administer in all. Shaw, Jardine and Fridjhon (1996) have suggested that high-frequency audiometry may be a useful addition to this package.

## The child with CAPD

The child with CAPD often presents a perplexing problem for parents, teachers and other professionals who are asked to evaluate and advise on the management of the child's communication difficulties and the ensuing effects on academic and social development (Willeford & Burleigh, 1985; Bench, 1992a). This child tends to be male, under-achieves academically and yet has normal-to-high intelligence. He has little or no peripheral hearing loss. His fine and gross motor skills are usually good, so that he can draw and paint adequately. He communicates well in simple, individual-to-individual conversations that have a straightforward grammatical and semantic structure. However, this child commonly has difficulty in following conversations that involve more complex sequencing of syntax and/or semantics. He often experiences problems in following conversations or instructions presented against a noisy background. His auditory memory span may be very short for his age (Page, 1985). He has problems with reading comprehension, especially with irregular verbs and embedded clauses and phrases. More generally, he presents with language learning difficulties.

It is thus of considerable interest that Tonnquist-Uhlén (1996) has recently described a study of auditory evoked potentials in 20 children with severe language impairment and low performance on a number of psychometric tests, including tests of auditory processing. Tonnquist-Uhlén found a high degree of pathological electroencephalograms and some pathological auditory brainstem responses in these children when compared with normally developing controls. Magnetic resonance imaging abnormalities were found in only two children. Overall, 17 of the 20 children showed a pathological outcome in one or more of the measures. The results suggested a dual pathophysiology, namely a specific auditory disorder and a non-specific general cerebral disorder. Whereas other studies had indicated abnormal electrophysiological and neuroimaging findings in such children, this work of Tonnquist-Uhlén showed particular promise for establishing individual diagnostic criteria.

Problems with CAPD may be suspected from age 3 or 4 years. However, auditory behaviour at such young ages shows considerable variability and hence questionable reliability in measurement, with high standard deviations in test norms. This situation may be ascribed to immaturity of relevant functions of the developing central nervous system. For example, such features as auditory memory span and articulatory memory rehearsal differ considerably between children and are not well-developed in early childhood (Henry, 1991), but increase from year to year as the child matures. Clearly, it will be difficult to make reasonably precise and stable measurements of such features of the central auditory system while that system continues to be 'plastic' (Bench, 1992a, p. 191). Therefore, although CAPD may emerge at an early age, it most frequently comes to professional attention in the beginning primary school years, often in association with failure to make acceptable progress in reading at age 7–8 years.

Satisfactory estimates of the prevalence of CAPD in children are widely acknowledged as hard to come by, because of confusion over, or imprecision in, terminology (Roeser & Downs, 1988). Also, mild cases of CAPD are inconspicuous and easily compensated for, especially by some more artful brighter children, when educational demands are minimal. Some of the more precise estimates come from the study of CAPD in special groups, such as emotionally disturbed children or juvenile delinquents. For example, CAPD has been found in up to half of a sample of juvenile delinquents (Smock, 1982). However, the prevalence of CAPD in the general child population is of wider interest. Some CAPD prevalence figures can be gleaned from the literature on learning disabilities. For instance, Oberklaid, Harris and Keir (1989) found evidence of auditory processing problems in 62 per cent of a sample of children referred with learning difficulties. As 5–10 per cent of schoolchildren have learning difficulties (Dockrell & McShane, 1992, p. 152), a working estimate of the prevalence of CAPD in children is thus around 3–6 per cent. This perhaps surprisingly high range confirms suspicions, frequently expressed in the literature, that CAPD problems in children are more prevalent than previously believed. Also, it accords with prevalence estimates (Dockrell & McShane, 1992, pp. 58, 88) of listening problems (6 per cent prevalence in 4-year-olds) and reading problems (6.6 per cent prevalence in 9–11-year-olds), to which it would be expected to relate.

## Otitis media and CAPD

Zinkus and Gottlieb (1980) and Page (1985), among others, have argued that early persistent and/or recurrent otitis media can lead to auditory processing difficulties. In this condition, resulting from malfunction of the Eustachian tube, the middle-ear cavity fills with fluid, producing what is called serous otitis media or otitis media with effusion. The condition may resolve spontaneously with time but persists in 50–70 per cent of cases two weeks after assessment and treatment, in 20–40 per cent after four weeks, in 10–20 per cent after eight weeks and in 10 per cent after 12 weeks (New South Wales Health Department, 1993). Some 5 per cent of children have the condition after 12 months (Zielhuis, Rach & van den Broek, 1989). About one child in three or four may be affected by such chronic otitis media (Moore & Best, 1988; Schilder et al., 1994). It is uncommon to find this condition, which has a first, major, prevalence peak at 6–18 months of age, and a second, less marked, prevalence peak around age 4 years, after the age of 6 or 7 years (New South Wales Health Department, 1993).

As otitis media with effusion typically results in a mild hearing loss, its chronic manifestation may be expected to interfere with speech perception over a period of time when hearing for speech is important for the development of speech-processing ability and for the development of language. A later consequence may be retarded educational progress. Overall, the linguistic and educational sequelae of chronic otitis media are not very great, being about one-third to one-half of a standard deviation in lowered performance on a range of tests, and tend to dissipate over time (Chalmers et al., 1989; Haggard & Hughes, 1991). However, the sequelae vary in magnitude and duration. Although most children who present with sequelae show only moderate, short-duration effects, some clinical reports indicate that a small proportion may experience more serious, persistent problems. In summary, although most studies agree that chronic effusive otitis media in the first three years of life is associated with delays in phoneme perception, some phonological contrasts, development of the lexicon and produced phonology, the evidence for the effects of chronic otitis media thereafter on auditory processing and on language and academic development is generally less compelling (Bench & Harrold, 1996).

## Clinical examples

Two clinical CAPD cases are now described, a 42-year-old mother and her 9-year-old son from a family in which the 44-year-old father reported no hearing problems of any kind, and an elder brother, aged 12 years, who had no peripheral or CAPD problems on audiological assessment.

### The son

At initial interview, the son attended with his mother, who reported that he had a slight, barely noticeable hearing loss and difficulties with reading, writing and spelling at school, where his teacher's instructions had sometimes to be repeated. However, his numerical skills were good. He had occasional problems in hearing in noisy situations. He had experienced middle-ear problems in his first 11 months of life, and had sustained a head injury in a fall at age 3 years, but with no apparent long-term damage. He suffered from asthma and was presently being treated for a lisp by a speech-language therapist. At a previous optometric assessment his colour vision was found to be normal, his distance vision was 6/6 bilaterally and he was slightly long-sighted. However, he had borderline focusing skills for close vision and divergent eye alignment, for which he was receiving training with eye exercises.

At audiological assessment the son produced the following results.

### Otoscopy and tympanometry

Both ear canals were clear with normal-appearing eardrums. Type A (normal) pressure/compliance curves were obtained bilaterally, with acoustic reflexes present bilaterally at 100 dB SPL for 500, 1000, 3000 and 4000 Hz tones and at 80 dB SPL for 3000 and 4000 Hz tones.

### Conventional pure tone audiometry

Hearing for pure tones over the range 250–8000 Hz was within normal limits bilaterally, but only just so (20 dB HTL) at 250 Hz. Speech-audiometry-in-quiet at 50 dB speech reference level (dB SRL) gave scores of 100 per cent for each ear.

The above tests indicated that the son's peripheral hearing and middle-ear functions were all within normal limits.

### CAPD tests

The son's score on the phonemic synthesis test was 56 per cent, around grade 1 level. On the SSW test he showed a non-significant Ear Effect, but a significant low/high Order Effect, suggestive of problems with phonemic decoding and language functions. His SSW-gram was of a Type A pattern, indicative of reading and spelling difficulties and, overall, the SSW test showed moderately depressed auditory processing ability. Further, he produced a significant number of reversals ($n = 10$), reporting test words in an incorrect order. His total auditory digit span score was 7, equivalent to that for a child aged 6.5 years. He scored 3 on digits-forward and 4 on digits backward, so his auditory memory problem was unlikely to have been with rehearsal. He obtained 64 per cent for right and left ears alone and 68 per cent binaurally for the speech-in-noise test, more than one standard deviation below the expected level for a child of his age.

### Outcome

The results of the son's peripheral hearing and middle ear-function tests raised no concerns, but the results of his CAPD tests, where he experienced difficulties with all four tests, indicated further evaluation and therapy. He was referred for speech and language therapy. Meanwhile, he and his mother were advised to bring to the attention of his teachers the suggestions in the 'Informal approaches' list of the 'Management of clients with CAPD' section following.

At speech and language therapy assessment two months later, his lisp had resolved. The Clinical Evaluation of Language Fundamentals-Revised (CELF-R) of Semel, Wiig and Secord (1989) showed a mix of language strengths and weaknesses. He had no problems with medium-length sentences, but showed particular difficulty in understanding and constructing long, complex sentences, where he presented with a 12-month delay. In assessment of his reading ability (Neale, 1988), he mispronounced some words and made a number of incorrect substitutions, losing the meaning as a result. His reading rate was slow. His overall reading age delay was 12 months. Additional testing showed that, although he could hear individual phonemes (e.g. /b/, /s/) and represent them visually with coloured blocks, he could not perceive them as individual sounds within syllables. He was further referred to a clinic for learning-disabled children.

## The mother

At initial interview, the mother presented as a self-referred client who suspected that she may have a CAPD problem after linking information she had gathered from our clinical laboratory about her son's CAPD with the difficulties which she had herself experienced with reading, memory and word confusions (e.g. hearing 'ship' as 'shape'). She had a busy lifestyle, working in business with her husband as well as running her household, but felt that her difficulties were possibly due to some CAPD problem rather than to stress. She reported great difficulty with reading, but had devised tactics to circumvent the need to read, such as taking photographs to give her visual information for a craft project. She also reported problems in remembering what she had been told, stating that, in listening to a long flow of speech, she managed only to perceive short sequences of the spoken message and had to guess at the meaning of the remainder of the message.

She stated that she had no special problems in hearing for non-speech material. For example, she experienced no trouble in hearing a telephone ring or in localising sounds, though she often set the radio volume higher than others. She experienced occasional slight tinnitus, heard as a 'soft buzz', more in one ear than the other, although she could not remember which. Her parents had worn hearing aids since the age of about 70, and her husband had commented that her family home, 25 years ago, was always a lot louder than he was accustomed to, suggesting that her parents had been hearing impaired from the age of about 40, and consequently that she had some family history of hearing impairment.

On audiological assessment, she produced the following results.

### Otoscopy and tympanometry

The ear canals were clear with normal-appearing tympanic membranes. Tympanograms were of Type A (normal pressure/compliance range) with acoustic reflexes elicited by 500, 1000, 3000 and 4000 Hz tones at 80 dB SPL (normal responses).

### Conventional pure tone audiometry

Responses were obtained bilaterally to pure tones between –5 and 5 dB HTL across the range 250 to 8000 Hz, well within normal limits. For speech-audiometry-in-quiet, 100 per cent correct responses were obtained bilaterally at 50 dB SRL, within normal expectations.

The above results indicate that the mother's peripheral hearing was within normal limits bilaterally. No test gave even a hint of a pathological problem for either ear.

### CAPD tests

The mother scored 92 per cent (close to the maximum score) on the phonemic synthesis test. However, her two errors were of the type indicated in her initial interview, such as reporting 'cot' for 'coat'. Her SSW test results were also within normal limits, although she showed a slight (non-significant) difficulty with ordering the stimulus words correctly in producing four reversals. With the auditory digit span test, she obtained a total score of 10 units, equivalent to that of a child of 8.5 years. Her performance on digits-forward was the same as on digits-backward (5 units), suggesting that her memory problem was due to other cause than weak rehearsal. For speech-audiometry-in-noise, she obtained scores of 80 per cent and 84 per cent for her right and left ears respectively and 84 per cent binaurally, below expected performance in all instances.

### Outcome

The mother's difficulties appeared to be in processing speech-in-noise and especially with auditory memory. She was referred to clinical psychology for further evaluation and treatment of her memory problem as the next stage. Additionally, she found it useful to attend speech-language therapy sessions with her son.

## Memory and coding problems in children with CAPD and language learning disabilities

Readers may wonder how CAPD in children comes to affect their academic progress, especially in such activities as vocabulary, reading, spelling and writing. A provisional answer is that, in their early years and for various reasons, possibly including mild intermittent conductive hearing loss caused by recurrent otitis media (Downs, 1985; Bench & Harrold, 1996), these children do not sufficiently attend to speech inputs. Hence the speech inputs to such children are weakly imprinted on, or are interrupted in their registration on, their auditory processing systems (cf. Welsh, Welsh & Healy, 1983).

The likely linguistic and psycholinguistic consequences are several and will interact in various complex ways. However, to take just one example, it appears that, as we have seen, children with CAPD commonly have problems in phonemic synthesis and analysis, analogous to the findings on acoustic cue discrimination and processing of computer-synthesised syllables in language-impaired children described by Tallal and Piercy (1978), Tallal and Stark (1981) and Tallal, Stark and Mellits (1985). Such children do not adequately develop the phonological processes, phonological awareness and other functions needed for the early stages of language development (Ellis & Young, 1988; Gathercole & Baddeley, 1990, 1993). As a result, they have difficulties with phoneme discrimination (differentiating one phoneme from another) and in matching the phonological forms of the speech sound system to phonological patterns previously experienced and held in long-term storage. Consequently they experience breakdowns in deriving meanings at the word and phrase levels, via the semantic system. Ultimately, they are assessed as language disordered.

James, van Steenbrugge and Chiveralls (1994) studied a group of six language-disordered children with CAPD, aged 8–10 years, who were matched with chronological and language age controls. These children were given auditorily presented tests for:

(a) immediate phonological memory;
(b) recall of phonologically similar and dissimilar words;
(c) effect of word length on recall;
(d) articulation rate;
(e) phoneme discrimination;
(f) lexical decision;
(g) word comprehension.

James et al. found that the children with CAPD had impaired semantic systems and impaired phonological working memory, together with inconsistent, but significant, phonological processing deficits. This outcome was in accordance with the poor phonological working memory found in language-disordered children (Gathercole & Baddeley 1990, 1993). James et al. were careful to point out that their findings were based on a small group of subjects. As such, the findings were best considered as indicative rather than compelling. Further, to be sure that CAPD in language-disordered children is associated with impaired semantic systems and impaired phonological memory required a comparison with a matched group of language-disordered children who do not have CAPD.

Bench and Maule (1997) have investigated similar issues to those explored by James et al. (1994), beginning by noting that children with CAPD not only have problems with certain listening tasks, but also have trouble with non-auditory tasks, such as reading or writing, when in noisy environments. It appears that CAPD affects learning in ways beyond disrupting the processing of auditory material. However, in processing non-auditory verbal information there is no auditory signal to be limited or distorted as it travels along the auditory pathways. It thus seems that, in some way, CAPD also affects the capacity to attend and to think, and that these cognitive activities are associated with the auditory pathways.

Now, when learning to read (by phonics), normally developing children typically process written verbal information via an articulatory- or auditory-based code known as internal speech or subvocal speech. Internal speech reflects the verbal language used for thought (Conrad, 1979, pp. 1–26). The nature of internal speech can be further explained as follows. Occasionally, we find ourselves reading under our breath, or even out loud, a passage of text that is difficult to follow, or sometimes we come across an unfamiliar word in our reading and try to pronounce it, syllable by syllable. In such instances internal speech has (just) become externalised.

Internal speech may also be explained by considering the memory systems with which it has been investigated, especially the memory subsystem of the phonological loop. As expounded by Baddeley (1992), the phonological loop contains a phonological memory store, able to hold traces of acoustic or speech-based material. These traces will fade away within about two seconds unless they are refreshed by subvocal rehearsal, namely, internal speech. In addition to preserving the memory trace through subvocal rehearsal, internal speech can register visual material by subvocal representation. For example, in reading, the visual stimulus of the written word is translated or recoded into the articulatory/auditory code of inner speech. Hence, the effect of background noise on reading is plausibly explained as interference with the subvocal naming of the written or printed words in inner speech. This conclusion is particularly convincing in view of the frequently stated link between aspects of reading and phonological processing (e.g. Bradley & Bryant, 1978; Snowling, 1981). A likely corollary of this situation is that the client who is a 'visual processor', and unable to recode visual stimuli into phonemic representations, would not be similarly affected by background noise.

Bench and Maule (1997) hypothesised that CAPD affects such academic tasks as reading because it leads to weak development of internal speech. If CAPD is associated with diminished ability to use phonemic information, disorders of auditory sequencing and impaired auditory memory (and consequently with impaired operation of the phonological loop), then use of internal speech in reading is likely to be impaired also.

To investigate this hypothesis, Bench and Maule made use of the phonological similarity effect, as employed by Conrad (1979) in his notable work with deaf school-leavers. The phonological similarity effect refers to the situation where, for example, visually presented homophone words (words that may look different, but would be similar if pronounced, such as 'do', 'through', 'screw') are less well recalled in a serial memory recall task than visually presented non-homophone words (words that may look similar, but would be different if pronounced, such as 'home', 'bare', 'lane').

The phenomenon apparently occurs because the phonological memory store depends on a purely phonological code, implying that similar words are stored on the basis of similar codes. Coding similarity will present fewer discriminating features between items, leading to impaired retrieval and poorer overt recall. So if, in a serial recall memory task, a client makes more errors on the homophone than the non-homophone lists, the likelihood is that the client is using an auditory or articulatory code, as do most normally developing children. If, however, the client makes more errors on the non-homophone than the homophone lists, it is likely that the client is using a visually-based code. Thus, exploration of the phonological similarity effect in children with CAPD could indicate whether such children use internal speech, a reduced or weakly developed form of internal speech or some other means to process verbal information.

A group of children, four female and 14 male, aged 8;2 (8 years 2 months) to 12;8 (mean 10;7) years, with diagnosed language learning (reading) disability (LLD) and a control group of normally developing children matched for age and gender, were first checked for hearing within normal limits and tested with a modified Katz CAPD test battery (see above). All members of the LLD group performed poorly on at least two of the four CAPD tests and, as a group, scored significantly worse on all four CAPD tests than the normal control group. Following checks that the children could read the test words (see below) without difficulty, they were given a memory pretest, following which a serial recall memory task was adjusted to be of equivalent difficulty for each child. The children were then asked to perform the serial memory recall task using lists of homophone (H) and non-homophone (NH) words, as described above. When errors on the H lists were calculated as a percentage of total errors on both H and NH lists, using the formula:

$$\text{Internal speech ratio (ISR)} = \frac{H}{H + NH} \times 100\%$$

the LLD group with CAPD problems scored a mean of 55.2 per cent whereas the normally developing controls scored 76.1 per cent. This difference was highly significant. The internal speech ratios are plotted by matched subject pairs according to age in Figure 9.2. The control children experienced considerably more difficulty with the H than the NH lists, a result indicating their use of internal speech. However, as a group, the LLD children with CAPD problems had only slightly more difficulty with the H than the NH lists, suggesting that they had no strong preference between an auditory/articulatory code on the one hand and a visual code on the other. There was no apparent age effect, indicating that the relative use of internal speech did not vary systematically with age.

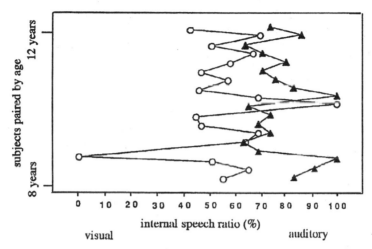

**Figure 9.2:** Internal speech ratios for 18 CAPD children (open circles) and their 18 matched controls (solid triangles) shown according to the age of each matched pair.(Reprinted with permission from Audiology)

These results are congruent with the explanation that, overall, the LLD/CAPD group could use phonological coding (cf. James, van Steenbrugge and Chiveralls, 1994) and internal speech, but to a lesser degree than the normally developing controls. The results support the contention that CAPD problems lead to relatively weak use of phonological coding and internal speech, and consequent reading difficulties, with an ensuing diagnosis of language learning disability.

## Some criticisms of the concept of central auditory processing disorders

From the discussion of the CAPD area so far, the reader will have understood that the area is very complex, and that it leads to complex outcomes. That the area is complex is clearly shown by the adoption of a test battery approach to investigations of CAPD by most of the researchers and clinicians involved. That the outcomes are complex is illustrated by the variety of disordered behaviours that seem to result from CAPD, and which can be manifest in initially rather alarming numbers of combinations.

The reader may also have gained the impression that some of the functions assessed are overlapping and that the underlying concepts are confused. If so, the reader is not alone. Bench (1992a, p. 193) referred to the use of 'woolly' concepts, which could be 'used to cloak mixed and disorderly findings of obscure aetiology'. Earlier, Davis and Rampp (1983) criticised the available tests for auditory processing disorders as woefully inadequate. These tests were of doubtful reliability and validity, often being gross measures, which, as they assessed several features at the same time, confused one disorder with another. To cite perhaps the most common difficulty, many, if not most, tests involved memory because the more complex auditory stimuli, with more than one compo-nent, must necessarily implicate memory. There is little doubt that these criticisms of Davis and Rampp continue to have force more than a decade later.

Influential writing by Rees (1981, pp. 94–120) has further called into question the use of some auditory processing tests and therapy in clinical use. She began by observing that there were two different positions from which the auditory processing explanation was used for failures in the development of articulation and language, and the acquisition of reading skills. The first position, commonly adopted by remedial workers, was that the complex behaviours involved in such abilities could be broken down into a set of subskills, which could be reduced further to under-lying perceptual-motor abilities. This position assumed that elements of language behaviour ('auditory discrimination', 'auditory sequencing' and 'auditory memory') could be separately identified and assessed, and remediated where necessary. It aimed to discover basic deficits that could be treated via therapeutic techniques, and paid little heed to theoretical or conceptual explanations. The second position had a medical orienta-tion and included work by audiologists. It was based on a diagnostic, site of lesion approach, where performance on certain auditory processing tests could be correlated with the presence of known lesions in the brain. The emphasis of this second position was on test development, rather than on therapeutic treatments.

Rees went on to note the very wide range and varied complexity of the tasks and presumed auditory processing skills, and the lack of a coherent supporting theory, concluding that 'auditory processing' referred to a non-existent simplicity and unity. She asked, for example, how a child's auditory memory span for digits could affect ability to learn language, and how following speech switched alternately between the ears could affect classroom learning. The reader may recall at this point that, earlier, we referred to the work of James, van Steenbrugge and Chiveralls (1994), which suggested that children with CAPD use phono-logical coding, though to a lesser extent than do normally developing children, and to the study of Bench and Maule (1997), which showed that memory for homophone and non-homophone words could explain, at least in part, the difference in reading ability between children who were developing normally and those with CAPD. Thus, research has moved on and some of Rees's comments are now rather dated. However, it is worth continuing to outline some of her criticisms because they illustrate several traps that may ensnare the neophyte. Also, they help to explain why traditional therapy in the area is often unsuccessful (e.g. Hammill & Larsen, 1974) and why more recent accounts of therapeutic approaches (e.g. Schneider, 1992, pp. 161–168) are more intriguing than compelling.

Rees criticised the large literature that sought to associate a variety of language and learning difficulties with disorders in the sequencing of auditory stimuli. She pointed out that different claims had been made at different times for different units (phonemes, syllables, words or sentences) as the units to be sequenced. This search for units was a feature of associationism, the argument that complex behaviour, such as language, can be reduced to indivisible entities beyond which analysis can go no further. However, research showed that no one kind of unit was any better than another. Studies of sequencing had to take account of the concomitant sequencing of all kinds of units in all their various patterns. To simply propose therapy in which the client is instructed to tap out a rhythm, or to imitate a sequence of letters or words, grossly underestimated the complex skills involved in sequences of speech and language. Further, the relationship between auditory sequencing and the comprehension of language was complex. For example, although word order is of great importance in comprehending the English language, its function is dependent on grammatical structure (e.g. 'The dog bit the man' versus 'The man was bitten by the dog').

Rees offered yet further criticisms. Auditory synthesis (and auditory closure) were intellectual, metalinguistic skills concerned with manipulating speech sounds into words rather than auditory abilities as such. Auditory memory was known to be of different types—sensory (echoic), short-term and long-term (and now working memory), which operated differently on different material with different outcomes—but such differences were insufficiently acknowledged, and so on.

Rees (1981, p. 118) concluded that test batteries that attempt to assess central auditory processing have established that some children differ in their ability to 'engage the speech processor in cases of limited redundancy, like competing speech. and (differ in their ability to) deal linguistically with distorted or unexpected versions of the input'. She argued, however, that future research should be more directed to an appropriate account of how central auditory processing deficiencies relate to the language disorders with which they are associated. As we have seen, such research is now under way.

## Criticisms of test stimuli

From the discussion so far, it will be apparent that much of the difficulty in teasing out the nature of auditory processing and its disorders arises because of the nature of the test stimuli. In particular, it is often unclear whether the test results are assessing an auditory disorder, a psychological or language disorder, or some combination of these. It might be supposed that the test stimuli used to measure auditory processing should be designed to be unaffected by language, and that non-language, non-speech stimuli should therefore be employed. Alternatively, if language-related stimuli are used, they should be so familiar and undemanding that the linguistic aspect will be of no account. This line of thought was adopted by Keith (1981b, pp. 63–4), who recommended that an auditory processing test:

- cannot be loaded with language comprehension items;
- cannot require linguistic manipulation of the signal;
- should not utilise (but when necessary should minimise) cross-sensory input (auditory-visual) or response modality (e.g. auditory-motor);
- should utilise non-linguistic signals;
- must be primarily a speech imitative task using non-meaningful material or speech stimuli so familiar to the person being tested that comprehension plays no role in the response.

The difficulty with such requirements is that it is not possible to be sure that all elements of language comprehension are excluded when using speech stimuli, even if such stimuli are nonsense material (e.g. nonsense syllables) or are highly overlearned. To process stimuli that are recognisable as speech stimuli is to process linguistic rather than auditory material (Rees, 1981, pp. 94–120). If the tester proposes instead to use only non-speech stimuli, such as tones or noise bands, then the results may be of limited utility. Although non-speech stimuli can be useful, as in tests exploring binaural interaction (e.g. Matkin & Hook, 1983), it seems necessary to use speech stimuli, even if modified, to study higher-level auditory processing. In this context, it is of interest to note that the early tests for CAPD (e.g. Bocca & Calearo, 1963) used speech stimuli, arguing that speech stimuli were needed because speech processing is a high-level auditory activity (cf. Studdert-Kennedy, 1976).

Some authors continue to cast doubt on the concept of CAPD and whether it constitutes a specific condition (e.g. Burd & Fisher, 1986; Peck, Gressard & Hellerman, 1991). However, as argued by Gordon and Ward (1995), meaning has to be given to auditory stimuli when they reach the cortical level, and auditory processing, like other cortical functions, can be disordered.

## CAPD and attention deficit disorder

Selective attention to meaningful information sources while simultaneously ignoring irrelevant stimuli is essential to adaptive functioning

(Lane & Pearson, 1982; Burack, 1994). The individual is bombarded with so much information from the environment that, unless the meaningful part of this information can be filtered for processing, the individual has little or no possibility of making sense of the environment or of behaving competently in it. It is clear that for CAPD tests to be conducted effectively, the client must attend to the test stimuli. A problem arises, however, in that poor control of selective attention is frequently attributed to clients with CAPD. We have previously remarked that these clients tend to tire easily, probably, in part at least, because attending to test stimuli under difficult conditions requires considerable mental effort. The alert clinician will be on the watch for signs of tiring, with consequent loss of attention, and will introduce rest periods to counter it.

Since the early 1980s an increasing number of reports have begun to appear about attention deficit disorder (ADD) and, more recently, attention deficit hyperactivity disorder (ADHD), with a focus on the behavioural problems of inattention and overactivity, although Keller (1992, pp. 107–114) reminded us that the symptoms (notably impulsivity, hyperactivity, inattention and distractibility) have been recorded since the early 1900s. The nature of the distinction between ADD and ADHD, and their relationship to learning disabilities, has been described by numerous authors (e.g. Silver, 1990; Cantwell & Baker, 1991; Epstein et al., 1991; Goodyear & Hynd, 1992).

Some authors (e.g. Burd & Fisher, 1986; Gascon, Johnson & Burd, 1986) pointed out that the criteria for CAPD and ADD had several features in common, including weak concentration, fidgeting, distractibility and poor academic work. Keller (1992), who presented a useful outline of the symptoms of ADD and CAPD, came to a similar conclusion. He stressed that great care was needed in making a differential diagnosis (see also Bellis, 1996, p. 93).

The use of stimulant medication has also indicated some similarities between ADD/ADHD on the one hand and CAPD on the other. Keith and Engineer (1991) found improvement in auditory attention in ADHD children treated with methylphenidate. More recently, Cook et al. (1993) reported a study of 15 boys aged 6–10 years who met criteria for ADD in comparison with 10 boys without ADD. In a placebo-controlled, double-blind study of the effects of methylphenidate, with all subjects assessed with a CAPD test battery, they found that 12 of the 15 boys with ADD, and none of the controls without ADD, met criteria for CAPD. The boys with ADD also responded to the medication, as assessed by measures of both ADD and CAPD. Cook et al. concluded that, because of the overlap in symptomatology, the meeting of criteria for both disorders, and the effects of medication on both ADD and CAPD measures, ADD and CAPD are closely related disorders. Importantly, they also concluded that the current diagnostic criteria for CAPD make it difficult to separate the two disorders on the basis of CAPD assessments alone. However, stimulant medication could alleviate the symptoms of both ADD and CAPD, and CAPD tests seemed useful in assessing the symptomatology of ADD and its response to medication.

The current consensus (Moss & Sheiffele, 1994; Riccio et al. 1994) is that by no means all children with CAPD demonstrate ADD or ADHD. Further, it will be recalled that Tonnquist-Uhlén (1996) reported that children with severe language impairment and auditory processing difficulties produced electrophysiological and neuroimaging results indicating dual pathology, a specific auditory disorder and a non-specific cerebral disturbance. It may be that Tonnquist-Uhlén's approach will assist the resolution of present problems of differential diagnosis between ADD/ADHD and CAPD.

Meanwhile, it is noteworthy that Keller (1992) suggested that the differential diagnosis of CAPD and ADD can be determined largely by whether the first professional consulted by the child's family is a psychologist or an audiologist. The present author, who is both a psychologist and an audiologist, makes no further comment.

## Management of clients with CAPD

A number of techniques and treatments have been suggested for clients with CAPD problems. Many of these suggestions are the result of empirical work in various clinics, and have yet to be fully evaluated in thoroughgoing research investigations. However, the following list of informal approaches is offered to the therapist as comprising techniques which seem worth adopting at the present time.

### Informal approaches

1. A cue to gain attention should be used before beginning the message proper (e.g. Say: 'I want to ask you a question' or touch the child on the shoulder).
2. Body movement should be reduced to assist in focusing attention ('Stop what you are doing and listen').
3. Oral instructions should be given in a strong, clear voice.
4. The child should be able to see the talker's lips, not simply to obtain lipreading cues but also to help focus attention.
5. Written instructions should be presented in clear text, using precise wording.
6. To ensure that the message has been understood, ask the child to repeat it (e.g. to a classmate).
7. If possible, give messages both verbally and visually (e.g. point to pictures in a catalogue or to items on kitchen shelves when giving directions about a shopping list).
8. Minimise competing stimuli, especially auditory stimuli. Keep the auditory environment as quiet as possible (encourage classmates to

speak quietly) when the child is working independently on maths problems, reading or writing (especially important in test-taking). Noise-reducing earplugs (obtained from pharmacies or audiologists) and preferential seating in the classroom, near the teacher or therapist, may be helpful.
9. Breaks should be given during long periods spent in listening activities to allow the child's auditory system to recover from fatigue.

## Management programmes

Many authors (e.g. Oberklaid et al., 1989; Katz, 1992; James et al., 1994; Bench & Maule, 1997) have noted that a large proportion of children with learning disabilities, especially language learning disabilities, experience CAPD. When such children are referred for audiological assessment, they usually present with peripheral hearing within normal limits, but perform poorly on CAPD tests. This finding suggests that auditory processing difficulties underlie the problems these children have with reading, writing and spelling, although, doubtless, other variables complicate the situation. The association of CAPD with the language learning disability suggests that training in grapheme to phoneme, and similar, tasks may provide a useful entry to therapy, particularly as there is evidence (Bench & Maule, 1997) that such children are relatively weak in processing the written word into its subvocal (auditory/articulatory) form.

The ADD: Auditory Discrimination in Depth Programme (Revised) of Lindamood and Lindamood (1975) is an example of such approaches to treatment. Its authors argued that, as letters represent speech sounds, the correspondence between sound sequences in spoken words and letter sequences in written words provides a base for independence in reading and spelling. Thus clients who cannot perceive contrasts between speech sounds or who have a poor notion of the order of sounds in syllables may learn to read and spell through rote memory rather than through understanding of the relationship between sound and symbol. Two basic problems are encountered. The first is a problem of association, where the client finds it hard to make the basic association between the letter name or form and the speech sound. Examples include problems in remembering letter names, how to write letters or the sound that the letter represents. The second problem lies in integrating sight words and sound–symbol associations, and using this knowledge in reading and spelling. The client can apparently make the associations, but not use them. The puzzle is how best to train the client to associate letter names, letter symbols and speech sounds, and to integrate this knowledge in reading and spelling. The ADD Programme attempts this task as a preconditioning or ancillary programme for reading, spelling and speech programmes. An important underlying rationale of the ADD Programme is the use of the motor-kinaesthetic system as an aid in learning the sounds and their symbol associations. The Programme thus augments use of the auditory system rather than focusing exclusively on it, aiming to teach the child to integrate auditory, visual and motor-kinaesthetic information.

### Phonemic analysis

A proportion, but not all, clients with reading and spelling difficulties may have a yet more basic problem: difficulty in discriminating phonemes from one another. However, this situation is recognised in the ADD Programme, which incorporates the Lindamood Auditory Conceptualization Test (Lindamood & Lindamood, 1971), a test which assesses ability in phonemic analysis.

The ADD Programme takes the client in small steps through a series of stages:

1. discriminating likenesses and differences between speech sounds;
2. perceiving sameness or difference, number and order of speech sounds, with both individual sounds and syllables;
3. perceiving minimal changes within and between syllables by paired comparisons;
4. associating speech sounds with letters;
5. using sound–symbol associations to spell sequences of sounds in spoken syllables into written symbols, and to read sequences of written symbols into spoken syllables;
6. to generalise these spelling and reading skills to real words, and to apply them to ordinary spelling and reading.

The ADD Program may be used with:

- kindergarten children, to build a base of auditory-perceptual skills in preparation for reading and spelling (stages 1–3) ;
- beginning readers and students of English as a second language;
- slow learners and clients with learning disabilities;
- clients at the intermediate and adult levels.

Further, this author suggests that stages 1–3 could be used in conjunction with the information provided by CAPD tests.

Tallal and Piercy (1975), Tallal and Stark (1981), Tallal, Stark and Mellitts (1985) and Elliot, Hammer and Scholl (1989) observed that some children with language learning disabilities were poor at perceiving rapid transitions in synthesised speech, indicating that these children had auditory perceptual problems. Such observations provide good evidence for the difficulties which stage 1 of the ADD Programme seeks to address. Further, Tallal et al. (1996) found that a particularly useful approach to therapy was to manipulate speech by amplifying and extending the duration of fast speech elements. These manipulations made the fast speech elements more salient and easier to perceive. Language learning-disabled children were given daily training in listening to such synthetic speech over a period of 4 weeks. They also participated daily in computer games, which trained their temporal processing of the speech adaptively. Significant improvements were obtained in speech discrimination and language comprehension after the 4-week period, and were substantially maintained on retesting after a further 6 weeks. Additional evaluation of long-term improvement is, however, required, and is awaited with interest. Meanwhile, the interim success of this approach supports the view that a basic problem for language learning-disabled children lies in difficulty with processing rapidly changing speech and other sensory elements (hence their auditory processing problems), which subsequently leads to the observed linguistic or cognitive deficits.

## Phonemic synthesis

Phonemic synthesis is a meta-phonological task in which individual phonemes are combined to produce a coarticulated speech sound (refer to Katz's Phonemic Synthesis Test (1983) described above). Katz and Harmon (1982) described a tape-recorded set of lessons with the following characteristics:

- reproducible, auditory-only stimuli produced by tape-recorded material;
- phoneme presentation in neutral form, minimising coarticulation;
- slow presentation rate; sequential organisation, with easier phoneme blends presented first;
- discovery learning in which clients are not informed of whether a response is right or wrong but learn through their auditory experiences;
- mastery learning to defined levels of skill before attempting the next level of difficulty;
- training only up to the syllable level.

## Frequency-modulated (FM) amplification

FM amplification, as used for 'radio hearing aids'(see also Chapter 7), offers the prospect of transmitting speech signals while reducing transmission of accompanying background noise. It is thus a device that merits consideration for those clients who have difficulty in discriminating speech from noise. The principle behind this use of FM hearing aids is that the microphone can be sited next to the talker's mouth via, for example, a headset, thus increasing the signal-to-noise ratio for the speech signal, while the client listener has much of the noise excluded by the earmould. This approach looks promising (e.g. Stach, Loiselle & Jerger, 1987), but is a relatively expensive option. The cost per client may be reduced if several clients can be fitted with such a system for classroom use.

The reader may well ask whether a more straightforward approach to the treatment of clients with speech-in-noise problems would be to reduce the ambient noise by the sound-treatment of classrooms, etc. There is much to be said in favour of such an approach for regular class-rooms, let alone rooms in which CAPD clients are taught. However, in practice, it will rarely be possible for the interested therapist or teacher to attain such a degree of control over present-day classrooms. Hence, this solution is not considered further here.

### Noise desensitisation

Noise desensitisation involves exposure to speech signals while the ambient noise is increased over a period of time, normally spread over several sessions. Katz, Yeung and Metwesky (1988) suggested that the speech signals be tape-recorded monosyllables (with low predictability) presented at a comfortable listening level. The speech is presented in quiet at the start, following which a minimally interfering noise (e.g. fan noise) is introduced, to be followed in turn by other increasingly loud and distracting noises (e.g. cafeteria noise). This technique offers no easy route to therapy because of the intense listening effort required, with the result that the client tires easily. Also, improvements in speech-in-noise tasks tends to fall off over time, unless maintenance programmes are introduced (Katz et al., 1988).

## Concluding comment

This brief account of approaches to the management of clients with CAPD is necessarily incomplete, but provides an indication of some techniques that are worth considering. The reader should nevertheless bear in mind that these techniques have yet to be fully evaluated in thoroughgoing research investigations across a number of clinical centres.

## Summary of key points

CAPD is a complex area representing a constellation of disorders, which, for particular clients, may be discrete or may occur in combination. The underlying physiology and neurology are imperfectly understood. A test battery approach is generally used in the clinical assessment of CAPD. Assessment of clients with CAPD is complicated by client problems with such intervening variables as intelligence, linguistic features, short-term memory, attention, metacognition, metalinguistics and motivation. Otitis media may lead to CAPD problems, but this relationship is not yet clearly established. Many children with (language) learning disabilities have CAPD problems. The distinction between CAPD and attention deficit disorder is unclear. Although management programmes are available for clients with CAPD, more research is needed on such programmes.

## Further reading

Katz J, Stecker, NA, Henderson D (1992) (Eds) Central auditory processing: a transdisciplinary view. St Louis, MO: Mosby. (This book addresses neuroanatomy and neural function in CAPD and provides discussion of how auditory processing disorders might be categorised and related to language disorders. A wide-ranging book.)

Pinheiro MP, Musiek FE (Eds) (1985) Assessment of central auditory dysfunction: foundations and clinical correlates. Baltimore, MD: Williams & Wilkins. (This book considers CAPD from a background of neuroanatomy. Results of CAPD tests are matched with the results of CAT scans and other physical evidence of neurological changes.)

# Chapter 10
# Integration

JANET DOYLE

This final chapter attempts to illustrate, by way of case examples, how some of the audiological features and principles discussed in earlier chapters may be integrated to inform the clinical practice of speech-language therapy. Certain key messages are reiterated.

## Case example 1

A 49-year-old man attending speech therapy because of a long history of stuttering had a hearing loss detected on routine pure tone hearing screening (the case shown in Table 5.4). A rescreen confirmed that although his hearing was probably normal at low and mid frequencies, a high-frequency loss could not be excluded as the levels of first response at 4000 Hz were 40 dB HTL in the right ear and 45 dB HTL in the left. He had a history of noise exposure. As a result of this identification on screening he was referred to an audiologist for hearing assessment. Speech therapy continued in the meantime, as the ability to converse in quiet appeared normal. The audiogram and other test results are shown in Figure 10.1.

The diagnostic audiogram confirmed the high frequency loss (Figure 10.1a), and documents a sensorineural loss consistent with cochlear damage due to chronic noise exposure. The configuration of the loss shows greatest impairment at 6000 Hz, with some recovery of hearing at 8000 Hz. Although no cause can be definitely assumed on the basis of a pure tone audiogram only, this configuration is very typical of noise-induced hearing loss (see Chapter 3). The audiogram shows a Q1–2–4 quadrant pattern (see Chapter 6). The relationship of the air- and bone-conduction thresholds indicates a purely sensorineural loss. The left and the right ears show similar levels of air-conduction hearing, therefore there does not appear to be any indication that this individual would have localisation problems. The audiogram has been obtained without the use of masking.

The tympanometry and acoustic reflex results for this individual (Figure 10.1b) are also consistent with a sensorineural hearing loss, because there is no evidence of abnormal mechanical functioning in either middle ear (see Chapters 2 and 4).

The results of a speech discrimination test (see Chapter 4) using AB words (Figure 10.1c) show that, at least in the test situation, this individual achieves near-perfect scores using hearing alone as long as the test words are presented in quiet. When competing speech noise is introduced there is more difficulty understanding the test words, and this is consistent with the Q1–2–4 audiogram pattern and the sensorineural nature of the hearing loss. This individual may of course achieve good understanding of spoken messages in real life, even in the presence of background noise, because of the advantage of linguistic context and via the use of speech-reading (see Chapter 8). The results of a speech audiometry test taken in the clinic cannot give definitive information about the degree of handicap the individual will experience. Other factors, including the communication abilities and habits of conversational partners, will influence what is experienced in the daily context.

All test results are fairly similar in the right and left ears. In general the test results and the client's history are consistent.

In this case the audiologist counselled the client about ear protection in the event of any further noise exposure and arranged for a hearing review in 12 months. After discussion it was decided that the client would do without technical assistance at this time.

### Case summary points

This individual had a bilateral hearing loss that was undetected until routine screening by the speech-language therapist. The tests results available after referral to an audiologist show a set of results that describe a sensorineural hearing loss consistent with noise-induced hearing loss. The level of handicap associated with such losses is highly variable, but such individuals would very commonly have difficulty hearing in background noise. Counselling about further noise exposure is important.

## Case example 2

A speech-language therapist was asked to assess a 73-year-old female resident of a nursing home who had had a number of transient ischaemic attacks. The staff were finding communication difficult with this resident. The client's level of insight was limited and her family was concerned that she was becoming more isolated within the community of the home. The client had two hearing aids, which were infrequently worn and appeared to be of little benefit. As part of a complete assessment of this client the speech-language therapist noted several important facts, which are shown in Figure 10.2.

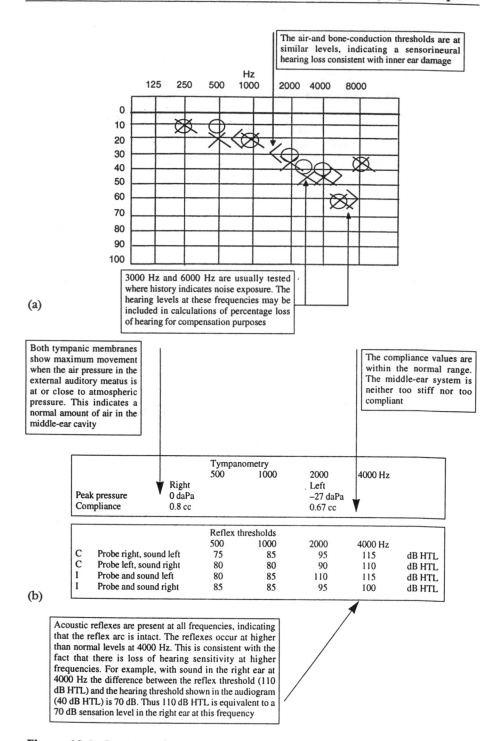

**Figure 10.1:** Case 1: Audiometric test results from a 49-year-old client presenting with stuttering. (a) Pure tone audiogram; (b) tympanometry and acoustic reflex results; (c) performance intensity functions for speech audiometry.

(contd)

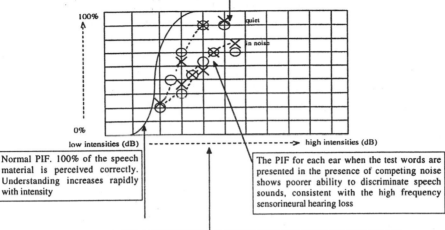

Both ears can correctly identify almost 100% of the test words, in this case AB words, when presented in quiet. The maximum score (AB max) occurs at slightly higher intensities than that required by an average listener with normal hearing for this test

Normal PIF. 100% of the speech material is perceived correctly. Understanding increases rapidly with intensity

The PIF for each ear when the test words are presented in the presence of competing noise shows poorer ability to discriminate speech sounds, consistent with the high frequency sensorineural hearing loss

The dB reference in such PIF functions might be HTL, SPL or SRL depending on the convention in a particular clinic (see Chapter 4)

Note: Sometimes the speech audiometry results are presented in tabular form, and in discrimination tests the maximum scores only may be recorded, as in for example:

|       | Right ear  | Left ear   |
|-------|------------|------------|
| Score | 92%        | 96%        |
| Level | 50 dB HTL  | 55 dB HTL  |

(c)

**Figure 10.1:** (contd)

---

*Impressions related to hearing*
Willing to communicate, but clearly not able to understand conversation at normal levels. Wearing left hearing aid today. Intermittent whistling from aid. Responds well when speaker talks directly into right ear.

*Screening test*
Auroscopic inspection showed wax in both ears.
Pure tone screening carried out at 40 dB HTL, 1000 Hz, 2000 Hz and 4000 Hz. No response until tone raised to at least 70 dB HTL at all test frequencies. No audiogram available.

*Troubleshooting of hearing aids*
Both aids were behind-the-ear style with appropriately visible controls. Batteries had power. Client and staff knew how to operate on-off volume controls. Feedback whistle did not appear due to leakage from tubing. Client was able to insert aids in ears. Close inspection showed moulds were loose-fitting. Client and staff were controlling feedback by turning aid down to low levels.

*Conclusions*
The most obvious explanation for hearing problems appeared to be inadequate gain from hearing aids due to using aids at low volume settings to control feedback whistle. The level of hearing loss indicated by the initial screening showed the client definitely required hearing-aid amplification. The feedback may have been caused by a combination of loose-fitting earmoulds and the presence of wax in the ear canal.

*Clinical decisions*
1. Arrange for medical examination of ears and wax removal.
2. Arrange for new earmoulds and put on waiting list for full hearing assessment.
3. Loan of binaural amplified listener (BAL) to facilitate communication.
4. Instruction for staff and family in use of BAL and rewording of messages.
5. After wax removal and new moulds assess perception ability using live voice and Ling Five Sound Test.

**Figure 10.2:** Case 2: Clinical findings for a 73-year-old client resident in a nursing home.

In this case the speech-language therapist's assessment included a check of the client's hearing (see Chapter 5) and her hearing aids (see Chapter 7). Although the aids were found to be functioning, the acoustic coupling to the client's ear was not optimal. The wax occlusion discovered in both ears meant that some of the amplified sound entering the ear canal was reflected back, causing feedback whistle and possibly adding a conductive component to an already significant hearing loss (see Chapters 3 and 7). As a means of getting amplified speech to the client until the wax could be removed and new earmoulds could be made, the speech-language therapist arranged the loan of a binaural amplified listener, a broad-band amplifier that is operated from a cassette tape-sized box and delivers sound to Walkman-like earphones. This assistive listening device is helpful where earmoulds cannot be worn or hearing aids are not available. It is also useful for demonstrating in a very rough way the benefit of amplification when the hearing loss is significant.

### Case summary points

The clinician in this case checked ears and hearing aids even though the presence of functioning aids might have been assumed to indicate that the client's hearing loss had been managed. The check revealed two problems, which could significantly affect the client's communication and could be resolved fairly readily. The availability of an assistive listening device allowed for communication in the meantime and facilitated the assessment of the client's cognitive abilities. The therapist arranged to work with nursing home staff and the client's family to improve communication, and planned a review of the client's situation after the obvious problems had been resolved.

# Case example 3

A 4-year-old boy who had recently been diagnosed with profound bilateral hearing loss following bacterial meningitis (see Chapter 3) had been referred for assistance with speech and language maintenance and development. The boy's parents were distressed and anxious to investigate all options to help their son. The child had been fitted with behind-the-ear hearing aids, which he had readily accepted wearing. Unaided and aided audiograms supplied by the hearing aid clinic are shown in Figure 10.3.

The unaided (HTL) audiogram (Figure 10.3a) was obtained with play audiometry (see Chapter 4). There is measurable hearing at 250 Hz, 500 Hz and 750 Hz in each ear, and at 1000 Hz a response at 110 dB HTL in the right ear only. The aided audiogram (Figure 10.3b), a result of testing in sound field conditions using warble tones (see Chapter 4), shows separate responses for the right and left ears, indicated by the

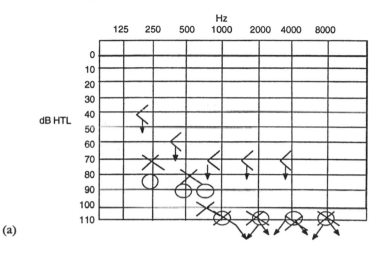

(a)

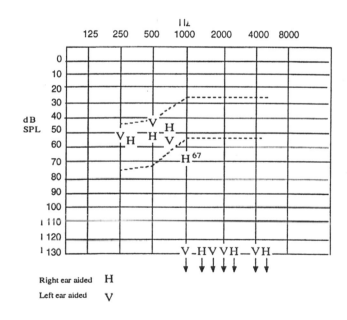

Right ear aided    H

(b)    Left ear aided    V

**Figure 10.3:** Case 3: Audiometric test results from a 4-year-old boy with post-meningitic hearing loss. (a) Unaided pure tone audiogram; (b) SPL audiogram showing aided responses; (c) tympanometry and acoustic reflex results.

(contd)

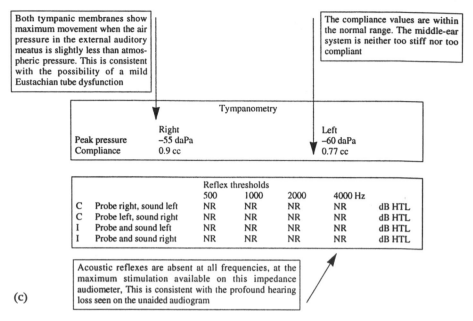

**Figure 10.3:** (contd)

symbols 'H' and 'V' respectively. At low frequencies there are aided responses in the speech area in each ear. There is also an aided response in the right ear for 1000 Hz, but higher than normal speech levels and/or reduced distance between speaker and listener would be required to perceive conversational speech sounds at this frequency by hearing alone. There was no measurable response at higher frequencies in either ear. Hearing has been tested at 750 Hz and 1500 Hz in this case. The unaided audiogram in this case has a Q3 only pattern. The loss is sensorineural. No response could be obtained at the maximum output of the audiometer for bone-conducted sounds. It is possible to translate the information from the dB HTL audiogram to the dB SPL audiogram and/or vice versa with a simple addition or subtraction (see Chapter 6).

Unaided, this child could not perceive speech, and would be likely to lose much of his own existing speech production ability because of lack of feedback from his own voice. The aided response is encouraging in that there is some perception of sounds up to 1000 Hz in at least one ear. This is favourable for the development and maintenance of normal prosody, the perception of the first format of all vowels and the use of coarticulatory cues to perceive many other speech sounds. The child has the advantage of presumably normal hearing over the first 3–4 years of life. He had well-established skills in using voice and in taking turns in conversation, and had language that was reportedly developing normally. The parents decided to build on this early foundation with an oral-aural approach, the use of hearing aids with FM capability (see Chapter 7) and intensive help from their speech-language therapist. It was further decided to review his progress in one year, with a view to cochlear implantation (see Chapter 7) if appropriate gains were not made.

Figure 10.3c shows the results of tympanometry and acoustic reflex testing (see Chapter 4). Tympanometry shows a minimal negative middle-ear pressure. Although in most cases this would be unremarkable, it was decided to monitor middle-ear function in this case, because of the significance of even a very slight conductive overlay, due for example to otitis media (see Chapter 3), on the profound sensorineural hearing loss. There were no measurable acoustic reflexes with either ipsilateral or contralateral stimulation (see Chapters 2 and 4). This is consistent with the level of the hearing loss, because the acoustic stimulus generally needs to be 70–100 dB above the individual's hearing threshold to elicit a response. In some cases with severe recruitment (see Chapter 3) the acoustic reflex may be elicited with lower sensation levels, but this is not so in this case.

### Case summary points

In this case the aided audiogram gives information more pertinent to potential for speech and language development than the unaided graph. Despite the profound hearing loss, aided results are encouraging for the maintenance of language skills already acquired, provided appropriate hearing aids are used and a communication-rich environment is encouraged. Articulation skills will almost certainly be more difficult to develop. The child's young age means that close monitoring for any intermittent conductive hearing problems is necessary as this could seriously compromise aided hearing levels. The quality of the child's residual hearing is difficult to ascertain at this time.

## Case example 4

A 29-year-old man with Down's syndrome was referred for voice therapy because of apparent vocal abuse. His social skills appeared to vary. Cooperative behaviours and responsiveness seemed to fluctuate. After initial assessment the speech-language therapist referred the client for otolaryngological investigation because of suspected vocal-fold nodules, and in the meantime began a programme of encouraging better voice use. The therapist also referred this client to the hospital hearing clinic for audiometry. The results of the hearing tests are shown in Figure 10.4.

The pure tone audiogram shows a bilateral hearing loss of approximately 30 dB. The overall level of the loss is shown by the air-conduction thresholds. Unmasked bone-conduction testing (see Chapters 2 and 4) shows that in at least one ear the cochlea has normal hearing. The client could not cope with the masking procedure (see Chapter 4) and so the audiogram is incomplete. On the basis of the audiogram alone it is possible that one or other ear has a sensorineural or mixed loss because of cross-hearing (see Chapter 4). The tympanometry and acoustic reflex results (Figure 10.4b) show that both ears had immobile tympanic membranes on this day, and that there were no acoustic reflexes. The lack of acoustic reflexes is likely to be due to the increased stiffness of the middle-ear system. The reflex arc may function to produce a contraction of the stapedial muscles, but a corresponding reflexive movement of the ossicular chain and tympanic membrane was absent. Given the hearing loss and the tympanograms, this result was consistent with middle-ear fluid such as would accompany some form of otitis media (see Chapter 3).

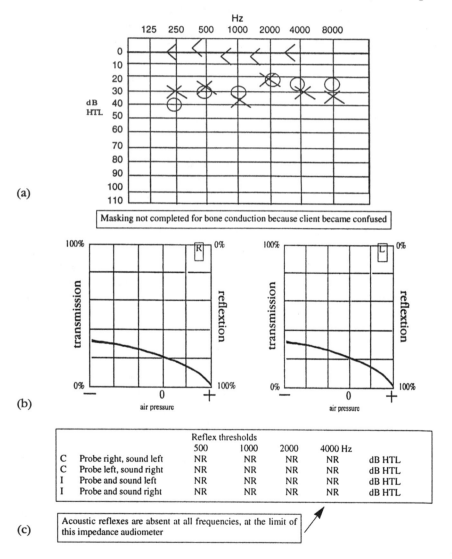

(a)

Masking not completed for bone conduction because client became confused

(b)

(c)

| | | Reflex thresholds | | | | |
|---|---|---|---|---|---|---|
| | | 500 | 1000 | 2000 | 4000 Hz | |
| C | Probe right, sound left | NR | NR | NR | NR | dB HTL |
| C | Probe left, sound right | NR | NR | NR | NR | dB HTL |
| I | Probe and sound left | NR | NR | NR | NR | dB HTL |
| I | Probe and sound right | NR | NR | NR | NR | dB HTL |

Acoustic reflexes are absent at all frequencies, at the limit of this impedance audiometer

**Figure 10.4:** Case 4: Audiometric test results from a 29-year-old man with Down's syndrome. (a) Pure tone audiogram; (b) tympanometry results; (c) acoustic reflex results.

The otolaryngologist confirmed vocal nodules and diagnosed bilateral non-purulent otitis media with effusion. It was agreed to establish regular monitoring of middle-ear function following ENT treatment. It was agreed that the client's variable social skills may be at least in part due to intermittent/fluctuating conductive hearing loss. Any relationship to the vocal problems was less clear.

### Case summary points

This client had an obvious voice disorder, which was the reason for referral. Given that the client also had Down's syndrome, it might have been assumed that variable responsiveness and social abilities were the result of intellectual handicap. However, routine audiometry showed a bilateral hearing loss of a level easily associated with the possibility of frustration during communication, and of a type that is often fluctuating in level and therefore associated with inconsistent auditory input. The speech-language therapist made an appropriate referral for hearing assessment and an otherwise asymptomatic hearing problem was detected.

## Summary of some key messages in this book

The preceding examples illustrate that many of the speech-language therapist's clients may have communication compromised by hearing problems, even when the presenting problem is language, intellectual disability, dysfluency or voice disorder. The importance of ascertaining the client's ability to hear is obvious. Routine pure tone screening can inform therapy and referral as well as detect problems not directly reported by the client. The troubleshooting of hearing aids is important whenever communication of an aided client appears to be less than expected, and the routine checking of aided function in hearing-impaired children is vital. Monitoring of middle-ear function is especially important in children with severe-to-profound hearing loss, and in other cases where there are significant challenges to effective communication via oral language.

Recent developments in hearing aids, assistive listening devices, tactile devices and cochlear implants have been rapid. Individuals requiring such technical assistance now have available an impressive range and quality of instruments, although in cases of severe-to-profound hearing loss considerable challenges remain.

Speech-reading is used by all sighted people to some degree and can be of significant benefit to persons with hearing impairment. The abilities of conversational partners, the acoustic environments in which communication takes place and the linguistic context of the spoken message all have significant interactions with the communication abilities of individual clients and should be considered in a thorough programme of therapy.

A large range of behavioural and electrophysiological tests are available to diagnose the site and nature of auditory problems. The most routinely used of these have been explained in this book. It is possible, because of central auditory processing problems, for example, to have normal results on routine tests of auditory function and still experience problems utilising hearing for communication. Inconsistency in test results or between client report and routine test results are cause for further investigation.

## Further reading and continuing education

Speech-language therapists will usually have access to continuing education via their professional associations, special interest groups and the various universities and hospitals involved in student training. However, it may be that aspects of practice involving the application of audiological principles are not often directly targeted in such programmes. Audiological societies and cross-discipline interest groups can be a source of information and update in such circumstances. Additionally, self-help groups and client associations (e.g. the Australian Tinnitus Association, the Acoustic Neuroma Association, the Down's Syndrome Association and many more) can offer valuable opportunities to keep up to date with aspects of audiology important to the practice of speech and language therapy. Access to a range of journals that provide readable treatments of clinically relevant studies in audiology, otolaryngology and education of the deaf is invaluable and this can often be arranged by special borrower status in various libraries. The basic treatment of audiology provided in this book is seen as providing a practical foundation on which the practising speech-language therapist will build. As the technical developments in audiology are rapid, it is advisable to maintain contact with the field and develop supporting networks of professionals in the audiology field. My own experience has shown me that much can be learned from clients, some of whom demonstrate remarkable persistence and creativity in their communication. They have taught me a lot.

# References

Abbas PJ, Brown CJ (1991) Assessment of the status of the auditory nerve. In Cooper, H (Ed.) Cochlear implants: a practical guide. London: Whurr Publishers, pp. 109–24.

Alcantara JI, Whitford LA, Blamey PJ, Cowan RSC, Clark GM (1990) Speech feature recognition by profoundly hearing-impaired children using a multiple channel electrotactile speech processor and aided residual hearing. Journal of the Acoustical Society of America 88: 1260–73.

Alcorn S (1932) The Tadoma method. Volta Review 34: 195–8.

Allard B, Welsh T (1990) Diagnostic value of vertical nystagmus recorded from ENG. Ear & Hearing 11: 62–5.

Allonen-Allie N, Florentine M (1990) Hearing conservation programs in Massachusetts' vocational/technical schools. Ear & Hearing 11: 237–9.

American National Standards Institute (1970) Specifications for audiometers (ANSI S 3.6-1969). New York: ANSI.

American National Standards Institute (1987) American national standard specifications for instruments to measure aural acoustic impedance and admittance (aural acoustic immittance) (ANSI S 3.39). New York: ANSI.

American Speech-Language-Hearing Association (1979) Committee on Audiometric Evaluation: Guidelines for acoustic immittance screening of middle ear function. Asha 21: 283–8.

American Speech-Language-Hearing Association (1985) Guidelines for identification audiometry. Asha 27: 47–52.

American Speech-Language-Hearing Association (1988) Telephone hearing screening. Asha 30: 53.

American Speech Language Hearing Association (1990a) Scope of practice: speech-language pathology and audiology. Asha 32(Suppl. 2): 1–2.

American Speech-Language-Hearing Association (1990b) Guidelines for audiometric symbols. Asha 32(Suppl. 2): 25–30.

American Speech-Language-Hearing Association (1990c) Guidelines for screening for hearing impairments and middle ear disorders. Asha 32(Suppl. 2): 17–24.

American Speech-Language-Hearing Association (1990d) Aids/HIV: implications for speech-language pathologists and audiologists. Asha 32: 46–487.

American Speech-Language-Hearing Association (1991) Issues in ethics: clinical practice by certificate holders in the profession in which they are not certified. Asha 33: 51.

American Speech-Language-Hearing Association (1992) Considerations in screening adults/older persons for handicapping hearing impairments. Asha 34: 81–7.

American Speech-Language-Hearing Association (1993) Preferred practice patterns for the professions of speech-language pathology and audiology. Asha 35(Suppl. 11): 3–96.

American Speech-Language-Hearing Association (1994a) Audiologic screening: ad hoc committee on screening for impairment, handicap, and middle ear disorders. Asha 36: 53–4.

American Speech-Language-Hearing Association (1994b) Joint committee on infant hearing 1994 position statement. Asha 36: 38–41.

American Speech-Language-Hearing Association (1995) Position statement and guidelines for acoustics in educational settings. Asha 37(Suppl. 14): 15.

American Speech-Language-Hearing Association Ad Hoc Committee on Screening for Hearing-impairment, Handicap and Middle Ear Disorders. (1995) American Journal of Audiology 4: 24–40.

American Speech-Language-Hearing Association Task Force on Central Auditory Processing Consensus Development (1997) Central auditory processing: current status of research and implications for clinical practice. American Journal of Audiology 5: 41–54.

Arnst D, Katz J (1982) The SSW Test: development and clinical use. San Diego, CA: College Hill Press.

Audiological Society of Australia (1997) Recommended audiometric symbols. In The ASA professional standards of practice of audiologists. Melbourne: Audiological Society of Australia.

Australian Association of Speech and Hearing (1994) Competency based occupational standards for speech pathologists. Melbourne: Australian Association of Speech and Hearing.

Axelsson A, Barrenas M-L (1992) Tinnitus in noise induced hearing loss. In Dancer A, Henderson D, Salvi RJ, Hamernik RP (Eds) Noise induced hearing loss. St Louis, MO: Mosby, pp. 269–76.

Baddeley AD (1992) Is working memory working? The fifteenth Bartlett lecture. Quarterly Journal of Experimental Psychology 44A: 1–32.

Bader JA (1992a) Development of auditory skills in children who are hearing impaired. In Hull RH (Ed.) Aural rehabilitation, 2nd edn. San Diego, CA: Singular Publishing, pp. 88–94.

Bader JA (1992b) Language development for children who are hearing impaired. In Hull RH (Ed.) Aural rehabilitation, 2nd edn. San Diego, CA: Singular Publishing, pp. 95–102.

Ballantyne D (1990) Handbook of audiological techniques. London: Butterworth-Heinemann.

Balthazor RJ, Cevette MJ (1978) An objective predictor of cochlear function in the speech clinic. Australian Journal of Human Communication Disorders 6:1, 69–74.

Bamford J, Saunders E (1991) Hearing impairment, auditory perception and language disability, 2nd edn. London: Whurr Publishers.

Baran JA, Musiek FE (1995) Central auditory processing disorders in children and adults. In Wall LG (Ed.) Hearing for the speech language therapist and health care professional. Boston, MA: Butterworth-Heinemann, pp. 415–40.

Barber HO (1983) Ménière's disease: symptomatology. In Oosterveld WJ (Ed.) Ménière's disease: a comprehensive appraisal. Chichester: J Wiley & Sons, pp. 25–34.

Barber HO, Stockwell CW (1980) Manual of electronystagmography, 2nd edn. St Louis, MO: Mosby.

Barrenas M-L, Lindgren F (1991) The influence of eye colour on susceptibility to temporary threshold shift in humans. British Journal of Audiology 25: 303–7.

Bauman N, Braemer M (1996) Using a CIC hearing aid in transcranial CROS fittings. The Hearing Journal 49: 27–46.

Beales PH (1987) Otosclerosis. In Booth JB (Ed.) Scott-Brown's otolaryngolgy: otology, 5th edn. London: Butterworths, pp. 301–39.

Beasley DS, Rintelmann AK (1979) Central auditory processing. In Rintelmann WF (Ed.) Hearing assessment. Baltimore, MD: University Park Press, pp. 321–49.

Bellis TJ (1996) Assessment and management of central auditory processing disorders in the educational setting: from science to practice. San Diego, CA: Singular Publishing.

Bellman S, Mahon M, Triggs E (1996) Evaluation of the E2L Toy test as a screening procedure in clinical practice. British Journal of Audiology 30: 286–96.

Bench RJ (1992a) Communication skills in hearing impaired children. London: Whurr Publishers.

Bench RJ (1992b) A note on the BKB/A sentences versus the BKB/A words: a further validation. Australian Journal of Audiology 14: 63–5.

Bench RJ (1993) Sequelae of recurrent otitis media: some issues of validity. Proceedings of the first national conference on childhood fluctuating conductive deafness/otitis media, pp. 123–9. Parkville, Victoria, October 1992.

Bench RJ, Bamford J (Eds) (1979) Speech-hearing tests and the spoken language of hearing-impaired children. London: Academic Press.

Bench RJ, Harrold E (1996) On the sequelae of recurrent otitis media (ROM): a review and a proposed model. Asia-Pacific Journal of Speech, Language & Hearing 1: 1–14.

Bench RJ, Maule RM (1997) The use of internal speech by children with auditory processing problems. Audiology, 36: 312–24.

Bench RJ, Doyle J, Greenwood KM (1987) A standardisation of the BKB/A Sentence Test for children in comparison with the NAL-CID Sentence Test and the CAL-PBM Word Test. Australian Journal of Audiology 9: 39–48.

Bench RJ, Doyle J, Daly N, Lind C (1993) The BKB/A Speechreading Test. Victoria, Australia: La Trobe University.

Bench RJ, Daly N, Doyle J, Lind C (1994) Standardisation of the BKB/A Speechreading Test I: speechreading under visual-only conditions. Australian Journal of Audiology 16: 107–17.

Bench RJ, Daly N, Doyle J, Lind C (1995) Choosing talkers for the BKB/A Speechreading Test: a procedure with observations on talker age and gender. British Journal of Audiology 29: 172–87.

Bennett M, Mowat L (1981) Validity of impedance measurements and referral criteria in school hearing screening programmes. British Journal of Audiology 15: 147–50.

Berg FS (1976) Educational audiology: hearing and speech management. New York, NY: Grune & Stratton.

Berger KW (1970) Vowel confusions in speech reading. Journal of Speech & Hearing 5: 123–8.

Berger KW (1972) Speechreading: principles and methods. Baltimore, MD: National Educational Press.

Berger KW, Popelka GR (1971) Extra-facial gestures in relation to speechreading. Journal of Communication Disorders 3: 302–8.

Bess FH (1985) The minimally hearing-impaired child. Ear & Hearing 6: 43–7.

Bess FH, Tharpe AM (1984) Unilateral hearing impairment in children. Pediatrics 15: 206–16.

Bess FH, Tharpe AM (1986) An introduction to unilateral sensori-neural hearing loss in children. Ear & Hearing 7: 3–13.

Bess FH, Humes LE (1990) Audiology: the fundamentals. Baltimore, MD: Williams & Wilkins.

Bess FH, Lichtenstein MJ, Logan SA (1991) Audiologic assessment in the elderly. In Rintelman WF (Ed.) Hearing assessment, 2nd edn. Austin, TX: Pro-Ed, pp. 511–48.

Bilger RC, Nuetzel JM, Rabinowitz WM, Rzeczkowski C (1984) Standardization of a test of speech perception in noise. Journal of Speech & Hearing Research 27: 32–48.

Blamey PJ, Clark GM (1985) A wearable multi-electrode electrotactile speech processor for the profoundly deaf. Journal of the Acoustical Society of America 77: 1619–20.

Blamey PJ, Clark GM (1987) Psychophysical studies relevant to the design of a digital electrotactile speech processor. Journal of the Acoustical Society of America 82: 116–25.

Blamey PJ, Cowan RSC (1992) The potential benefit and cost-effectiveness of tactile devices in comparison to cochlear implants. In Summers IR (Ed.) Tactile devices for the hearing impaired. London: Whurr Publishers, pp. 187–217.

Bluestone CD, Klein JO (1990) Otitis media, atelectasis, and Eustachian tube dysfunction. In Bluestone CD, Stool SE (Eds) Pediatric otolaryngology. Philadelphia, PA: Saunders, pp. 320–486.

Bluestone CD, Paradise J, Berry QC, Wittel R (1972) Certain effects of cleft palate repair on Eustachian tube function. Cleft Palate Journal 9: 183–93.

Bocca E, Calearo C (1963) Central hearing processes. In Jerger J (Ed.). Modern developments in audiology. New York & London: Academic Press.

Bocca E, Calearo C, Cassinari V (1954) A new method for testing hearing in temporal lobe tumors: a preliminary report. Acta Otolaryngolica 44: 219–21.

Bolanowski SJ Jr, Gescheider GA, Verrillo RT, Checkowsky CM (1988) Four channels mediate the mechanical aspect of touch. Journal of the Acoustical Society of America 84: 1680–94.

Booth JB (1981) Surgical management of deafness in adults: the external and middle ear. In Beagley HA (Ed.) Audiology and audiological medicine, vol. 1. Oxford University Press, pp. 482–505.

Boothroyd A (1968) Developments in speech audiometry. Sound 2: 3–10.

Boothroyd A (1993) Speech perception, sensori-neural hearing loss and hearing aids. In Studebaker G, Hochberg I (Eds) Acoustical factors affecting hearing aid performance. Boston, MA: Allyn & Bacon, pp. 277–99.

Boothroyd A, Erickson FN, Medwetsky L (1994) The hearing aid input: a phonemic approach to assessing the spectral distribution of speech. Ear & Hearing 15: 432–42.

Brackett D (1985) The role of the speech-language therapist with hearing-impaired infants. Ear & Hearing 6: 36–8.

Bradac JJ (1990) Language attitudes and impression formation. In Giles H, Robinson WP (Eds) Handbook of language and social psychology. New York, NY: John Wiley & Sons, pp. 387–412.

Bradley L, Bryant P. (1978) Difficulties in auditory organization as a possible cause of reading backwardness. Nature 271: 746–7.

Bridges-Webb C (1993) Otitis media in general practice: do we hear the questions? Proceedings of the first national conference on childhood fluctuating conductive deafness/otitis media, pp. 31–3. Parkville, Victoria, October 1992.

British Society of Audiology (1981) Speech audiometric terminology. British Journal of Audiology 15: 143.

British Society of Audiology (1989) British Society of Audiology—recommended format for audiogram forms. British Journal of Audiology 23: 265–6.

British Society of Audiology (1992). Technical note: Recommended procedure for tympanometry. British Journal of Audiology 26: 255–7.

Brooks DN (1982) Acoustic impedance studies on otitis media with effusion. International Journal of Pediatric Otorhinolaryngology 4: 89–94.

Brooks DN, Geoghgan PM (1992) Non-organic hearing loss in young persons: Transient episode or indicator of deep seated difficulty. British Journal of Audiology 26: 347–50.

Brooks DN (1996) The time course of adaptation to hearing aid use. British Journal of Audiology 30: 55–62.

Bruhn M (1960) The Mueller-Waller method of lipreading for the hard of hearing, 7th edn. Washington, DC: Volta Bureau.

Bunger AM (1961) Speech reading: Jena method: A textbook with lesson plans in full development for hard of hearing adults and discussion of adaptations for hard of hearing and deaf children, 4th edn. Danville, IL: Interstate Press.

Burack JA (1994) Selective attention deficits in persons with autism: preliminary evidence of an inefficient attentional lens. Journal of Abnormal Psychology 103: 535–43.

Burd L, Fisher W (1986) Central auditory processing disorder or attention deficit disorder? Journal of Developmental & Behavioral Pediatrics 7: 215–6.

Byrne D (1977) The speech spectrum – some aspects of its significance for hearing aid selection and evaluation. British Journal of Audiology 11: 40–6.

Byrne D, Noble W, LePage B (1992) Effects of long term bilateral and unilateral fitting of different hearing aid types on the ability to locate sounds. Journal of the American Academy of Audiology 3: 269–382.

Byrne D, Noble W, Sinclair S (1996) Effects of earmould type on auditory localisation: reverse slope sensori-neural hearing losses. National Acoustic Laboratories Research and Development Annual Report 1995–96. Sydney: Australian Hearing Services, pp. 13–14.

Caitlin FI (1981) Otologic diagnosis and treatment of disorders affecting hearing. In Martin FN (Ed.) Medical audiology: disorders of hearing. Englewood Cliffs, NJ: Prentice-Hall, pp. 174–92.

Calearo C, Lazzaroni A (1957) Speech intelligibility in relation to the speed of the message. Laryngoscope 67: 305–19.

Calvert DR (1986) Speech in perspective. In Luterman DM (Ed.) Deafness in perspective. San Diego, CA: College Hill Press.

Cantwell DP, Baker L (1991) Association between attention deficit-hyperactivity disorder and learning disorders. Journal of Learning Disabilities 24: 78–86.

Cevette MJ, Balthazor RJ (1977) Measuring middle ear function in the speech clinic. Australian Journal of Human Communication Disorders 5:2 142–8.

Chalmers D, Stewart I, Silva P, Mulvena A (1989) Otitis media with effusion in children – The Dunedin study. London: MacKeith Press.

Chung DY, Willson GN, Gannon RP, Mason K (1982) Individual susceptibility to noise. In Hammernik RP, Henderson D, Salvi R (Eds) New perspectives on noise-induced hearing loss. New York: Raven Press, pp. 511–19.

Clezy G (1984) An early auditory-oral intervention program. In Ling D (Ed.) Early intervention for hearing-impaired children: oral options. San Diego, CA: College Hill Press, pp. 65–117.

Clezy G (1993) Learning from mainland China. Human Communication 2(2): 25–7.

Coates J (1993) Women, men and language, 2nd edn. London: Longman.

Coats AC (1981) The summating potential and Ménière's disease. Archives of Otolaryngology 107: 199–208.

Cohen A (1981) Etiology and pathology of disorders affecting hearing. In Martin FN (Ed.) Medical audiology: disorders of hearing. Englewood Cliffs, NJ: Prentice Hall, pp. 123–44.

Coltheart K, Lesser R (1991) Psycholinguistic assessments of language processing in aphasia. Hove: Lawrence Erlbaum & Associates.

Compton CL (1991) Clinical management of assistive technology users. In Studebaker GA, Bess FH, Beck LB (Eds) The Vanderbilt hearing aid report II. Parkton, MD: York Press, pp. 301–18.

Conrad R (1979) The deaf school child. London: Harper & Row.

Cook JR, Mausbach T, Burd L, Gascon G, Slotnick H, Patterson B, Johnson R, Hankey B, Reynolds B (1993) A preliminary study of the relationship between central auditory processing disorder and attention deficit disorder. Journal of Psychiatry and Neuroscience 18: 130–7.

Cooper H (1991) Selection of candidates for cochlear implantation: an overview. In Cooper H (Ed.) Cochlear implants: a practical guide. London: Whurr Publishers, pp. 92–100.

Cornett RO (1972) Cued speech. In Fant G (Ed.) Speech communication ability and profound deafness. Washington, DC: Alexander Graham Bell Association, pp. 213–22.

Cornett RO (1985) Diagnostic factors bearing on the use of cued speech with hearing-impaired children. Ear & Hearing 6: 33–5.

Cox RM, Alexander GC (1995) The abbreviated profile of hearing aid benefit. Ear & Hearing 16: 176–86.

Dalebout S (1995a) Disorders of hearing in children. In Wall LG (Ed.) Hearing for the speech-language pathologist and health care professional. Boston, MA: Butterworth-Heinemann, pp. 39–70.

Dalebout S (1995b) Identification and evaluation of hearing loss in infants and new born children. In Wall LG (Ed.) Hearing for the speech language pathologist and the health care professional. Boston, MA: Butterworth-Heineman, pp. 103–40.

Daly N, Bench RJ, Chappell H (1996a) Observer-based speech variables which contribute to the visual intelligibility of talkers. Journal of Speech & Hearing Research (Submitted).

Daly N, Bench RJ, Chappell H (1996b) Gender differences in speechreadability. Journal of the Academy of Rehabilitative Audiology 29: 1–14.

Daly N, Bench RJ, Chappell H (1996c) Interpersonal impressions, gender stereotypes, and visual speech. Journal of Language and Social Psychology 15: 468–78.

Damasio A, Damasio H (1983) The anatomic basis of pure alexia. Neurology 33: 1573–83.

Danhauer JL, Crawford SE, Edgerton BJ (1984) English and bilingual speakers' performance on a Nonsense Syllable Test (NST) of speech sound discrimination. Journal of Speech & Hearing Disorders 49: 164–9.

Davies B, Penniceard RM (1980) Auditory function and receptive vocabulary in Down's syndrome children. In Taylor IG, Markides A (Eds) Disorders of auditory function III. London: Academic Press, pp. 51–8.

Davis SM, Rampp DL (1983) Normal and disordered auditory processing skills: a developmental approach. Audiology 8: 45–58.

De Filippo CL (1982) Memory for articulated sequences and lipreading performance of hearing-impaired observers. Volta Review 84(3): 134–46.

De Filippo CL (1990) Speechreading training: believe it or not! Asha 32 (April), 46–8.

De Filippo CL, Scott BL (1978) A method for training and evaluating the reception of ongoing speech. Journal of the Acoustical Society of America 63: 1186–92.

De Filippo CL, Sims DG (1988). New reflections on speechreading. Volta Review 90. Washington, DC: Alexander Graham Bell Association for the Deaf

Demorest ME, Bernstein LE (1992) Sources of variability in speechreading sentences: a generalizability analysis. Journal of Speech & Hearing Research 35: 876–91.

Denes PB, Pinson EN (1973) The speech chain: the physics and biology of spoken language. New York: Bell Telephone Laboratories.

Derlacki EL (1984) Otosclerosis. In Northern J (Ed.) Hearing disorders. Boston, MA: Little Brown & Co., pp. 111–8.

Dillon H, Ching T (1995) What makes a good speech test? In Plant G, Spens K-E (Eds) Profound deafness and speech communication. London: Whurr Publishers, pp. 305–44.

Dillon H, James A, Ginis J (1997) The Client Oriented Scale of Improvement (COSI) and its relationship to several other measures of benefit and satisfaction provided by hearing aids. Journal of the American Academy of Audiology 8: 27–43.

Dineen R, Doyle J, Bench RJ (1997a) Audiological and psychological characteristics of a group of tinnitus sufferers, prior to commencement of tinnitus management training. British Journal of Audiology 31: 27–38.

Dineen R, Doyle J, Bench RJ (1997b) Managing tinnitus: a comparison of different approaches to tinnitus management training. British Journal of Audiology 31: 331–44.

Dobie RA (1992) The relative contribution of occupational noise and aging in individual cases of hearing loss. Ear & Hearing 13: 19–27.

Dockrell J, McShane J (1992) Children's learning difficulties: a cognitive approach. Oxford: Blackwell.

Dodd B (1987). The acquisition of lip-reading skills by normally hearing children. In Dodd B, Campbell R (Eds) Hearing by eye: the psychology of lipreading. Hillsdale, NJ: Lawrence Erlbaum Associates, pp. 163–75.

Dolan TG, Maurer JF (1996) Noise exposure associated with hearing aid use in industry. Journal of Speech & Hearing Research 39: 251–90.

Dornan D, Del Dot J (1996) The speech and language pathologist in a paediatric cochlear implant program: a case study. Australian Communication Quarterly, Winter: 20–2.

Downs DW, Crum MA (1978) Processing demands during auditory learning under degraded listening conditions. Journal of Speech & Hearing Research 21: 702–14.

Downs MP (1985) Effects of mild hearing loss on auditory processing. Otolaryngologic Clinics of North America 18: 337–44.

Doyle J (1989) Hearing screening: misunderstood, a misnomer, or both? Australian Communication Quarterly 8: 10–12.

Doyle J (1995) Issues in teaching clinical reasoning to students of speech and hearing sciences. In Higgs J, Jones M (Eds) Clinical reasoning skills. Oxford: Butterworth-Heinemann, pp. 224–34.

Doyle J, Healey JE (1981) Questions of efficacy in identification audiometry. Australian Journal of Audiology 3(2): 59–64.

Doyle J, Thomas SA (1988) Clinical decision-making in audiology: the case for investigating what we do. Australian Journal of Audiology 10: 45–56.

Doyle J, Oakes T (1993) The appropriateness of tympanometry in screening for developmentally significant hearing loss in children. Australian Communication Quarterly, Summer: 15–17.

Doyle J, Wong LN (1996) The mismatch between aspects of hearing impairment and hearing disability/handicap in adult/elderly Cantonese speakers: some hypotheses concerning cultural and linguistic influences. Journal of the American Academy of Audiology 7(6): 442–6.

Dudic, MA, Duff MA (1977) The effect of appropriate facial expressions on speechreading ability. In Berger KW (Ed.) Research studies in speechreading. Kent, OH: Herald Publishing House, pp. 8–13.

Dufresne RM, Alleyne BC, Reesal MR (1988) Asymmetric hearing loss in truck drivers. Ear & Hearing 9: 41–2.

Dunham M, Friedman H (1990) Audiologic management of bilateral external auditory canal atresia with the bone conducting implantable hearing device. Cleft Palate Journal 27: 369–73.

Durrant JD, Lovrinic JH (1984) Bases of hearing science, 2nd edn. Baltimore, MD: Williams & Wilkins.

Dwyer J (1993) Educational difficulties associated with childhood fluctuation conductive loss: a survey of 301 primary school children. Proceedings of the first national conference on childhood fluctuating conductive deafness/otitis media, pp. 163–9. Parkville, Victoria, October 1992.

El-Refaie A, Parker DJ, Bamford JM (1996) Otoacoustic emission versus ABR screening: The effects of external and middle ear abnormalities in a group of SCBU neonates. British Journal of Audiology 30: 3–8.

Eldert MA, Davis H (1951) The articulation function of patients with conductive deafness. Laryngoscope 61: 891–909.

Elliot LL, Hammer MA, Scholl ME (1989) Fine-grained auditory discrimination in normal children and children with language-learning problems. Journal of Speech & Hearing Research 32: 112–9.

Elliot M, Doyle J (1993) The performance of monolingual and bilingual Italian speakers on standard tests of speech discrimination. Australian Journal of Human Communication Disorders 21(2): 65–73.

Ellis AW, Young AW (1988) Human cognitive neuropsychology. London: Erlbaum.

Epstein MM, Shaywitz SE, Shaywitz BA, Woolston JL (1991) The boundaries of attention deficit disorder. Journal of Learning Disabilities 24: 78–86.

Erber NP (1982) Auditory training. Washington, DC: AG Bell Association for the Deaf.

Erber NP (1985) Telephone communication and hearing impairment. London: Taylor and Francis.

Erber NP (1988) Communication therapy for hearing impaired adults. Abbotsford, Melbourne: Clavis Publishing.

Erber NP (1992) Adaptive screening of sentence perception in older adults. Ear & Hearing 13: 58–60.

Erber NP (1996) Communication therapy for adults with sensory loss, 2nd edn. Clifton Hill: Clavis.

Erber NP, Alencewiciz CM (1976) Audiologic evaluations of deaf children. Journal of Speech & Hearing Disorders 41: 256–67.

Erber NP, Lind SC (1994) Communication therapy: theory and practice. In Gagné JP, Tye-Murray N (Eds) Research in audiological rehabilitation: current trends and future directions (Monograph). Journal of the Academy of Rehabilitative Audiology 27: 267–87.

Erber NP, Lamb NL, Lind C (1996) Factors that affect the use of hearing aids by older people: a new perspective. American Journal of Audiology 5: 11–8.

Erlandsson SI, Rubinstein B, Axelsson A, Carlsson SG (1991) Psychological dimensions in patients with disabling tinnitus and craniomandibular disorders. British Journal of Audiology 25: 15–24.

Everingham C (1996) Classroom communication skills in cochlear implant children. Australian Communication Quarterly, Winter: 30–5.

Ewing AWG (1957) Speech audiometry for children. In Ewing AWG (Ed.) Education guidance and the deaf child. Washington, DC: The Volta Bureau, pp. 278–96.

Fant G (1973) Speech sounds and features. Cambridge, MA: MIT Press.

Ferre JM (1987) Pediatric central auditory processing disorder: considerations for diagnosis, interpretation, and remediation. Journal of the Academy of Rehabilitative Audiology 20: 73–81.

Ferre JM, Wilber LA (1986) Normal and learning disabled children's central auditory processing skills: an experimental test battery. Ear & Hearing 7: 336–43.

Fishman PM (1983) Interaction: the work women do. In Thorne B, Kramarae C, Henley N (Eds) Language, gender and society. Rowley, MA: Newby House Publishers, pp. 89–101.

Fletcher SG (1987) Visual feedback and lip-positioning skills of children with and without impaired hearing. Journal of Speech & Hearing Research 29: 231–9.

Flowers A, Costello R (1970) Flowers–Costello Test of Central Auditory Abilities. Dearborn, MI: Perceptual Learning Systems.

Fowler EP (1936) A method for the early detection of otosclerosis: a study of sounds well above threshold. Archives of Otolaryngology 24: 731–41.

Frank T, Petersen DR (1987) Accuracy of a 40 dB HL Audioscope™ and audiometer screening for adults. Ear & Hearing 8: 180–3.

Fria TJ (1985) Threshold estimation with early latency auditory potentials. In Katz J (Ed.) Handbook of clinical audiology, 3rd edn. Baltimore, MD: Williams & Wilkins, pp. 549–64.

Fritsch MH, Sommer A (1991) Handbook of congenital and early onset hearing loss. New York, NY: Igaku-Shoin.

Fryauf-Bertschy H, Tyler RS, Kelsay DM, Gantz BJ (1992) Performance over time of congenitally deaf and postlingually deafened children using a multi-channel cochlear implant. Journal of Speech & Hearing Research 35: 913–20.

Gagné J-P (1994) Visual and audiovisual speech perception training: basic and applied research needs. In Gagné J-P, Tye-Murray, N (Eds) Research in audiological rehabilitation: current trends and future directions (Monograph). Journal of the Academy of Rehabilitative Audiology 27: 133–59.

Gagné J-P, Tye-Murray NE (1994) Research in audiological rehabilitation: current trends and future directions (Monograph Supplement). Journal of the Academy of Rehabilitative Audiology 27.

Gagné J-P, Tugby KG, Michaud J (1991) Development of a Speech Test on the Utilization of Contextual Cues (STUCC): preliminary findings with normal-hearing subjects. Journal of the Academy of Rehabilitative Audiology 24: 157–70.

Gagné J-P, Masterton V, Munhall KG, Bilida N, Querengesser C. (1994) Across talker variability in auditory, visual and audiovisual speech intelligibility for conversational and clear speech. Journal of the Academy of Rehabilitative Audiology 27: 135–58.

Gailey L (1987) Psychological parameters of lip-reading skill. In Dodd B, Campbell R (Eds) Hearing by eye: the psychology of lip-reading. Hillsdale, NJ: Erlbaum.

Gans D, Gans KD (1993) Development of a hearing test protocol for profoundly involved multi-handicapped children. Ear & Hearing 14: 128–40.

Garrard KR, Smith Clark B (1985) Otitis media: the role of speech-language pathologists. Asha 27: 35–9.

Garstecki DC (1976) Situational cues in visual speech perception. Journal of the American Audiological Society 2: 99–106.

Garstecki DC (1994) Assistive devices for the hearing-impaired. In Gagné J-P, Tye-Murray N (Eds) Research in audiological rehabilitation: current trends and future directions (Monograph Supplement). Journal of the Academy of Rehabilitative Audiology 27: 113–32.

Garstecki DC, O'Neil JJ (1980) Situational cue and strategy influence on speechreading. Scandinavian Audiology 9: 147–51.

Gascon GG, Johnson R, Burd L (1986) Central auditory processing and attention deficit disorders. Journal of Child Neurology 1: 27–33.

Gatehouse S, Killion M (1993) HABRAT: Hearing Aid Brain Rewiring Accomodation Time. Hearing Instruments 44: 29–32.

Gathercole SE, Baddeley AD (1990) Phonological memory deficits in language disordered children: is there a causal connection? Journal of Memory & Language 29: 336–60.

Gathercole SE, Baddeley AD (1993) Working memory and language. Hove: Erlbaum.

Geldard FA (1972) The human senses. New York, NY: John Wiley.

Gershal J, Kruger B, Giraudi-Perry D, Chobot J, Rosenberg M, Shapiro IM, Diano A, Kopet J, Shelov S (1985) Accuracy the Welch Allyn Audioscope and traditional hearing screening for children with known hearing loss. The Journal of Pediatrics 106: 15–20.

Gilad O, Glorig A (1979) Presbycusis: the ageing ear. Parts I & II. Journal of the American Auditory Society 4: 195–217.

Ginsberg IA, White TP (1985) Otologic considerations in audiology. In Katz J (Ed.) Handbook of clinical audiology, 3rd edn. Baltimore, MD: Williams & Wilkins, pp. 15–38.

Ginsberg IA, Hoffman SR, Stinziano GD, White TP (1979) Stapedectomy: in depth analysis of 2405 cases. Laryngoscope 88: 1999–2016.

Gold T (1980) Speech production in hearing-impaired children. Journal of Communication Disorders 13: 397–418.

Golding M, Lilly DJ, Lay JW (1996) A Staggered Spondaic Word (SSW) Test for Australian use. Australian Journal of Audiology 18: 81–8.

Goldman R, Fristoe M, Woodcock RW (1974) Goldman–Fristoe–Woodcock Auditory Skills Test Battery. Circle Pines, MN: American Guidance Service.

Goldstein MH, Stark RE (1976) Modifications of vocalisations of preschool deaf children by vibrotactile and visual displays. Journal of the Acoustical Society of America 59: 282–6.

Goodhill V, Harris I (1979) Sudden hearing loss syndrome. In Goodhill V (Ed.) Ear diseases, deafness and dizziness. New York, NY: Harper & Rowe, pp. 664–81.

Goodyear P, Hynd GW (1992) Attention-deficit disorder with (ADD/H) and without (ADD/WO) hyperactivity: behavioural and neuropsychological differentiation. Journal of Clinical Child Psychology 21: 273–303.

Gordon N, Ward S (1995) Abnormal response to sound, and central auditory processing disorder. Developmental Medicine and Child Neurology 37: 645–52.

Grandori F, Lutman ME (1996) Neonatal hearing screening programs in Europe: towards a consensus development conference. Audiology 35: 291–5.

Gray RF (1991) Cochlear implants: The medical criteria for patient selection. In Cooper H (Ed.) Cochlear implants: a practical guide. London: Whurr Publishers, pp. 146–54.

Green DS (1978) Pure tone air conduction testing. In Katz J (Ed.) Handbook of clinical audiology, 2nd edn. Baltimore, MD: Williams & Wilkins, pp. 98–109.

Gyo K, Saiki T, Yanagihara N (1996) Implantable hearing aid using a piezoelectric ossicular vibrator: a speech audiometric study. Audiology 35: 271–6.

Haggard M, Hughes E (1991) Screening children's hearing: a review of the literature and the implications of otitis media. London: HMSO.

Hall JW (1992) Handbook of auditory evoked responses. Boston, MA: Allyn & Bacon.

Hallam RS (1989) Living with tinnitus. Wellingborough: Thorsons Publishers.

Hammill DD, Larsen SC (1974) The effectiveness of psycholinguistic training. Exceptional Children 41: 5–14.

Hammond V.(1987) Diseases of the external ear. In Booth JB (Ed.) Scott-Brown's otolaryngology: otology, 5th edn. London: Butterworths, pp. 156–71.

Hart CW, Geltman-Cokely C, Schupbach J, Dal Canto MC, Coppleson LW (1989) Neurotologic findings in a patient with acquired immune deficiency syndrome. Ear & Hearing 10: 68–76.

Haskins HA (1964) Kindergarten PB word lists. In Newby HA (Ed.) Audiology. New York: Appleton-Century-Crofts.

Healey JE, Doyle J (1980) Self-perception of hearing loss and its application for mass hearing. Australian Journal of Audiology 2(2): 48–55.

Hellstrom PA, Dengerik HA, Axlesson A (1992) Noise levels from toys and recreational articles for children and teenagers. British Journal of Audiology 26: 267–70.

Henry LA (1991) Development of auditory memory span: the role of rehearsal. British Journal of Developmental Psychology 9: 493–511.

Hill M, Dellaflora R, Dillon H, Jordt J, Birtles G, Byrne D, Hartley D (1996) Aided speech audiogram. Paper presented to the 12th National Scientific Conference and Workshops of the Audiological Society of Australia. Brisbane, 29 April–2 May.

Hirsch IJ, Davis H, Silverman SR, Reynolds EG, Eldert E, Benson RW (1952) Development of materials for speech audiometry. Journal of Speech & Hearing Disorders 15: 321–37.

Holmes J (1993) New Zealand women are good to talk to: an analysis of politeness strategies in interaction. Journal of Pragmatics 20: 91–116.

Horvath BM (1985) Variation in Australian English. Cambridge: Cambridge University Press.

House WF, Berliner KI (1991) Cochlear implants: from idea to clinical practice. In Cooper H (Ed.) Cochlear implants: a practical guide. London: Whurr Publishers, pp. 9–33.

Hovind H, Parving A (1987) Detection of hearing impairment in early childhood. Scandinavian Audiology 16: 187–93.

Hubbard TW, Paradise JL, McWilliams BJ, Elster BA, Taylor FH (1985) Consequences of unremitting middle-ear disease in early life. Otologic, audiologic and developmental findings in children with cleft palate. New England Journal of Medicine 312: 1529–34.

Hudgins CV, Numbers F (1942) An investigation of the intelligibility of the speech of the deaf. Genetic Psychological Monographs 25: 289–392.

Humes LE (1991) Understanding the speech-understanding problems of the hearing-impaired. Journal of the American Academy of Audiology 2: 59–69.

Hunter MF, Kimm L, Caferelli Dees D, Kennedy CR, Thornton ARD (1994) Feasibility of otoacoustic emission detection followed by ABR as a universal neonatal screening test for hearing impairment. British Journal of Audiology 28: 47–51.

Hyde ML, Davidson MJ, Alberti PW (1991) Auditory test strategy. In Jacobson JT, Northern JL (Eds.) Diagnostic audiology. Austin TX: Pro Ed, pp. 295–322.

Ijsseldijk FJ (1988) Speechreading tests for the deaf: a review and methodological considerations and recommendations. Journal of the British Association of Teachers of the Deaf 12: 3–15.

International Electrotechnical Commission (1979) IEC 645-1979. Standard for audiometers. Geneva: IEC.

International Electrotechnical Commission (1991) IEC 1027. Aural impedance/ admittance instruments. Geneva: IEC.

Jackson PL (1988) The theoretical minimal unit for visual speech perception: visemes and coarticulation. In De Filippo CL, Sims DG (Eds) New reflections on speechreading. Volta Review 90( 5): 99–115. Washington, DC: Alexander Graham Bell Association for the Deaf.

James D, van Steenbrugge W, Chiveralls K (1994) Underlying deficits in language disordered children with central auditory processing difficulties. Applied Psycholinguistics 15: 311–28.

Jastreboff PJ, Hazell JWP (1993) A neurophysiological approach to tinnitus: Clinical implications. British Journal of Audiology 27: 7–17.

Jeffers J, Barley M (1971) Speechreading (lipreading). Springfield, IL: Charles C. Thomas.

Jerger J (1960) Bekesy audiometry in the analysis of auditory disorders. Journal of Speech & Hearing Research 3: 275–87.

Jewett DL, Williston JS (1971) Auditory-evoked far fields averaged from the scalp of humans. Brain 94: 681–96.

Jirsa RE (1992) The clinical utility of the P3AERP in children with auditory processing disorders. Journal of Speech & Hearing Research 35: 903–12.

John JEJ, Gemmill J, Howarth NN, Kitzinger M, Sykes M (1976) Some factors affecting the intelligibility of deaf children's speech. In Taylor IG, Markides A (Eds) Disorders of auditory function II. London: Academic Press, pp. 187–96.

Johnson JJ, Bagi P, Elberling C (1983) Evoked emission from the human ear III: Findings in neonates. Scandinavian Audiology 12: 17–24.

Kalikow DM, Stevens KN, Elliot LL (1977) Development of a test of speech intelligibility in noise using sentence materials and controlled predictability. Journal of the Acoustical Society of America 61: 1337–51.

Kankkunen A (1982) Preschool children with impaired hearing. Acta Otolaryngologica 391(Suppl.): 1–124.

Kaplan HF (1992) The impact of hearing impairment and counseling adults who are deaf or hearing impaired. In Hull RH (Ed.) Aural rehabilitation, 2nd edn. San Diego, CA: Singular Publishing, pp. 135–48.

Kaplan H, Bally SJ, Garretson C (1987) Speechreading: a way to improve understanding, 2nd edn. Washington, DC: Gallaudet University Press.

Katz J (1968) The SSW test: an interim report. Journal of Speech & Hearing Disorders 33: 132–46.

Katz J (1978) SSW workshop manual. Buffalo, NY: Allentown Industries.

Katz J (1983) Phonemic synthesis. In Lasky EZ, Katz J (Eds) Central auditory processing disorders: problems of speech, language and learning. Baltimore, MD: University Park Press.

Katz J (1992) Classification of auditory processing disorders. In Katz J, Stecker NA, Henderson D (Eds) Central auditory processing: a transdisciplinary view. St Louis, MO: Mosby.

Katz J (Ed.) (1994) Handbook of clinical audiology, 4th edn. Baltimore, MD: Williams & Wilkins.

Katz J, Pack G (1975) New developments in differential diagnosis using the SSW test. In Sullivan M (Ed.) Central auditory processing disorders. Omaha, NE: University of Nebraska Press.

Katz J, Harmon C (1982) Phonemic synthesis. Allen, TX: Developmental Learning Materials.

Katz J, Yeung E, Metwesky L (1988) SSW C-I-R manual for calculations, interpretation, and recommendation of SSW test results. Amherst, NY: Jimm Co.

Katz J, Stecker NA, Henderson D (Eds) (1992) Central auditory processing: a transdisciplinary view. St Louis, MO: Mosby.

Kei J, Chan T, Ma MC, Ng L, Lowe C, Lai DM, Ng YH, Kwan E (1991) Cantonese speech audiometry for children of Hong Kong. Australian Journal of Audiology 13: 41–5.

Keith RW (Ed.) (1977) Central auditory dysfunction. New York, NY: Grune & Stratton.

Keith RW (Ed.) (1981a) Central auditory and language disorders in children. Houston, TX: College Hill Press.

Keith RW (1981b) Audiological and auditory language tests of central auditory function. In Keith RW (Ed.) Central auditory and language disorders in children. Houston, TX: College Hill Press.

Keith RW (1983) Interpretation of the Staggered Spondee Word (SSW) test. Ear & Hearing 4: 287–92.

Keith RW (1986) SCAN: a screening test for auditory processing disorders. San Antonio, TX: The Psychological Corporation/Harcourt Brace Jovanovich.

Keith RW, Engineer P (1991) Effects of methylphenidate on the auditory processing abilities of children with attention deficit hyperactivity disorder. Journal of Learning Disabilities 24: 630–6.

Keith RW, Pensak ML (1991) Central auditory function. Otolaryngologic Clinics of North America 24: 371–9.

Keller WD (1992) Auditory processing disorder or attention deficit disorder? In Katz J, Stecker NA, Henderson D (Eds) Central auditory processing: a transdisciplinary view, 1. St Louis, MO: Mosby, pp. 107–14.

Kelsall DC, Shallop JK, Burnelli T (1995) Cochlear implantation in the elderly. American Journal of Otology 16. 609–15.

Kemker FJ, Zarajczyk DR (1989) Audiological management in patients with cleft palate. In Bzoch KR (Ed.) Communication disorders related to cleft lip and palate. Boston, MA: College Hill, pp. 174–84.

Kemp DT (1978) Stimulated acoustic emissions from within the human auditory system. Journal of the Acoustical Society of America 64: 1386–91.

Kemp DT, Ryan S, Bray P (1990) A guide to the effective use of otoacoustic emissions. Ear & Hearing 11: 93–105.

Kettlety A (1987) The Manchester high pitch rattle. British Journal of Audiology 21: 73–4.

Kileny PR (1985) Evaluation of vestibular function. In Katz J (Ed.) Handbook of clinical audiology, 3rd edn, Baltimore, MD: Williams & Wilkins, pp. 582–603.

Kileny PR, Zwolan TA, Zimmerman-Phillips S, Kemink JL (1992) A comparison of round window and transtympanic electric stimulation in cochlear implant candidates. Ear & Hearing 13: 295–99.

Kinzie CE, Kinzie R (1936) Lip-reading for children. Washington, DC: Volta Bureau.

Kirk S, McCarthy J, Kirk W (1968) Illinois Test of Psycholinguistic Abilities, revised edn. Urbana, IL: University of Illinois Press.

Klee TM, Davis-Dansky E (1986) A comparison of unilaterally hearing-impaired children and normal-hearing children on a battery of standardised language tests. Ear & Hearing 7: 27–37.

Knight JJ (1987) Some aspects of speech tests in non-European languages. In Martin M (Ed.) Speech audiometry. London: Taylor & Francis, pp. 279–85.

Koay CB, Sutton GJ (1996) Direct hearing aid referrals: a prospective study. Clinical Otolaryngology 21: 142–6.

Kricos PB, Lesner SA (1982) Differences in visual intelligibility across talkers. Volta Review 84: 219–25.

Kricos PB, Lesner SA (1985) Effect of talker differences on the speechreading of hearing-impaired teenagers. Volta Review 87: 5–14.

Kricos PB, Lesner SA (Eds) (1995) Hearing care for the older adult. Boston, MA: Butterworth-Heinemann.

Kværner KJ, Engdahl B, Aursnes J, Arnesen AR, Mair IWS (1996) Transient-evoked otoacoustic emissions: helpful tool in the detection of pseudohypacusis. Scandinavian Audiology 25: 173–7.

Lane DM, Pearson DA (1982) The development of selective attention. Merrill-Palmer Quarterly 28: 317–37.

Lasky EZ, Katz J (1983a) Perspectives on central auditory processing. In Lasky EZ, Katz J (Eds) Central auditory processing disorders: problems of speech, language and hearing disorders. Baltimore, MD: University Park Press, pp. 3–10.

Lasky EZ, Katz J (1983b) Central auditory processing disorders: problems of speech, language, and learning. Baltimore, MD: University Park Press.

Lassman FM, Aldridge J (1985) General medical considerations in audiology. In Katz J (Ed.) Handbook of clinical audiology, 3rd edn. Baltimore, MD: Williams & Wilkins, pp. 54–63.

Leder SB, Spitzer JB (1990) A perceptual evaluation of the speech of adventitiously deaf adult males. Ear & Hearing 11: 169–75.

Lesner SA (1988) The talker. In De Filippo CL, Sims DG (Eds) Volta Review Monographs: Special Issue on Speechreading 90(5): 89–98.

Lesner SA, Kricos PB (1981) Visual vowel and diphthong perception across speakers. Journal of the Academy of Rehabilitative Audiology 14: 252–8.

Lesner SA, Klingler MS (1995) Considerations in establishing an optimum assistive listening devices center. Journal of the Academy of Rehabilitative Audiology 28: 60–7.

Lesner SA, Sandridge S, Kricos P (1987) Training influences on visual consonant and sentence recognition. Ear & Hearing 8: 283–7.

Lichtenstein MN, Bess FH, Logan SA (1988) Validation of screening tools for identifying hearing impaired elderly in primary care. Journal of the American Medical Association 259: 2875–8.

Lindamood C, Lindamood P (1971) Lindamood Auditory Conceptualization Test. Allen, TX: Developmental Learning Materials.

Lindamood CH, Lindamood PC (1975) The ADD Program: Auditory Discrimination in Depth, revised edn. Columbus, OH: Macmillan/McGraw-Hill.

Ling D (1976) Speech and the hearing impaired child: theory and practice. Washington, DC: The Alexander Graham Bell Association for the Deaf.

Ling D (1984) Early intervention for hearing-impaired children: oral options. San Diego, CA: College Hill Press.

Ling D (1992) Speech development for children who are hearing impaired. In Hull RH (Ed.) Aural rehabilitation, 2nd edn. San Diego, CA: Singular Publishing, pp. 103–19.

Ling D, Ling A (1978) Aural habilitation. Washington, DC: The Alexander Graham Bell Association for the Deaf.

Lipscomb DM, Taylor AC (Eds) (1978) Noise control: handbook of principles and practices. New York, NY: Van Nostrand Reinhold Company.

Lloyd L, Spradlin J, Reid M (1968) An operant audiometric procedure for difficult-to-test patients. Journal of Speech & Hearing Disorders 33: 236–45.

Lukas RA, Genchur-Lukas J (1985) Spondaic word tests. In Katz J (Ed.) Handbook of clinical audiology. Baltimore, MD: Williams & Wilkins, pp. 383–403.

Luria AR (1966) Higher cortical functions in man. New York, NY: Basic Books.

Lybarger SF (1985) Earmoulds. In Katz J (Ed.) Handbook of clinical audiology, 3rd edn. Baltimore, MD: Williams & Wilkins, pp. 885–910.

Lyxell B, Rönnberg J (1989) Information processing skills and speechreading. British Journal of Audiology 23: 339–47.

Macrae JH (1968) TTS and recovery from TTS after use of powerful hearing aids. Journal of the Acoustical Society of America 43: 1445–6.

Macrae JH (1991) Permanent threshold shift associated with overamplification by hearing aids. Journal of Speech & Hearing Research 34: 403–14.

Macrae JH (1992) Computer programs for determining extended percentage loss of hearing. Australian Journal of Audiology 14: 13–8.

Margolis RH (1993) Detection of hearing impairment with the acoustic stapedial reflex. Ear & Hearing 14: 3–10.

Markides A (1983) The speech of hearing impaired children. Manchester: Manchester University Press.

Martin FN (1975) Introduction to audiology. Englewood Cliffs, NJ: Prentice-Hall.

Martin FN (1985) The pseudohypacousic. In Katz J (Ed.) Handbook of clinical audiology, 3rd edn. Baltimore, MD: Williams & Wilkins, pp. 742–85.

Martin M (Ed.) (1987) Speech audiometry. London: Taylor & Francis.

Matkin ND, Hook PE (1983) A multidisciplinary approach to central auditory evaluations. In Lasky EJ, Katz J (Eds) Central auditory processing disorders. Baltimore, MD: University Park Press.

Mauk GW, While KR, Montensen LB, Behens TR (1991) The effectiveness of screening programs based on high risk characteristics in early identification of hearing impairment. Ear & Hearing 12: 312–9.

McCandles GA, Thomas GK (1974) Impedance audiometry as a screening procedure for middle ear disease. Transactions of the American Academy of Opthalmology and Otolaryngology, ORL 78: 98–102.

McGarr NS, Osberger MJ (1978) Pitch deviancy and intelligibility. Journal of Communication Disorders 11: 239–47.

McGarr NS, Harris KS (1983) Articulatory control in a deaf speaker. In Hochberg IE, Levitt H, Osberger MJ (Eds) Speech of the hearing-impaired: research, training and personal preparation. Baltimore, MD: University Park Press, pp. 75–95.

McGurk H, MacDonald J (1976) Hearing lips and seeing voices. Nature 264: 746–8.

McKenzie AR, Rice CG (1990) Binaural hearing aids for high frequency hearing loss. British Journal of Audiology 24: 329–34.

McMillan MO, Willette SJ (1988) Aseptic techniques: a procedure for preventing disease transmission in the practice environment. Asha 30: 35–7.

McPherson B (1990) Hearing loss in Australian Aborigines: a critical evaluation. Australian Journal of Audiology 12: 67–78.

McPherson B, Knox E (1992) Hearing loss in urban Aboriginal and Tories Strait Islander schoolchildren. Australian Aboriginal Studies 2: 60–70.

McPherson B, Smyth V (1997) Hearing screening for school children with otitis media using otoacoustic emission measures. Asia Pacific Journal of Speech, Language & Hearing 2: 69–82.

Meadow-Orlans KP (1985) Social and psychologic effects of hearing loss in adulthood: a literature review. In Orlans H (Ed.) Adjustment to adult hearing loss. San Diego, CA: College Hill Press, pp. 35–57.

Melnik W (1995) Noise and hearing loss. In Wall LG (Ed.) Hearing for the speech language therapist and health care professional. Boston, MA: Butterworth-Heinemann, pp. 401–13.

Menyuk P (1992) Relationship of otitis media to speech processing and language development. In Katz J, Stecker N, Henderson D (Eds) Central auditory processing: a transdisciplinary view. St Louis, MO: Mosby, pp. 187–97.

Meyer-Bish C (1996) Epidemiological evaluation of hearing damage related to strongly amplified music (personal cassette players, discotheques, rock concerts)—high definition audiometric survey on 1364 subjects. Audiology 35: 121–42.

Miller LA (1977) The effect of facial expressions on speechreading performance. In Berger KW (Ed.) Research studies in speechreading. Kent, OH: Hearlad Publishing House, pp. 14–8.

Mohay H (1983) The effects of cued speech on the language development of three deaf children. Sign Language Studies 38: 25–49.

Monley P (1994) Hearing impairment in the Western Australian intellectually handicapped population. Australian Journal of Audiology 16: 89–98.

Monsen RB (1978) Towards measuring how well deaf children speak. Journal of Speech & Hearing Research 21: 197–219.

Moore B (1996) The promise of digital hearing. ENT News 5(2): 17.

Moore DC (1993) Conductive hearing loss in a group of young Melbourne children: prevalence and some effects. Proceedings of the first national conference on childhood fluctuating conductive deafness/otitis media. Parkville, Victoria, October 1992.

Moore DC, Best GF (1988) Fluctuating conductive hearing loss in young children: incidence and effects. Victoria, Australia: Deafness Foundation (Victoria).

Moore S (1996) Adult cochlear implantees: the speech pathologist's role in rehabilitation. Australian Communication Quarterly, Winter: 36–40.

Morgan DE, Dirks DD, Bower DR (1979) Suggested threshold sound pressure levels for frequency modulated (warble) tones in the sound field. Journal of Speech & Hearing Disorders 44: 37–54.

Morris P (1993) Children with pre-existing difficulties: cleft lip and palate. Proceedings of the first national conference on childhood fluctuating conductive deafness/otitis media, p. 186. Parkville, Victoria, October 1992.

Moss WL, Sheiffele WA (1994) Can we differentially diagnose an attention deficit disorder without hyperactivity from a central auditory processing problem? Child Psychiatry & Human Development 25: 85–96

Mueller HG (1985) In Katz J (Ed.) Handbook of clinical audiology. Baltimore, MD: Williams & Wilkins, pp. 355–82.

Mueller HG, Ebinger KA (1996) CIC hearing aids: potential benefits and fitting strategies. Seminars in Hearing 17: 61–80.

Mueller HG, Killion M (1990) An easy method for calculating the Articulation Index. The Hearing Journal 43 (9): 14–7.

Musiek FE (1985) Application of central auditory tests: an overview. In Katz J (Ed.) Handbook of clinical audiology, 3rd edn. Baltimore, MD: Williams & Wilkins, pp. 321–36.

Musiek FE, Geurink NA, Kietel SA (1982) Test battery assessment of auditory perceptual dysfunction in children. Laryngoscope 92: 251–7.

National Institutes of Health (1993) Early identification of hearing impairment in infants and young children. NIH Consensus Statement 11: 1–24.

Neale MD (1988) Neale Analysis of Reading Ability – Revised. Melbourne: Australian Council for Educational Research.

Neate DM (1972) The use of tactile vibration in the teaching of speech to severely and profoundly deaf children. The Teacher of the Deaf 70: 136–46.

Nelson SM, Berry RI (1984) Ear disease and hearing loss among Navajo children: a mass survey. Laryngoscope 94: 310–23.

New South Wales Health Department Working Party (1993) Guidelines on the management of paediatric middle ear disease. Medical Journal of Australia, 159(Suppl. 4): S1–4.

Nitchie EB (1912) Lipreading: principles and practice. New York, NY: FA Stokes & Co.

Nitchie EB (1915) The use of homophenous words. Volta Review 18: 3.

Northern JL, Downs MP (1991) Hearing in children. Baltimore, MD: Williams & Wilkins.

Nowell RC (1985) Psychology of hearing impairment. In Katz J (Ed.) Handbook of clinical audiology, 3rd edn. Baltimore, MD: Williams & Wilkins, pp. 776–87.

Nozza RJ, Bluestone CD, Kardatzke D, Bachman R (1992) Towards the validation of aural acoustic immittance measures for diagnosis of middle ear effusion in children. Ear & Hearing 13: 442–53.

Oberklaid F, Harris C, Keir E (1989) Auditory dysfunction in children with school problems. Clinical Pediatrics 28: 397–403.

Oller DK, Ellers RE, Vergaro K, La Voie E (1986) Tactual vocoders in a mulitsensory program training speech production and reception. Volta Review 88: 21–36.

Olsen WO, Matkin ND (1979) Speech audiometry. In Rintelmann WF (Ed.) Hearing assessment. Baltimore, MD: University Park Press, pp. 133–206.

Osborn R, Doyle J (1983) A hearing screening procedure for use in the speech pathology clinic. Australian Journal of Human Communication Disorders 11(2): 77–84.

Owens E, Schubert ED (1977) Development of the California consonant test. Journal of Speech and Hearing Research 20: 463–74.

Oyer HJ, Franckmann JP (1975) The aural rehabilitation process: a conceptual framework analysis. New York, NY: Holt, Rinehart & Winston.

Page JM (1985) Central auditory processing disorders in children. Otolaryngologic Clinics of North America 18: 323–35.

Palmer C (1992) Assistive devices in the audiology practice. American Journal of Audiology 1: 37–51.

Paparella MM, MacDermott JC, de Sousa LCA (1982) Ménière's disease and the peak audiogram. Archives of Otolaryngology 108: 555–9.

Paparella MM, Adams GL, Levine SC (1989) Diseases of the middle ear and mastoid. In Adams GL, Bois LR, Hilger PA (Eds) Bois fundamentals of otolaryngology: A textbook of ear, nose and throat diseases. Philadelphia, PA: Saunders, pp. 90–122.

Parving A, Salomon G (1996) The effect of neonatal universal screening in a health surveillance perspective – a controlled study of two health authority districts. Audiology 35: 158–68.

Pascoe DP (1980) Clinical implications of nonverbal methods of hearing aid selection and fitting. Seminars in Speech, Language and Hearing 1: 217–29.

Patuzzi R (1992) Effect of noise on auditory nerve responses. In Dancer AL, Henderson D, Salvi RJ, Hamernik RP (Eds) Noise-induced hearing loss. St Louis, MO: Mosby, pp. 45–59.

Paul-Brown D (1994) Clinical record keeping in audiology and speech-language pathology. Asha 36: 40–2.

Pavlovic CV (1988) Articulation index predictions of speech intelligibility in hearing aid selection. Asha 30(6): 63–5.

Pavlovic CV (1989) Speech spectrum considerations and speech intelligibility predictions in hearing aid evaluations. Journal of Speech & Hearing Disorders 54: 3–8.

Pavlovic CV (1993) Problems in the prediction of speech recognition performance of normal-hearing and hearing-impaired individuals. In Studebaker G, Hochberg I (Eds) Acoustical factors affecting hearing aid performance. Boston, MA. Allyn & Bacon, pp. 221–34.

Pavlovic CV, Studebaker GA, Sherbecoe RL (1986) An articulation index based procedure for prediction of the speech recognition performance of hearing-impaired individuals. Journal of the Acoustical Society of America 80: 50–7.

Payne EE, Paparella MM (1976) Otitis media. In Northern J (Ed.) Hearing disorders. Boston, MA: Little Brown & Co., pp. 119–28.

Peck DH, Gressard RP, Hellerman GP (1991) Central auditory processing in the school-aged child: is it clinically relevant? Developmental & Behavioral Pediatrics 12: 324–6.

Pender DJ (1992) Practical otology. Philadelphia, PA: JB Lippincott Co.

Penn TO, Abbott ES (1997) Public health and newborn hearing screening. American Journal of Audiology 6: 11–6.

Perkins WH, Kent RD (1986) Textbook of functional anatomy of speech, language and hearing. London: Taylor & Francis.

Pinheiro MP, Musiek FE (Eds) (1985) Assessment of central auditory dysfunction: foundations and clinical correlates. Baltimore, MD: Williams & Wilkins.

Plant G (1991) The development of speech tests in Aboriginal languages. Australian Journal of Audiology 13: 30–40.

Plant G, Moore A (1992) The Common Objects Token (COT) Test: a sentence test for profoundly hearing-impaired children. Australian Journal of Audiology 14: 76–83.

Plant G, Spens K-E (Eds) (1995) Profound deafness and speech communication. London: Whurr Publishers.

Pollard J, Tan L (1993) They can't talk: can they hear? Proceedings of the first national conference on childhood fluctuating conductive deafness/otitis media, pp. 143–50. Parkville, Victoria, October 1992.

Poltl S, Hickson L (1990) Hearing status in elderly hospital inpatients. Australian Journal of Audiology 12: 79–83.

Popelka GR, Berger KW (1971) Gestures and visual speech perception. American Annals of the Deaf 116: 424–36.

Praeger DA, Stone DA, Rose DN (1987) Hearing loss screening in the neonatal intensive care unit: Auditory brain stem response versus Crib-O-Gram – a cost effectiveness analysis. Ear & Hearing 8: 213–6.

Primus MA (1991) Repeated infant thresholds in operant and non-operant audiometric procedures. Ear & Hearing 12: 119–22.

Proctor A (1995) Tactile aid usage in young deaf children. In Plant G, Spens K-E (Eds) Profound deafness and speech communication. London: Whurr Publishers, pp. 111–46.

Qvarnberg Y, Valtonen H (1995) Bacteria in middle ear effusion in children treated with tympanostomy: a 10 year series. Acta Otolaryngologica 115: 653–7.

Ramsden R, Graham J (1995) A safe and cost effective treatment for profoundly deaf adults and children. British Medical Journal 331: 1588.

Rawson VJ, Bamford J (1995) Selecting the gain for radio microphone (FM) systems: theoretical considerations and practical limitations. British Journal of Audiology 29: 161–71.

Reed CM (1995) Tadoma: an overview of research. In Plant G, Spens K-E (Eds) Profound deafness and speech communication. London: Whurr Publishers, pp. 40–55.

Reed M (1959) A verbal screening test of hearing. Proceedings of the III World Congress of the Deaf. Wiesbaden, Germany.

Rees NS (1981) Saying more than we know: is auditory processing disorder a meaningful concept? In Keith RW (Ed.) Central auditory and language disorders in children. San Diego, CA: College Hill Press, pp. 94–120.

Reeves D, Mason L, Prosser H, Kiernan C (1994) Direct referral systems for hearing aid provision. London: HMSO.

Rendell RJ, Williams G, Vinton M, Croucher L (1992) Why patients choose to purchase a hearing aid privately. British Journal of Audiology 26: 325–7.

Riccio CA, Hynd GW, Cohen MJ, Hall J, Molt L (1994) Comorbidity of central auditory processing disorder and attention-deficit hyperactivity disorder. Journal of the American Academy of Child & Adolescent Psychiatry 33: 849–57.

Richardson J (1992) Cost-utility analyses in health care: present status and future issues. In Daley J, McDonald I, Willis E (Eds) Research health care: designs, dilemmas, disciplines. London: Routledge.

Robinshaw HM (1995) Early intervention in hearing impairment: differences in the timing of communicative and linguistic development. British Journal of Audiology 29: 315–34.

Roeser RJ, Northern J (1981) Screening for hearing loss and middle ear disorders. In Roeser RJ, Downs MP (Eds) Auditory disorders in schoolchildren: the law, identification and remediation. New York: Thieme-Stratton, pp. 120–50.

Roeser RJ, Downs MP (1988) Auditory disorders in school children. Stuttgart: Thieme Medical Publishers.

Roeser RJ, Soh J, Dunckel DC, Adams R. (1977) Comparison of tympanometry and otoscopy in establishing pass/fail criteria. Journal of the American Audiology Society 3: 20–5.

Rönnberg J (1990) Cognitive and communication function: the effects of chronological age and 'handicap age'. European Journal of Cognitive Psychology 2: 253–73.

Rönnberg J (1995) What makes a skilled speechreader? In Plant G, Spens K-E (Eds) Profound deafness and speech communication. London: Whurr Publishers, pp. 393–416.

Rosen S, Corcoran T (1982) A videorecorded test of lipreading for British English. British Journal of Audiology 16: 245–54.

Rosenhall V, Pedersen K, Svanborg A (1990) Presbycusis and noise-induced hearing loss. Ear & Hearing 11: 257–63.

Ross M (Ed.) (1994) Communication access for persons with hearing loss: compliance with the American with Disabilities Act. Baltimore, MD: York Press.

Ross M, Lerman J (1970) A picture identification test for hearing impaired children. Journal of Speech & Hearing Research 13: 44–53.

Roush J, Tait CA (1985) Pure tone and acoustic immittance screening of pre-school aged children: an examination of referral criteria. Ear & Hearing 6: 245–50.

Rowe SJ (1991) An evaluation of ABR audiometry for the screening and detection of hearing loss in ex-SCBU infants. British Journal of Audiology 25: 259–74.

Sade J (1979) Secretory otitis media and its sequelae. New York, NY: Churchill Livingstone.

Sakai CS, Mateer CA (1984) Otological and audiological sequelae of closed head trauma. Seminars in Hearing 5: 157–73.

Samuelsson S, Rönnberg J (1991) Script activation in lipreading. Scandinavian Journal of Psychology 32: 124–43.

Sanders DA (1971) Aural rehabilitation. Englewood Cliffs, NJ: Prentice-Hall.

Sandridge SA (1995) Beyond hearing aids: use of auxiliary aids. In Kricos PB, Lesner SA (Eds) Hearing care for the older adult: audiologic rehabilitation. Boston, MA: Butterworth-Heinemann, pp. 127–66.

Sangster JF, Gerace TM, Seewal, RC (1991) Hearing loss in elderly patients in a family practice. Canadian Medical Association Journal 144: 981–4.

Saunders GH, Field DL, Haggard MP (1992) A clinical test battery for obscure auditory dysfunction (OAD): development, selection and use of tests. British Journal of Audiology 26: 33–42.

Shaw GM, Jardine CA, Fridjhon P (1996) A pilot investigation of high-frequency audiometry in obscure auditory dysfunction. British Journal of Audiology 30: 233–7.

Schilder AGM, Snik AFM, Straatman H, van den Broek P (1994) The effect of otitis media with effusion at preschool age on some aspects of auditory perception at school age. Ear & Hearing 15: 224–30.

Schneider D (1992) Audiologic management of central auditory processing disorders. In Katz J, Stecker NA, Henderson D (Eds) Central auditory processing: a transdisciplinary view. St Louis, MO: Mosby.

Schow RL (1991) Considerations in selecting and validating an adult/elderly hearing screening protocol. Ear & Hearing 12: 337–48.

Schow R, Smedley T, Longhurst T (1990) Self assessment and impairment in adult/elderly hearing screening: recent data and new perspectives. Ear & Hearing 11(Suppl.): 17S–27S

Schubert ED (1980) Hearing: its function and dysfunction. New York, NY: Springer-Verlag/Wein.

Schuknecht HF (1974) Pathology of the ear. Cambridge, MA: Harvard University Press.

Schwartz DM, Schwartz RH (1978) Acoustic impedance and otoscopic findings in young children with Down's syndrome. Archives of Otolaryngology 104: 652–6.

Schwartz K (1997) From clinic to conference room: speech pathology in the corporate sector: Asha 39(June/July): 42–6.

Semel E, Wiig EH, Secord W (1989) The CELF-R Screening Test. San Antonio, TX: The Psychological Corporation.

Shah N (1981) Surgical treatment of conductive deafness in children. In Beagley HA (Ed.) Audiology and audiological medicine, vol. 2. Oxford University Press, pp. 694–703.

Shelly P, Hansen SA (1983) The use of vibrotactile aids with preschool hearing impaired children: case studies. Volta Review 85: 14–26.

Shulman JB (1979) Traumatic diseases of the ear and temporal bone. In Goodhill V (Ed.) Ear diseases, deafness and dizziness. New York, NY: Harper & Rowe, pp. 504–16.

Silman MB, Silverman CA (1991) Auditory diagnosis: principles and applications. San Diego, CA: Academic Press.

Silver LB (1990) Attention deficit-hyperactivity disability or a related disorder? Journal of Learning Disabilities 23: 394–7.

Skinner MW, Binzer SM, Holden LK, Holden TA (1995) Hearing changes in adults with cochlear implants. Seminars in Hearing 16: 228–38.

Slater R, Terry M (1987) Tinnitus: a guide for suffers and professionals. London: Croom Helm.

Smith CR (1975) Residual hearing and speech production in deaf children. Journal of Speech & Hearing Research 18: 795–811.

Smith J, Tipping V, Bench RJ (1987) Discrimination of Boothroyd words by Greek and English speakers. Australian Journal of Audiology 9: 87–91.

Smock S (1982) Central auditory skills in juvenile delinquents. Unpublished Master's thesis, Colorado State University.

Smoski WJ, Brunt MA, Tannahill JC (1992) Listening characteristics of children with central auditory processing disorders. Language, Speech & Hearing Services in Schools 23: 145–52.

Snowling MJ (1981) Phonemic deficits in developmental dyslexia. Psychological Research 43: 219–34.

Soderlund G (1995) Tactiling and tactile aids: a user's viewpoint. In Plant G, Spens K-E (Eds) Profound deafness and speech communication. London: Whurr Publishers, pp. 25–39.

Spitzer JB (1983) A central auditory evaluation protocol: a guide for training and diagnosis of lesions of the central system. Ear & Hearing 4: 221–31.

Squires S, Dancer J (1986) Auditory versus visual practice effects in the intelligibility of words in everyday sentences. Journal of Auditory Research 26: 5–10.

Stach B, Loiselle L, Jerger J (1987) Clinical experience with personal FM assistive listening devices. Hearing Journal 40: 24–30.

Standards Association of Australia (1983) Audiometers (AS 2586). Sydney, NSW: Standards House.

Stephens D, Board T, Hobson J, Cooper H (1996) Reported benefits and problems experienced with bone-anchored hearing aids. British Journal of Audiology 30: 215–20.

Storey L, Dillon H (1996) Selection of hearing aid maximum power output (MPO). National Acoustic Laboratories Research and Development Annual Report 1995–96. Sydney: Australian Hearing Services, pp. 9–10.

Stratton WD (1974) Intonation feedback for the deaf through a tactile display. Volta Review 76: 26–35.

Studdert-Kennedy M (1976) Speech perception. In Lass NJ (Ed.)Contemporary issues in experimental phonetics. New York, NY: Academic Press.

Studebaker GA, Zachman TA (1970) Investigation of the acoustics of earmould vents. Journal of the Acoustical Society of America 47: 1107–15.

Sumby WH, Pollack I (1954) Visual contribution to speech intelligibility in noise. Journal of the Acoustical Society of America 26: 212–5.

Summerfield Q (1983) Some preliminaries to a comprehensive account of audio-visual speech perception. In Dodd B, Campbell R (Eds) Hearing by eye: the psychology of lipreading. Hillsdale, NJ: Erlbaum, pp. 3–51.

Summers IR (Ed.) (1992) Tactile aids for the hearing impaired. London: Whurr Publishers.

Suzuki T, Ogiba Y (1961) Conditioned orientation response audiometry. Archives of Otolaryngology 74: 84–90.

Tallal P, Piercy M (1975) Developmental aphasia: the perception of brief vowels and extended stop consonants. Neuropsychologia 13: 69–74.

Tallal P, Piercy M (1978) Defects of auditory perception in children with developmental aphasia. In Wyke M (Ed.) Developmental dysphasia. New York, NY: Academic Press.

Tallal P, Stark RE (1981) Speech acoustic-cue discrimination abilities of normally developing and language impaired children. Journal of the Acoustical Society of America 69: 568–78.

Tallal P, Stark RE, Mellits ED (1985) Identification of language-impaired children on the basis of rapid perception and production skills. Brain & Language 25: 314–22.

Tallal P, Miller SL, Bedi G, Byma G, Wang X, Nagarajan SS, Schreiner C, Jenkins WM, Merzenich MM (1996) Language comprehension in language-learning impaired children improved with acoustically modified speech. Science 271: 81–4.

Teele DW, Teele J (1984) Detection of middle ear effusion by acoustic reflectometry. Journal of Pediatrics 104: 832–8.

Teele DW, Klein JO, Rosner BA (1980) Epidemiology of otitis media in children. Annals of Otology, Rhinology & Laryngology 89: 5–6.

Teele DW, Klein JO, Rosner BA (1989) Epidemiology of otitis media during the first seven years of life in children in Greater Boston. Journal of Infectious Disease 160: 83–94.

Thomas A, Herbst KG (1980) Deafness and psychological disorder. In Taylor IG, Markides A (Eds) Disorders of auditory function III. London: Academic Press, pp. 321–8.

Toe D (1990) Understanding hearing aids: a child case study. Taralye Bulletin 8(1): 9–21. (Available from the Advisory Council for Children with Impaired Hearing (Vic), 137 Blackburn Road, Blackburn, 3130 Australia.)

Tonnquist-Uhlén I (1996) Topography of auditory evoked cortical potentials in children with severe language impairment. Scandinavian Audiology 44 (Suppl.): 1–40.

Trine MB, Hirsch JE, Margolis RH (1993) The effect of middle ear pressure on transient evoked otoacoustic emissions. Ear & Hearing 14: 401–7.

Turner RG (1988) Techniques to determine test protocol performance. Ear & Hearing 9: 177–89.

Turner RG (1990) Recommended guidelines for infant hearing screening: analysis. Asha 32: 57–61, 66.

Turner RG (1991) Making clinical decisions. In Rintelmann NF (Ed.) Hearing assessment, 2nd edn. Austin TX: Pro-Ed, pp. 679–738.

Turner RG, Neilson DW (1984) Application of clinical decision analysis to audiological tests. Ear & Hearing 5: 125–33.

Turner RG, Frazer GJ, Shepard NT (1984) Formulating and evaluating audiological test protocols. Ear & Hearing 5: 321–30.

Turner RG, Shepard NT, Frazer GJ (1984) Clinical performance of audiological and related diagnostic tests. Ear & Hearing 5: 187–94.

Tye-Murray N (1991) The establishment of open articulatory postures by deaf and hearing talkers. Journal of Speech & Hearing Disorders 34: 453–9.

Tyler RS, Baker LJ (1983) Difficulties experienced by tinnitus sufferers. Journal of Speech & Hearing Disorders 48: 150–4.

Utley J (1946) A test of lipreading ability. Journal of Speech & Hearing 11: 109–16.

van Buunen RA, Feston JM, Houtgast T (1996) Peaks in the frequency response of hearing aids: Evaluation of the effects on speech intelligibility and sound quality. Journal of Speech & Hearing Research 39: 239–50.

Ventry IM, Schiavetti N (1986) Evaluating research in speech pathology and audiology, 2nd edn. New York: Macmillan.

Ventry IM, Weinstein BE (1983) Identification of elderly people with hearing problems. Asha 25: 37–42.

Vernon J (1987) Common errors of masking for the relief of tinnitus. In Feldman H (Ed.) Proceedings of the 4th International Tinnitus Seminar. Karlsruhe: Harsch Verlag, pp. 229–38.

Vernon J, Greist S, Press L (1990) Attributes of tinnitus and the acceptance of masking. American Journal of Otolaryngology 11(1): 44–50.

Verrillo RT (1979) Change in vibrotactile thresholds as a function of age. Sensory Processes 3: 49–59.

Verrillo RT (1982) Age related changes in the sensitivity to vibrations. Journal of Gerontology 35: 185–93.

Verrillo RT, Gescheider GA (1992) Perception via the sense of touch. In Summers IR (Ed.) Tactile aids for the hearing impaired. London: Whurr Publishers, pp. 1–36.

Vesterager V (1994) Combined psychological and prosthetic management of tinnitus: a cross sectional study of patients with severe tinnitus. British Journal of Audiology 28: 1–11.

Vorrath J (1993) Otitis media treatment options: their upsides and downsides. Proceedings of the first national conference on childhood fluctuating conductive deafness/otitis media, pp. 25–9. Parkville, Victoria, October 1992.

Vrabec JT, Lambert PR, Arts HA, Ruth RA (1995) Promontory stimulation following translabyrinthine excision of acoustic neuroma with preservation of the cochlear nerve. American Journal of Otology 16: 643–7.

Walden BE, Prosek RA, Montgomery AA, Scherr CK, Jones CJ (1977) Effects of training on the visual recognition of consonants. Journal of Speech & Hearing Research 20: 130–45.

Walden BE, Erdman SA, Montgomery AA, Schwartz DM, Prosek RA (1981) Some effects of training on speech recognition by hearing-impaired adults. Journal of Speech & Hearing Research 24: 207–16.

Walker G, Lamb II (1989) Measuring the components of conductive and mixed hearing losses in children: a case study. Australian Journal of Audiology 11: 21–5.

Walker G, Dillon H, Byrne D (1984) Sound field audiometry: recommended stimuli and procedures. Ear & Hearing 5: 13–21.

Wall LG (Ed.) (1995) Hearing for the speech language therapist and health care professional. Boston, MA: Butterworth-Heinemann.

Warren Y, Dancer J, Monfils B, Pittenger J (1989) The practice effect in speechreading distributed over five days: same versus different CID sentence lists. Volta Review 91: 321–5.

Watson TJ (1967) The education of hearing-impaired children. Springfield, IL: Charles Thomas.

Wechsler D (1980) Wechsler Intelligence Scale for Children – Revised. New York, NY: Psychological Corporation.

Weinstein BE (1986) Validity of a screening protocol for identifying elderly people with hearing problems. Asha 28: 41–5.

Weinstein BE, Ventry IM (1983) A protocol for identifying elderly people with hearing problems. Asha 25: 37–42.

Weisenberger JM (1995) Tactile aids and cochlear implants. In Wall LG (Ed.) Hearing for the speech-language pathologist and health care professional. Boston, MA: Butterworth-Heinemann, pp. 311–35.

Welsh LW, Welsh JJ, Healy MP (1983) Effect of sound deprivation on central hearing. Laryngoscope 93: 1569–75.

Wenthold RJ, Schneider ME, Kim HN, Dechesne (1992) Putative biochemical processes in noise-induced-hearing-loss. In Dancer AL, Henderson D, Salvi RJ, Hamernik RP (Eds) Noise-induced hearing loss. St Louis, MO: Mosby, pp. 28–37.

Whitehead RL (1983) Some respiratory and aerodynamic patterns in the speech of the hearing-impaired. In Hochberg IE, Levitt H, Osberger MJ (Eds.) Speech of the hearing-impaired. research, training and personnel preparation. Baltimore, MD: University Park Press, pp. 97–116.

Wilber LA (1985) Calibration: pure tone, speech and noise signals. In Katz J (Ed.) Handbook of clinical audiology, 3rd edn. Baltimore, MD: Williams & Wilkins.

Willeford JA (1977) Assessing auditory behavior in children: a test battery approach. In Keith RW (Ed.) Central auditory dysfunction. New York, NY: Grune & Stratton.

Willeford JA, Burleigh JM (1985) Handbook of central auditory processing disorders. Orlando, FL: Grune & Stratton.

Williams A (1982) The relationship between two visual communication systems: reading and lipreading. Journal of Speech & Hearing Research 25: 500–3.

Williams CE (1970) Some psychiatric observations on a group of maladjusted deaf children. Journal of Child Psychology and Psychiatry 11: 1–18.

Willot JF (1991) Aging and the auditory system: anatomy, physiology and psychophysics. San Diego, CA: Singular Publishing.

Wilson WR, Walton WK (1974) Identification audiometry accuracy: evaluation of a recommended programme for school age children. Language, Speech & Hearing Services in Schools 5: 132–42.

Wilson WR, Folosom RC, Widen JE (1983) Hearing impairment in Down's syndrome. In Mencher GT, Gerber SE (Eds) The multiply handicapped hearing impaired child. New York, NY: Grune & Stratton, pp. 259–99.

Wright DC, Frank T (1992) Attenuation values for a supra-aural earphone for children and adults. Ear & Hearing 13: 454–9.

Wright R (1987) Basic properties of speech. In Martin M (Ed.) Speech audiometry. London: Taylor & Francis, pp. 1–32.

Yakovlev PI, LeCours AR (1967) The myelogenic cycles of regional maturation in the brain. In Minkowski A (Ed.) Regional development of the brain in early life. Oxford: Blackwell Scientific, pp. 3–70.

Young CV (1985) Developmental disabilities. In Katz J (Ed.) Handbook of clinical audiology, 3rd edn. Baltimore, MD: Williams & Wilkins, pp. 689–706.

Zeitoun H, Lesshafft C, Begg PA, East DM (1995) Assessment of a direct referral hearing aid clinic. British Journal of Audiology 29: 13–21.

Zielhuis GA, Rach GH, van den Broek PV (1989) Screening for otitis media with effusion in preschool children. Lancet i: 311–4.

Zinkus P, Gottlieb M (1980) Pattern of perceptual and academic deficits related to early chronic otitis media. Pediatrics 66: 246–53.

# Appendix A
# Causes of hearing loss

Notes: This list is not exhaustive. Some individuals develop sensori-neural hearing loss of unknown cause. Some individuals experience a combination of conductive and sensori-neural hearing loss. The following conditions are not all invariably associated with hearing loss.

## Conditions associated with conductive hearing loss

Bullous myringitis (inflammation of outer layer of tympanic membrane).

Cancers (eg. acquired skin cancer, congenital tumours).

Cholesteatoma (congenital or acquired).

Cleft lip and palate.

Congenital deformities of the external and/or middle ear (eg. atresia, microtia, fixation of stapes)

Down Syndrome.

External otitis (caused by various bacteria, viruses and fungi, eg. herpes simplex, aspergillus fumigatus, candida albicans).
Foreign bodies in external ear canal

Head injury (depends on nature of injury).
Otitis media (various in severity, chronicity, and cause)
Otosclerosis.
Mastoiditis.

Treacher Collins syndrome.

Tympanic membrane perforation

Wax occlusion

## Conditions associated with sensori-neural hearing loss

Bacterial meningitis

Birth trauma (eg. anoxia).

Cerebral palsy
Cochlea Otosclerosis

Congenital deformities of the cochlea.

Cytomegalovirus.

Genetically inherited loss.

Head injury (depends on nature of injury).

Jervell and Lange-Nielsen syndrome.

Labyrinthitis.

Maternal Rubella

Measles

Ménière's disease

Multiple sclerosis

Mumps

Noise exposure

Ototoxic drugs

Pendred's syndrome

Presbyacusis

Syphilis

Toxoplasmosis

Tumours (eg. Schwannoma of the VIIIth nerve, various brain tumours).

Turner syndrome

Usher's syndrome (retinitis pigmentosa)

Vascular disorders.

# Appendix B
# Audiometric symbols

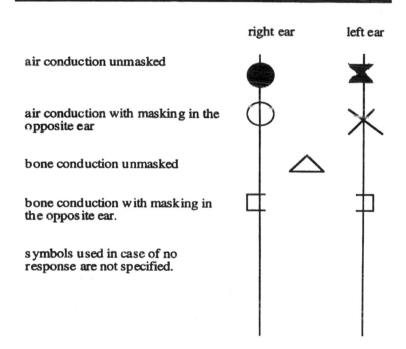

British Society of Audiology Audiometric Symbols

|  | right ear | left ear |
|---|---|---|
| air conduction unmasked | | |
| air conduction with masking in the opposite ear | | |
| bone conduction unmasked | | |
| bone conduction with masking in the opposite ear. | | |
| symbols used in case of no response are not specified. | | |

Note: The BSA recommend that separate audiograms are used for each ear. The calibration reference for the dB HL (dB HTL) scale is not specified on BSA audiograms because it is assumed that there is still some variance in the standard used.

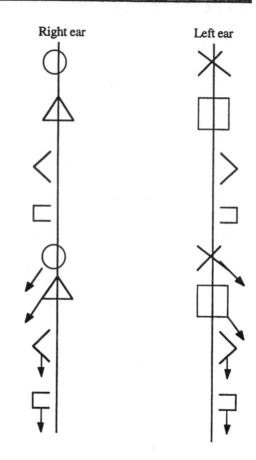

American Speech Language Hearing Association
Audiometric Symbols

|  | Right ear | Left ear |

air conduction

air conduction
with masking in
the opposite ear

bone conduction

bone conduction
with masking in
the opposite ear

Symbols used
when there is no
response at the
maximum
output of the
audiometer.

Note: ASHA recommends that the results
from both ears are graphed on a single
audiogram. The calibration standard for the
dB HL (dB HTL) scale is ANSI 1969.

| Audiological Society of Australia Audiometric Symbols |
|---|

|  | right ear | left ear |
|---|---|---|
| air conduction unmasked |  |  |
| air conduction with masking in the opposite ear |  |  |
| bone conduction unmasked |  |  |
| bone conduction with masking in the opposite ear. |  |  |
| air conduction aided | H | V |
| air conduction aided when ear not specified |  |  |
| air conduction sound field |  |  |
| symbols used in case of no response |  |  |

# Index